Mental Health Self-Help

Louis D. Brown · Scott Wituk
Editors

Mental Health Self-Help

Consumer and Family Initiatives

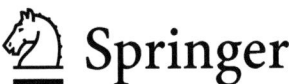

Editors
Louis D. Brown
Prevention Research Center
The Pennsylvania State University
135 E, Nittany Ave
Suite 402
State College, PA 16801
USA
ldb12@psu.edu

Scott Wituk
Center for Community Support
 and Research
Wichita State University
1845 Fairmount, Box 201
Wichita, KS 67260-0201
USA
scott.wituk@wichita.edu

ISBN 978-1-4419-6252-2   e-ISBN 978-1-4419-6253-9
DOI 10.1007/978-1-4419-6253-9
Springer New York Dordrecht Heidelberg London

Library of Congress Control Number: 2010931246

© Springer Science+Business Media, LLC 2010
All rights reserved. This work may not be translated or copied in whole or in part without the written permission of the publisher (Springer Science+Business Media, LLC, 233 Spring Street, New York, NY 10013, USA), except for brief excerpts in connection with reviews or scholarly analysis. Use in connection with any form of information storage and retrieval, electronic adaptation, computer software, or by similar or dissimilar methodology now known or hereafter developed is forbidden.
The use in this publication of trade names, trademarks, service marks, and similar terms, even if they are not identified as such, is not to be taken as an expression of opinion as to whether or not they are subject to proprietary rights.

Printed on acid-free paper

Springer is part of Springer Science+Business Media (www.springer.com)

Dedicated to mental health consumers and family members who inspired us, Greg Meissen who mentored us, and our families who supported us.

Acknowledgments

We would like to thank the thousands of research participants who have enabled the study of mental health self-help to progress. This book serves as a distillation of their input. We would also like to express our gratitude towards all of the chapter authors, who politely endured and accommodated our sometimes relentless requests for revisions. The quality of the finished product reflects their outstanding efforts. Finally, we would like to thank Springer for making this book possible and Sharon Panulla for shepherding us through the book publication process.

Contents

1 **Introduction to Mental Health Self-Help** 1
Louis D. Brown and Scott Wituk

Part I   Frameworks for Research and Practice

2 **Theoretical Foundations of Mental Health Self-Help** 19
Louis D. Brown and Alicia Lucksted

3 **Participatory Action Research and Evaluation with Mental Health Self-Help Initiatives: A Theoretical Framework** 39
Geoffrey Nelson, Rich Janzen, Joanna Ochocka, and John Trainor

Part II   MHSH Groups

4 **The Contributions of Mutual Help Groups for Mental Health Problems to Psychological Well-Being: A Systematic Review** 61
Nancy Pistrang, Chris Barker, and Keith Humphreys

5 **Online Self-Help/Mutual Aid Groups in Mental Health Practice** 87
J. Finn and T. Steele

6 **An Overview of Mutual Support Groups for Family Caregivers of People with Mental Health Problems: Evidence on Process and Outcomes** 107
Wai-Tong Chien

Part III   Consumer-Delivered Services

7 **Consumer-Run Drop-In Centers: Current State and Future Directions** 155
Louis D. Brown, Scott Wituk, and Greg Meissen

8 Certified Peer Specialists in the United States Behavioral Health System: An Emerging Workforce 169
Mark S. Salzer

9 The Development and Implementation of a Statewide Certified Peer Specialist Program 193
Emily A. Grant, Nathan Swink, Crystal Reinhart, and Scott Wituk

Part IV MHSH Policy

10 Finding and Using Our Voice: How Consumer/Survivor Advocacy is Transforming Mental Health Care 213
Daniel Fisher and Lauren Spiro

11 How Governments and Other Funding Sources Can Facilitate Self-Help Research and Services 235
Crystal R. Blyler, Risa Fox, and Neal B. Brown

Part V Technical Assistance

12 Consumer and Consumer-Supporter National Technical Assistance Centers: Helping the Consumer Movement Grow and Transform Systems 265
Susan Rogers

13 A Statewide Collaboration to Build the Leadership and Organizational Capacity of Consumer-Run Organizations (CROs) 287
Oliwier Dziadkowiec, Crystal Reinhart, Chi Connie Vu, Todd Shagott, Ashlee Keele-Lien, Adrienne Banta, Scott Wituk, and Greg Meissen

Part VI Self-Help/Professional Collaboration

14 Helping Mutual Help: Managing the Risks of Professional Partnerships 303
Deborah A. Salem, Thomas M. Reischl, and Katie W. Randall

15 The Contribution of Self-Help Groups to the Mental Health/Substance Use Services System 335
Thomas J. Powell and Brian E. Perron

Index 355

Contributors

Adrienne Banta Center for Community Support and Research, Wichita State University, Wichita, KS, USA, anbanta@wichita.edu

Chris Barker Department of Clinical, Educational and Health Psychology, University College London, London, UK, c.barker@ucl.ac.uk

Crystal R. Blyler SAMHSA Center for Mental Health Services, Rockville, MD, USA, crystal.blyler@samhsa.hhs.gov

Louis D. Brown Prevention Research Center, The Pennsylvania State University, State College, PA, USA, ldb12@psu.edu

Neal B. Brown Community Support Programs Branch, SAMHSA Center for Mental Health Services, Rockville, MD, USA, neal.brown@samhsa.hhs.gov

Wai-Tong Chien The School of Nursing, Faculty of Health & Social Sciences, The Hong Kong Polytechnic University, Hong Kong SAR, China, chinwaton@yahoo.com.hk; hschien@inet.polyu.edu.hk

Oliwier Dziadkowiec Center for Community Support and Research, Wichita State University, Wichita, KS, USA, oliwier.dziadkowiec@wichita.edu

Jerry Finn Social Work Program, University of Washington, Tacoma, WA, USA, finnj@u.washington.edu

Daniel Fisher National Empowerment Center, Lawrence, MA, USA, daniefisher@gmail.com

Risa Fox SAMHSA Center for Mental Health Services, Rockville, MD, USA, risa.fox@samhsa.hhs.gov

Emily A. Grant Center for Community Support and Research, Wichita State University, Wichita, KS, USA, emily.grant@wichita.edu

Keith Humphreys Department of Psychiatry, Stanford University Stanford, CA, USA, knh@stanford.edu

Rich Janzen Center for Community Based Research, Kitchener, ON, Canada, rich@communitybasedresearch.ca

Ashlee Keele-Lien Center for Community Support and Research, Wichita State University, Wichita, KS, USA, ashlee.keele-lien@wichita.edu

Alicia Lucksted Center for Mental Health Services Research, Division of Services Research, Department of Psychiatry, University of Maryland School of Medicine, Baltimore, MD, USA, aluckste@psych.umaryland.edu

Greg Meissen Department of Psychology, Wichita State University, Wichita, KS, USA, greg.meissen@wichita.edu

Geoffrey Nelson Department of Psychology, Wilfrid Laurier University, Waterloo, ON, Canada, gnelson@wlu.ca

Joanna Ochocka Centre for Community Based Research, Kitchener, ON, Canada, joanna@communitybasedresearch.ca

Brian E. Perron School of Social Work, University of Michigan, Ann Arbor, MI, USA, beperron@umich.edu

Nancy Pistrang Department of Clinical, Educational and Health Psychology, University College London, London, UK, n.pistrang@ucl.ac.uk

Thomas J. Powell School of Social Work, University of Michigan, Ann Arbor, MI, USA, tpowell@umich.edu

Katie W. Randall Washington State Department of Social and Health Services, Olympia, WA, USA, weavek@dshs.wa.gov

Crystal Reinhart Center for Prevention Research & Development, University of Illinois at Urbana-Champaign, Champaign, IL, USA, reinhrt@illinois.edu

Thomas M. Reischl Prevention Research Center of Michigan, University of Michigan School of Public Health, Ann Arbor, MI, USA, reischl@umich.edu

Susan Rogers National Mental Health Consumers' Self-Help Clearinghouse, Philadelphia, PA, USA, srogers@mhasp.org

Deborah A. Salem Department of Health Behavior & Health Education, University of Michigan School of Public Health, Ann Arbor, MI, USA, debbysalem@gmail.com

Mark S. Salzer Department of Psychiatry, University of Pennsylvania, Philadelphia, PA, USA, mark.salzer@uphs.upenn.edu

Todd Shagott Center for Community Support and Research, Wichita State University, Wichita, KS, USA, tpshagott@gmail.com

Lauren Spiro National Coalition of Mental Health Consumer/Survivor Organizations, Washington, DC, USA, laurenspiro1@gmail.com

T. Steele MSW student, University of Washington, Tacoma, USA, steelet@u.washington.edu

Nathan Swink Center for Community Support and Research, Wichita State University, Wichita, KS, USA, npswink@wichita.edu

John Trainor Department of Psychiatry, University of Toronto, Toronto, ON, USA, john_trainor@camh.net

Chi Connie Vu James Bell Associates, Washington, DC, USA, vu@jbassoc.com

Scott Wituk Center for Community Support and Research, Wichita State University, Wichita, KS, USA, scott.wituk@wichita.edu

About the Editors

Louis D. Brown is a community psychologist and research faculty member of The Pennsylvania State University. His research examines how people engage in and benefit from self-help/mutual support initiatives. As a research associate at the Penn State Prevention Research Center, Dr. Brown also studies community health partnerships and the implementation of evidence-based programs to promote healthy youth development.

Scott Wituk, PhD, is the director of the Center for Community Support and Research (CCSR) at Wichita State University. Previously he served as the research coordinator at CCSR. In these positions he has conducted community-based research projects with self-help groups, coalitions, nonprofits, and other community-based organizations. He has over 30 peer-reviewed publications and book chapters and numerous professional presentations.

About the Authors

Adrienne Banta has a bachelors of science in psychology from Wichita State University. She currently works at the Center for Community Support and Research as a research assistant. Her research interests include evaluating consumer-run organizations, as well as conducting needs assessments and program evaluations for a variety of other nonprofit organizations.

Chris Barker is a reader in clinical psychology at University College London. He received his PhD in clinical psychology from UCLA. His research focuses on the communication of psychological helping and support, in a variety of clinical and community contexts, and he also publishes on research methodology.

Crystal R. Blyler is a social science analyst for the U.S. Substance Abuse and Mental Health Services Administration (SAMHSA). She was the co-program leader for the Consumer-Operated Services Program (COSP), a multi-site randomized trial of consumer-operated services, and the government project officer for the development of a Consumer-Operated Services Evidence-Based Practice KIT. Prior to joining SAMHSA in 1999, she received a PhD in experimental psychopathology from Harvard University and worked as a schizophrenia researcher.

Neal B. Brown, M.P.A. has been a national leader on policy and program issues in mental health and since 1983 has directed the Federal Community Support Program (CSP), a national program and movement designed to promote and advocate for community treatment, rehabilitation, employment, and opportunities for individuals with psychiatric disabilities. He also currently directs a national initiative focused on transforming and reforming state and community mental health systems to better emphasize consumer direction, empowerment, and recovery.

Wai-Tong Chien is associate professor in the School of Nursing, Faculty of Health and Social Sciences, The Hong Kong Polytechnic University of Hong Kong S.A.R., China. He has published widely on mental health issues and psychosocial interventions for clients with physical and mental health problems and their family members, using both quantitative and qualitative research methods. He has also committed to the development of education curriculum, licensure, and practice guidelines of psychiatric/mental health nursing in the Nursing Council of Hong Kong.

Oliwier Dziadkowiec is a doctoral student in the Department of Community Psychology at Wichita State University and is a research associate at the Center for Community Support and Research. His research interests include evaluation of the impact of consumer-run organizations and other consumer-based initiatives, the impact of social capital on various health related outcomes, as well as the use of systemic methods in public health and public policy research.

Jerry Finn, PhD is currently a professor in the Social Work Program, University of Washington, Tacoma. Dr. Finn has 30 years of teaching experience in social work that includes courses in human behavior, research, practice, and information technology and human services at the bachelors and masters levels, and has served on doctoral committees. In addition he has published many scholarly articles and two edited books, primarily in areas related to the impact of information technology on human services. In addition, Dr. Finn has provided training and consultation to human service agencies in the areas of digital divide intervention, child welfare programs, consumer satisfaction, online hotlines, and program evaluation.

Daniel Fisher, MD, PhD has devoted his life to bringing hope and recovery to the lives of those labeled mental illness through his work as a board-certified, community psychiatrist who works at Riverside Community Care, a neurochemist who worked on neurotransmitters at the NIMH, an advocate who has recovered from schizophrenia and directs the National Empowerment Center, and as a member of the White New Freedom Commission on Mental Health.

Risa Fox is a public health advisor for the U.S. Substance Abuse and Mental Health Services Administration. She is the GPO on an Interagency Agreements with the Department of Educational, National Institute on Disability and Rehabilitation for two currently funded adult Rehabilitation, Research, and Training Centers. Ms. Fox is the program director for the Consumer & Consumer-Supporter National Technical Assistance Centers on Consumer/Peer-Run Programs and previous GPO of the Statewide Consumer Network Grantee Program. She previously held positions at the National Institute of Mental Health working with the Community Mental Health Centers (CMHCs) Program and worked with CMHS at regional and local levels. She is a licensed psychiatric social worker and holds an MS degree from Columbia University.

Emily A. Grant is a doctoral student in the Department of Community Psychology at Wichita State University and conducts research and evaluation at the Center for Community Support and Research. Her current research interests include evaluation of the certified peer specialist program in Kansas and integration of certified peer specialists into the mental health system.

Keith Humphreys is a professor of psychiatry and behavioral sciences at Stanford University and a VA senior research career scientist. A clinical/community psychologist by training, his research focuses on the prevention and treatment of addictive disorders, and on the extent to which subjects in medical research differ from patients seen in everyday clinical practice. Since 2004, he has also volunteered as a consultant and teacher in the multinational effort to rebuild the psychiatric care system of Iraq, for which he recently won the American Psychological Association's Award for Distinguished Contribution to the Public Interest. Dr Humphreys has been extensively involved in the formation of federal drug control policy.

Rich Janzen is research director at the Centre for Community Based Research and a doctoral candidate in community psychology at Wilfrid Laurier University. Rich has been involved in over 70 participatory action research projects, most focusing on issues of cultural diversity or mental health. Rich lives in Waterloo, Ontario.

Ashlee Keele-Lien is a doctoral student in the community psychology program at Wichita State University. Her research interests involve empowerment within marginalized communities. Her current research is focused on mental health consumer perceptions of Certified Peer Specialists.

Alicia Lucksted is a clinical-community psychologist and assistant professor of psychiatry at the University of Maryland School of Medicine, Center for Mental Health Services Research. Her work focuses on applied research to improve mental health services for people with serious mental illnesses, self-help interventions among mental health consumers and their family members, qualitative methods in mental health services research, and consumer views of mental health services.

Greg Meissen is professor of psychology at Wichita State University, has had faculty appointments at Harvard Medical School and Boston University, and served on the Surgeon General's Council on Self-Help and Public Health. In 1985 he brought the newly founded Self-Help Network to WSU where he served as director until 2008 as it grew into the nationally recognized Center for Community Support and Research where he was involved in projects focused on capacity building of community and faith-based organizations, development of self-help and mutual support organizations particularly mental health consumer-run organizations, and initiatives to promote community leadership. This work was funded by grants he was awarded from numerous agencies including the National Institute of Mental Health, Substance Abuse and Mental Health Services Administration, Center for Mental Health Services Research, and WT Grant Foundation, and he has published this research in such outlets as the New England Journal of Medicine, American Journal of Community Psychology, Social Work, Journal of Applied Behavioral Science, Journal of Community Psychology and Psychiatric Services.

Geoffrey Nelson is professor of psychology at Wilfrid Laurier University, Waterloo, Ontario, Canada. He has served as senior editor of the Canadian Journal of Community Mental Health and Chair of the Community Psychology Section of the Canadian Psychological Association. Professor Nelson was the recipient in 1999 of the Harry MacNeill award for innovation in community mental health from the American Psychological Foundation and the Society for Community Research and Action of the American Psychological Association.

Joanna Ochocka (PhD sociology) is executive director of the Centre for Community Based Research and adjunct faculty member in the Department of

Sociology at University of Waterloo and in the MA and PhD program in community psychology at Wilfrid Laurier University in Waterloo, Ontario, Canada. Joanna is one of the leaders in the use of participatory action research approach and she practices community-based research as a tool to mobilize people for social change. Joanna's research and action have focused on community mental health for people with serious mental health issues, on cultural diversity and immigration, and on community supports for marginalized populations.

Brian E. Perron is an assistant professor at the University of Michigan, School of Social Work. He received his PhD in social work from Washington University in 2007. His research focuses on problems associated with psychiatric and substance use disorders.

Nancy Pistrang is a reader in clinical psychology at University College London. She received her PhD in clinical psychology from UCLA, after which she worked as a clinical psychologist in the British National Health Service before taking up her present position. Her research focuses on psychological helping in everyday relationships, including peer support, communication in couples, and mutual support groups.

Thomas J. Powell, MSW, PhD is professor of social work, University of Michigan. His research interests are in the area of mental health services for people with serious mental illness. He has a particular interest in self-help, support, and advocacy groups with a special emphasis on how these mutual help resources can be coordinated with professional care.

Katie W. Randall received her MA in community psychology from Michigan State University in 2000. She worked as a research investigator for the Washington Institute for Mental Health Research and Training at the University of Washington and Washington State University from 2001–2007. In this position, she contracted with the Mental Health Division of Washington State to conduct mental health services research and evaluation. She currently works for the Washington State Department of Social and Health Services as a management analyst where she provides assistance with planning, performance management, and accountability.

Crystal Reinhart is a doctoral student in the Community Psychology program at Wichita State University. Ms. Reinhart's doctoral research is focused on mental health consumer-run organizations, and her research interests have also included Certified Peer Specialists and other consumer initiatives. She is currently working on substance abuse prevention and teen parenting at the Center for Prevention Research and Development at the University of Illinois.

Thomas M. Reischl is an associate research scientist in the Department of Health Behavior and Health Education at University of Michigan's School of Public Health. He received a PhD in psychology from the University of Illinois and has held previous faculty appointments at Michigan State University, the University of New Hampshire, and the University of Waikato (New Zealand). In his current position, he serves at the Director of Evaluation for the Prevention Research

Center of Michigan and conducts evaluation research studies of community-based public health programs, violence prevention programs, family support programs, consumer-controlled (self/mutual help) programs, and public-health preparedness programs.

Susan Rogers is director of the National Mental Health Consumers' Self-Help Clearinghouse, a mental health consumer-run national technical assistance center funded by a grant from the U.S. Department of Health and Human Services, Substance Abuse and Mental Health Services Administration, Center for Mental Health Services. She is also director of special projects of the Mental Health Association of Southeastern Pennsylvania. She has 33 years of experience as a writer and editor, and she has been active in the mental health consumer/survivor movement since 1984.

Deborah A. Salem received her PhD from the University of Illinois at Urbana-Champaign. Her research has focused on mutual help for individuals with serious mental illness, adoption of innovation, and organizational development. After 17 years on the faculty in the Department of Psychology at Michigan State University, she is currently teaching as a lecturer at the University of Michigan and doing research consultation.

Mark S. Salzer received his PhD in clinical/community psychology at the University of Illinois at Urbana-Champaign. He is an associate professor in the Department of Psychiatry at the University of Pennsylvania and an investigator in the Mental Illness Research, Education, and Clinical Center based at the Philadelphia VA Medical Center. Dr. Salzer's research focuses on the delivery of effective community mental health and rehabilitation services to individuals with psychiatric disabilities, with a particular focus on identifying and eliminating barriers to full community participation, promoting effective utilization of mainstream community resources, and enhancing the development and effectiveness of support initiatives (e.g., peer, employment, education, and natural supports).

Todd Shagott recently received his doctorate degree from the Community Psychology Program at Wichita State University. His interests are in evaluation, behavior setting theory, and working with nonprofit organizations. Most recently his research evaluated how the setting characteristics of consumer-run organizations promoted positive health behaviors.

Lauren Spiro, MA, is director of the National Coalition of Mental Health Consumer/Survivor Organizations, and co-director of the Education for Social Inclusion Project funded by the Substance Abuse and Mental Health Services Administration. She has traveled a liberating journey to wellness from her being labeled with 'chronic schizophrenia' to devoting her life's works to building emotionally healthy communities. She co-founded two nonprofit corporations and as the director of the National Coalition of Mental Health Consumer/Survivor Organizations, she advances the values, vision, policies, and legislative priorities of mental health consumers in Washington, D.C. and across the country.

T. Steele is currently a graduate student in social work at the University of Washington Tacoma. She holds a BA in communication with an emphasis in communication technology and society from the University of Washington Seattle.

Nathan Swink received a masters degree in 2007 at Wichita State University in Wichita, KS, where he is currently pursuing a PhD in community psychology. His research focuses on ways the underlying assumptions and cognitive processing styles of individuals take form in communities. Living downtown, he is both physically and politically active in Wichita communities.

John Trainor has had a long-standing interest in self-help and consumer/survivor-run organizations. He led the initial development of over 40 of these groups in Ontario, Canada in the 1990s. He has also worked internationally and supported the development of groups in the Baltic states and Sri Lanka.

Chi Connie Vu received her MA in community psychology from Wichita State University in 2006. She has 5 years of experience in applied social science research design, program evaluation, grant writing, and capacity building technical assistance. As a senior staff member at James Bell Associates (JBA), Ms. Vu currently provides evaluation technical assistance to discretionary grant programs funded by the Administration for Children and Families. Prior to joining JBA, Ms. Vu was a research associate at the Wichita State University Center for Community Support and Research where she conducted research for a jointly funded National Institute of Mental Health and Substance Abuse and Mental Health Services Administration project on promoting effective practices among mental health consumer-run organizations.

Chapter 1
Introduction to Mental Health Self-Help

Louis D. Brown and Scott Wituk

Abstract Mental health self-help (MHSH) refers to any mutual support-oriented initiative directed by people with mental illness or their family members. These initiatives have become increasingly widespread over the years and today MHSH initiatives outnumber traditional mental health organizations in the United States (Goldstrom et al., 2006). The goal of this book is to provide research-based insight into the development of effective MHSH initiatives. This chapter explores the defining characteristics of MHSH and reviews its historical development. Building on this foundation, the chapter examines several factors contributing to the growth and popularity of MHSH, along with an exploration of factors impeding the use of MHSH. Following is a discussion of future directions for research and practice. Finally, the chapter provides a summary of the topics covered by each subsequent chapter.

This book brings together leading research across many different types of mental health self-help (MHSH) initiatives. Drawing from both existing research and experiential knowledge, each chapter provides insight into the development of effective MHSH initiatives. These insights will be useful to leaders of MHSH initiatives, mental health researchers, state and local administrators, and professionals who work with consumer and family-driven initiatives. Furthermore, students planning careers in mental health can use this book to understand an important approach to recovery from mental illness that is growing in popularity and utilization. Finally, leaders of MHSH initiatives can use the evaluation studies reviewed in this book to provide evidence for the effectiveness of MHSH.

Overall, the edited volume contains fifteen chapters addressing the development of effective MHSH initiatives. In addition to this introductory chapter, which outlines the field of MHSH, the book provides chapters exploring mutual-help groups for mental health problems, mutual-help groups for caregivers, consumer-run drop-in centers, online self-help, and consumer advocacy initiatives. Technical assistance

---

L.D. Brown (✉)
Prevention Research Center, The Pennsylvania State University, 135 E, Nittany Ave, Suite 402, State College, PA 16801, USA
e-mail: ldb12@psu.edu

organizations and peer support specialist initiatives are examined separately at the national level, with additional chapters on these two topics providing a more in-depth exploration of their implementation at the state level. The book also provides two chapters discussing collaboration with the professional mental health system, two chapters discussing theoretical frameworks for MHSH practice and research, and one chapter sharing the perspective of funding organizations interested in supporting MHSH. Before providing a more detailed summary of each chapter, the following sections explore (1) the terminology of MHSH, (2) the history of MHSH, and (3) factors influencing the use of MHSH.

1.1 MHSH Terminology

The term self-help broadly refers to any self-directed undertaking aimed at personal improvement. In this book, however, we specifically focus on collaborative efforts directed by mental health service consumers or their family members. These initiatives typically target mental health promotion goals such as enhanced coping and progress toward recovery. The degree to which mental health professionals influence organizational decision making varies substantially; however consumers and family members control final decision making. Considerable variation exists within these definitional boundaries and this book considers some of the most popular types of MHSH, including mutual-help groups (also known as self-help/mutual aid/mutual support groups), consumer-run drop-in centers, certified peer specialist programs, technical assistance organizations, advocacy organizations, and online self-help mutual aid groups. Other types of initiatives exist and several terms in the literature describe MHSH initiatives, including

- mutual-help groups (e.g., Corrigan et al., 2005)
- mutual support groups (e.g., Chien, Norman, & Thompson, 2006)
- mutual aid groups (e.g., Kelly, Salmon, & Graziano, 2004)
- self-help groups (e.g., Burti et al., 2005)
- consumer-run organizations (e.g., Brown, Shepherd, Wituk, & Meissen, 2007)
- consumer/survivor initiatives (e.g., Nelson, Lord, & Ochocka, 2001)
- consumer drop-in centers (e.g., Mowbray, Robinson, & Holter, 2002)
- consumer-operated self-help centers (e.g., Swarbrick, 2007)
- self-help agencies (e.g., Segal & Silverman, 2002)
- peer-run organizations (e.g., Clay, 2005)
- consumer-run businesses (e.g., Kimura, Mukaiyachi, & Ito, 2002)
- self-help programs (e.g., Chamberlin, Rogers, & Ellison, 1996)
- consumer-delivered services (e.g., Salzer & Shear, 2002)
- consumer-run services (e.g., Goldstrom, 2006).

Although the broad variety MHSH initiatives do not fit neatly into a small number of categories, two organizational characteristics that help to classify MHSH initiatives are organizational structure and organizational focus. Locating a MHSH initiative on the continuum of organizational structure and the continuum of organizational focus provides insight into the nature of its operations and the outcomes of its efforts.

Self-help groups exemplify the unstructured end of the organizational structure continuum, which is also characterized by the informal nature of interpersonal relations and a reliance on volunteer contributions from group members for all group activities. Highly structured MHSH initiatives that rival the organizational complexity of psychiatric hospitals and other formal agencies operated by paid staff do not yet exist. However, consumer-operated services such as certified peer specialist training programs and crisis residential services rely on paid staff and maintain substantially more structure than self-help groups. Some MHSH initiatives, such as consumer-run drop-in centers, rely on a mixture of paid and volunteer support and typically fall in the middle of the continuum of organizational structure.

It is important to understand the strengths and weaknesses of different organizational structures because the structure of a MHSH initiative typically evolves over time and needs to be strategically managed. As MHSH initiatives grow, they are likely to face pressure to adopt a more formal organizational structure. However, adding organizational structure to manage growth can have devastating unintended consequences as the advantages of unstructured initiatives are lost (Smith, 2000).

Unstructured groups lack role differentiation, which enables informal, highly personalized interactions between group members that are typically warmer, more encouraging, and more accepting (Wuthnow, 1994). Smaller initiatives are also better able to promote the investment and involvement of all participants because all contributions are needed and consensus-driven decision making is feasible. The lack of hierarchy and bureaucracy encourages mutual support, intimacy, and sharing. Relying exclusively on internal funding also ensures independent control over organizational activities and prevents cooptation by external funding agencies (Brown et al., 2007).

Although small informal organizations manifest several characteristics that promote MHSH success, developing organizational structure also has several advantages. Large organizational size and hierarchical role differentiation enables economies of scale, which are more efficient at the production of goods and the provision of services (Milofsky, 1988). Obtaining external funding allows MHSH initiatives to pursue activities and programs that cannot be accomplished otherwise. The role specialization and clear chain of command that accompany a structured organization can help promote efficient, goal-focused interactions and rapid organizational decision making. Training and certification requirements help to ensure paid staff members possess the skills necessary to fulfill role expectations. Although these characteristics of structured organizations are frequently necessary for MHSH initiatives to become effective service providers, they can also weaken the effectiveness of mutual support, which thrives in unstructured settings. Furthermore, there is concern that paying consumers to help other consumers will reproduce power inequities that currently exist in the professional mental health system. Regardless, using consumers as service providers can help to address the poverty-level conditions experienced by many mental health consumers and may help to build stronger therapeutic alliances (Solomon, 2004).

Organizational focus is another characteristic that can aid the classification of MHSH initiatives. Initiatives with an internal focus on helping members fall at one end of the continuum and externally focused initiatives that target changes in mental health policy and the broader community fall at the opposite end of the continuum. MHSH has traditionally focused on internal change, with members helping one another progress toward recovery. In fact, initiatives that are purely focused on external change are not traditionally conceptualized as part of self-help (Humphreys, 2004). However, initiatives that maintain both internal and external goals remain under the MHSH umbrella. For example, consumer-run drop-in centers often make presentations in the community to enhance education about mental illness. Consumer coalitions that directly target mental health policy changes also frequently invest in improving the leadership skills of their members. Understanding the focus of a MHSH initiative enables the specification of appropriate indicators of success. Success for internally focused initiatives may be indicated by the enhanced well-being of participants whereas the success of externally focused initiatives may be improvements in mental health policy or reduced stigma toward mental illness in the community.

1.2 History of MHSH

Over the past century, mental health treatment has seen drastic transformations and today a new philosophy is emerging in community mental health called the empowerment-community integration paradigm (Nelson et al., 2001). Table 1.1 provides a historical context for understanding the evolution of mental health treatment and how the empowerment-community integration paradigm differs from traditional treatment paradigms (Nelson et al., 2001).

One of the earliest approaches to mental health treatment is the medical-institutional paradigm, which became dominant in the nineteenth century. This paradigm emphasized the use of psychiatric hospitals constructed to treat patients who had little, if any, control in determining their treatment. During the 1960s, the community treatment-rehabilitation paradigm emerged, providing alternatives to institutionalization that included supportive housing, clubhouses, case management, and other services designed to provide clients life skills so they would require reduced amounts of professional care, especially hospitalization. While a significant advance, a number of issues in the community treatment-rehabilitation paradigm remain, including a focus on individual deficits leading to continued stigma and an imbalance of control between professionals and consumers (Carling, 1995; Nelson et al., 2001). Studies have found that the community treatment-rehabilitation paradigm helped many people have a physical presence in the community while remaining socially and psychologically unintegrated (Mowbray, Greenfield, & Freddolino, 1992; Sherman, Frenkel, & Newman, 1986).

Table 1.1 Changing paradigms in community mental health

Traditional paradigms		Emerging paradigm
Medical-institutional	Community treatment-rehabilitation	Empowerment-community integration
Lack of consumer voice and choice	Consumers have input but professional retains control	Self-directed collaboration with professionals
Dependence on professionals	Dependence on professionals	Autonomous consumer-run organizations
Patient role	Client role	Citizen role
Professional role as expert	Professional role as expert	Professional role focuses on collaboration and enabling
Professional services	Professional, paraprofessional, and volunteer services	Self-help/mutual support, informal supports
Institutional locus	Community-based locus	Integration into community settings and social support networks
Stigma, focus on illness	Stigma, focus on psychosocial deficits	Focus on strengths, potential for growth and recovery

Note: From Nelson et al. (2001)

The empowerment-community integration paradigm is now beginning to emerge in response to many of the weaknesses inherent in the community treatment-rehabilitation paradigm. This new conceptualization of mental health treatment emphasizes the importance of community integration, where people are a valued part *of the community*, not just *in the community* (Nelson, Walsh-Bowers, & Hall, 1998). The paradigm additionally emphasizes empowerment, where individuals actively participate in and gain control over their lives. Increasing both empowerment and community integration requires a change in the roles of both mental health consumers and professionals. People with mental illness must play the role of citizens rather than patients and professionals must play the role of "resource-collaborator" rather than "expert-technician" (Constantino & Nelson, 1995). This philosophical shift toward autonomy and self-sufficiency in the treatment of mental health problems provides important support for the use of MHSH, which has a rich history of its own.

The oldest MHSH initiatives are Recovery International and GROW. Recovery International was founded by Abraham Low, MD in 1937 as a therapy group that gradually multiplied, became fully consumer-controlled in 1952, and now hosts over 500 self-help groups internationally, along with telephone and online meetings (Recovery International, 2009). GROW is another international network of self-help groups that was founded in 1957 by consumers who developed their own 12-step program based on the Alcoholics Anonymous model. Through the "self-help revolution" (Norcross, 2000), numerous other groups have followed their footsteps, including Schizophrenics Anonymous, National Alliance for Mental Illness, the Depression and Bipolar Support Alliance, and Emotions Anonymous. Although other types of MHSH are becoming more common, internally focused, minimally structured self-help groups remain the most prevalent from of MHSH (Goldstrom et al., 2006).

The mental health patient's liberation movement has also played an influential role in the promotion of MHSH. The movement began in the 1970s after deinstitutionalization, when "ex-inmates" who fiercely rejected the professional mental health system began to organize, developing self-help initiatives and advocating for consumer rights (Chamberlin, 1990). The ideology promoted by these groups has increasingly gained mainstream acceptance and their work continues to influence MHSH. Chapters 10 and 12 review some of the advocacy and policy work of MHSH initiatives that continue to promote self-help, consumer rights, empowerment, and a recovery orientation in the mental health system.

Parents of people with mental illness also started self-help groups and in 1979, several groups combined to form NAMI, the national alliance on mental illness, which has groups in over 1000 communities. In addition to organizing self-help groups, NAMI organizes peer-led classes intended to help family members cope with the stress of caring for a family member with mental illness. With over $10,000,000 in contributions in 2007, NAMI is also involved in shaping mental health policy at the state and federal levels, educating the public about mental illness, and fighting stigma (www.nami.org).

Along with the burgeoning interest in MHSH among consumers and family members, elements of the professional mental health system have embraced the use of MHSH and promoted it as a means to achieve recovery (Solomon, 2004). In addition to supporting the use of volunteer-driven MHSH initiatives, the mental health system has also provided funding for the provision of consumer and family run programs. Examples of MHSH initiatives that use funding include consumer-run drop-in centers (Chapter 7), certified peer specialist training programs (Chapter 8 and 9), and consumer technical assistance centers (Chapter 12).

Increased consumer participation in the public mental health system has accompanied the growth in consumer-delivered services. As described in Chapter 10 by Daniel Fisher and Lauren Spiro, consumer voice in the decision-making processes of professional mental health organizations is growing. Additionally, consumers are becoming increasingly involved in the development of their treatment plan (Nelson et al., 2001). Further, professional mental health organizations such as the Veterans Health Administration (2004) are frequently hiring consumers as service providers. Finally, the services of peer support specialists are now Medicaid-reimbursable in a number of states (Sabin & Daniels, 2003).

1.3 Factors Influencing the Use of MHSH

Growth in the power of the consumer movement, as described in the previous section, stands as a critical factor promoting the use of MHSH. However, several other factors are also important to consider. MHSH can provide participants with several benefits at no cost that professional services are less capable of providing. For example, MHSH may provide friendships, empowering leadership roles, and spiritual inspiration. Participants who obtain these benefits are not only likely to continue participation but may also share their experiences with others who may decide to join. Through word of mouth, many self-help initiatives flourish.

Several factors also impede the use of self-help. The stigma associated with mental illness inhibits participation from individuals who do not want to further identify and affiliate with mental illness (Brown, 2009). Some potential participants also view self-help participation as a sign of weakness, for people who are overly emotional and sensitive. Furthermore, professionals sometimes view self-help with suspicion, unsure of whether participants provide sound advice. Groups that depend entirely on word of mouth may be isolated and liable to falter without external supports such as referrals from mental health professionals. Unresolved internal conflicts may also cause some members to discontinue participation or for the entire initiative to disband (Mohr, 2004).

1.4 Book Overview and Chapter Summaries

This book is organized into six sections. The first section, Frameworks for Research and Practice, has two chapters which review the theoretical foundations of MHSH and a framework for participatory action research with MHSH. The second section reviews three different types of MHSH groups – groups for people with mental health problems, online groups, and groups for caregivers of people with mental health problems. Consumer-delivered services are the topic of the third section, with chapters on consumer-run drop-in centers and certified peer specialists programs. The fourth section focuses on MHSH policy, examining consumer advocacy initiatives and the interface between funding sources and MHSH. Technical assistance is the topic of the fifth section, with one chapter examining US national consumer technical assistance centers and the other chapter describing a statewide collaboration to develop a network of consumer-run organizations. The sixth and final section explores the interface between MHSH initiatives and the professional mental health system, with emphasis placed on the strategic management of partnerships with professionals. The following six subsections provide a more detailed summary of the chapters that fall into each topic.

1.4.1 Frameworks for Research and Practice

Chapter 2, "Theoretical Foundations of Mental Health Self-Help," reviews the theoretical perspectives commonly applied to mental health self-help (MHSH). Louis Brown and Alicia Lucksted first examine *Recovery* and *community integration,* which are multifaceted constructs often used to conceptualize the outcomes of participation in MHSH. Second, the authors present several perspectives on MHSH setting characteristics that influence individual outcomes, including *sense of community, behavior setting theory,* and *empowerment theory.* Third, the authors summarize theoretical perspectives providing insight into how individuals benefit from their interactions with self-help settings, including the *helper-therapy principle*, *experiential knowledge*, *social comparison theory*, and *social support theories*. Finally, the *Role Framework* provides a theoretical model that helps to integrate and extend these different perspectives in the literature.

The third chapter, "Participatory Action Research and Evaluation with Mental Health Self-help Groups and Organizations: A Theoretical Framework" poses a series of questions researchers face when collaborating with MHSH. Geoff Nelson and associates address each of these questions by providing a framework for self-helpers, researchers, and others as they develop research projects. Their framework addresses six elements: (a) values, (b) participation and power sharing, (c) social programming, (d) knowledge construction, (e) knowledge utilization, and (f) practice. Embedded throughout the chapter are lessons learned and recommendations for future research and evaluation with MHSH initiatives.

1.4.2 MHSH Groups

Three chapters on MHSH groups examine three different types of groups – groups for people with mental health problems, online groups, and groups for caregivers of people with mental health problems. Authors Nancy Pistrang, Chris Barker, and Keith Humphreys focus on groups for people with mental health problems in Chapter 4, titled, "The contributions of mutual-help groups for mental health problems to psychological well-being: A systematic review." The chapter first outlines how mutual-help groups fit into the broader picture of mental health self-help initiatives, and discusses some issues involved in conducting effectiveness research on mutual-help groups. The methods and results of the review are then presented. The studies reviewed provide limited but promising evidence that mutual-help groups benefit people with three types of problems: chronic mental illness, depression/anxiety, and bereavement. The strongest findings come from two randomized trials showing that the outcomes of mutual-help groups were equivalent to those of substantially more costly professional interventions.

In Chapter 5, "Online self-help/mutual aid groups in mental health practice," Jerry Finn and T. Steele review the expanding use of online self-help mutual aid groups. Finn and Steele describe how this form of MHSH provides a number of advantages to consumers since they are not bound to time, place, or social presence. The authors describe research that supports the benefits in areas of health, mental health, addictions, stigmatized identities, trauma and violence recovery, and grief support. Finn and Steele also consider some of the challenges associated with this type of MHSH, including the potential for disinhibited communication, privacy concerns, and misinformation. Future development of online support through social networking sites and virtual communities will become new resources for consumers. In order for online MHSH to be a resource, mental health professionals and others will need to be positioned to help maximize benefits and guard against their potential weaknesses.

Wai-Tong Chien examines mutual support groups for family caregivers in Chapter 6, "An overview of mutual support groups for family caregivers of people with mental health problems: Evidence on process and outcomes." The chapter summarizes the literature from a systematic search and assesses the evidence on the effectiveness and therapeutic ingredients of mutual support groups for helping family caregivers of people with severe mental health problems. Many studies reported different benefits of group participation such as increasing knowledge about the illness and enhancing coping ability and social support. However, the review points out there is a lack of research examining the long-term effects of mutual support groups on families' and consumers' psychosocial health conditions. In addition, Chien discusses lessons learned from development and evaluation on family-led support groups including the major principles in establishing and strengthening a support group, barriers to group development and families who are likely to attend and benefit from group participation.

1.4.3 Consumer-Delivered Services

This section reviews two types of consumer-delivered services that typically require external funding – consumer-run drop-in centers and certified peer specialist programs. In Chapter 7, "Consumer-run drop-in centers: Current state and future directions," Louis Brown, Scott Wituk, and Greg Meissen examine this popular form of MHSH that remains largely volunteer driven. In addition to organizing recreational activities, drop-in centers can host self-help groups, bring in speakers from the community, offer classes to members, organize public awareness campaigns about mental illness, volunteer in the community, and work with professionals, administrators, and lawmakers to improve the public mental health system. Brown, Wituk, and Meissen review research on several different facets of these organizations including their activities, organizational structure, evidence base, funding support, and community relations. Strategies to enhance the organizational effectiveness and peer support of consumer-run drop-in centers are outlined with attention to enhancing empowerment and recovery.

This book also provides two chapters examining the recent emergence of certified peer support specialists at the national and state levels. Chapter 8, "Certified peer specialists in the US behavioral health system: An emerging workforce" by Mark Salzer, describes the development of Certified Peer Specialists (CPSs), who receive specialized training and certification to provide Medicaid-reimbursable peer support and mutual aid. The chapter provides a historical overview and discusses this movement as a significant evolutionary step in the involvement of peers-as-staff in the traditional service system, programs, and workforce. A review of current knowledge about Certified Peer Specialist (CPS) training programs is offered along with research findings on the benefits associated with participating in such training on well-being, knowledge, and employment. Additionally, national findings pertaining to CPS wages, hours worked per week, and number of persons they support, as well as job titles and work activities is presented. Evidence of continuing implementation barriers, emerging policy, program, and practice issues are discussed, as well as high priority future research topics.

Additional insight into the development and implementation of a statewide CPS program is provided by Emily Grant and her colleagues in Chapter 9. The chapter describes a Certified Peer Specialist (CPS) Program that emerged in Kansas in 2007. Grant and her co-authors trace the roots of the CPS program from Georgia to Kansas with particular focus on the benefits and crucial facets of the programs thought to be linked to program success. In addition, the chapter reports on findings from surveys conducted with over 100 Kansas CPSs. Reported findings include a description of job activities and services, workplace integration, satisfaction, and organizational support. Findings indicate that Kansas CPSs are being received well by many mental health centers, report high job satisfaction, and perceived positive organizational support. Limitations of current research and suggestions for future research are also discussed.

1.4.4 MHSH Policy

This section explores how consumers are shaping mental health policy and how governmental policy can effectively support MHSH. Chapter 10, titled, "Finding and Using Our Voice: How Consumer/Survivor Advocacy is Transforming Mental Health Care," discusses how consumers are influencing mental health policy. Authors Daniel Fisher and Lauren Spiro describe three components that are critical to the development and sustainability of the consumer/survivor movement and its national advocacy voice, including

- A consensus by the movement that recovery, wellness, and complete community integration are attainable goals for persons labeled with mental illness in contrast to the traditional negative prognosis of maintenance during a lifelong disability.
- Training programs in advocacy designed and carried out by consumer/survivors, such as Finding Our Voice.
- Building the National Coalition of Mental Health Consumer/Survivor Organizations which amplifies the voice of consumer/survivors at the state and federal level.

Their chapter includes a detailed description of these components, providing examples of each, and how they continue to contribute to the future of the consumer/survivor voice.

Chapter 11, "How governments and other funding sources can facilitate self-help research and services" provides a much needed description of the role of government and other funding sources in contributing to and supporting MHSH initiatives. Crystal Blyler, Risa Fox, and Neal Brown provide examples of the types of activities in which governments and other funding sources can engage to facilitate and support self-help research and services. Specific ideas for potential funding of self-help research and service are presented and future directions for self-help research and services are discussed. Through these examples, the authors point out how the efforts of the federal Community Support Program have contributed to the growth of self-help over the past 30 years.

1.4.5 Technical Assistance

The technical assistance section of the book provides two chapters that examine how technical assistance has been a critical support for MHSH at the state and national levels. Chapter 12, by Susan Rogers, examines consumer and consumer-supporter national technical assistance centers in the United States. These technical assistance centers (TACs) foster self-help/recovery-oriented approaches in the mental health system. The chapter examines TACs' history, their goals and objectives, the challenges and barriers they face, and their efforts to overcome those challenges and barriers. The chapter includes interviews with leaders of the TACs as well as some of the individuals and group leaders they have served, and with the TACs' government project officer.

Oliwier Dziadkowiec and his colleagues provide Chapter 13, "A statewide collaboration to build the leadership and organizational capacity of consumer-run organizations (CROs)." The chapter begins with the history of the national consumer movement and the history of CROs in Kansas. Following is an in-depth commentary about the collaborative relationship between the Center for Community Support and Research (CCSR) and Kansas CROs. The chapter describes the unique relationship between CCSR and Kansas CROs, partnerships that have developed, and activities to build the leadership and organizational capacity of CROs. Additionally, there is an overview of research studies conducted by CCSR and others to asses the impact and capacity needs of CROs. The chapter concludes with a focus on the future of CROs and the consumer movement in Kansas.

1.4.6 Self-Help/Professional Collaboration

The final section of the book provides two chapters that examine the collaboration between MHSH initiatives and the professional mental health system. In Chapter 14, Deborah Salem, Thomas Reischl, and Katie Randall address the recent trend for mutual-help organizations to form collaborative partnerships with professionally run organizations. Their chapter, "Helping Mutual Help: Managing the Risks of Professional Partnerships" reviews a multi-method case study of a partnership between Schizophrenia Anonymous (SA) and the Mental Health Association of Michigan (MHAM) over a 14-year period. Results are discussed with regard to the lessons learned for managing mutual-help/professional partnerships. The authors draw on organizational theories and risk management principles to discuss strategies by which mutual-help organizations can benefit from partnerships with other types of organizations, while minimizing unintended changes to their basic beliefs, processes, and structures.

The fifteenth and final chapter, by Thomas Powell and Brian Perron, calls attention to the immense amount of support and services provided by MHSH. Their chapter, "The contribution of self-help groups to the mental health/substance use services system," contends that many MHSH initiatives are largely misunderstood by professionals and not coordinated with professional services. Their chapter reviews previous epidemiological surveys that have documented the profiles of self-help users, the amount of self-help use, and the association between self-help use and professional services. The chapter also discusses the organizational supports necessary for effective collaboration between self-help groups and professional services. While the boundaries between mental health services and self-help groups must be respected, both parties have much to gain by entering into more extensive community partnerships.

1.5 Future Research Directions in MHSH

A key research question facing MHSH is to understand the extent to which MHSH is helpful and the conditions under which it succeeds. These effectiveness questions are best answered with randomized controlled trials (RCTs). However, RCTs are difficult to execute effectively in MHSH settings because MHSH initiatives are highly dependent upon self-selection. As consumer and family-driven initiatives, researchers and professionals cannot control their use, which makes the use of random assignment difficult.

One strategy that may make random assignment more feasible in a practice context is to use an intensive engagement intervention when assigning individuals to the treatment condition. A simple referral is frequently too weak of an engagement intervention because people often do not comply with the recommendation. However, previous research has found the use of a sponsor outreach intervention to be an effective strategy for increasing the likelihood that referral will lead to attendance (Powell, Hill, Warner, Yeaton, & Silk, 2000; Sisson & Mallams, 1981). Another strategy for enhancing engagement may be to supplement any in-person or phone contacts from professionals and group members with mailings and emails. Evaluations that use these engagement techniques can serve as both excellent outcome evaluations and tests of the effectiveness of different outreach tactics. Research that provides insight into the engagement process is of great practical value because the most prominent needs of self-help groups center on member involvement, attendance, and recruitment (Meissen, Gleason, & Embree, 1991).

Numerous other research strategies are equally promising. For example, longitudinal observational field studies can study the trajectories of different people who encounter MHSH initiatives. Findings can provide insight into patterns of engagement and disengagement. If enough groups are included in these studies, they will be able to examine how group differences influence participation, outcomes, and sustainability. Such studies can aid the development of guidelines for ideal group characteristics that promote participation, group sustainability, and individual benefit.

Qualitative research also has the potential to make important contributions to our understanding of MHSH. For example, in-depth interviews and focus groups can provide important insight into the creation of useful self-help group philosophies and effective outreach materials. Interviews with self-help leaders and professionals who support self-help groups can help build understanding of how professionals can best interact with and support MHSH. Given the lack of theoretical guidance in approaching these topics, they are ripe for development through qualitative techniques.

1.6 Future Directions for MHSH Practice

The influence of MHSH is likely to continue expanding in the foreseeable future, and could lead to dramatic changes in the mental health system. The use of consumers as providers of mental health services is a radical departure from the traditional mental health system. If they prove to be similarly effective in providing services as mental health professionals, service providers who do not hire consumers risk facing legitimate charges of discrimination.

Another area of potentially tremendous growth in MHSH is the use of online self-help mutual aid groups. These groups lack participation barriers such as transportation and scheduling, which makes participation substantially easier for a large portion of the population.

Regardless of how paid and online peer support develops, currently existing volunteer-driven MHSH groups are likely to persist because the people who create them continue to need them.

1.7 Conclusion

This 15-chapter edited volume organizes and synthesizes the current knowledge base on MHSH. Consideration of the issues addressed can help to enhance MHSH effectiveness. Although many questions about the development of effective MHSH initiatives remain, the tides of opinion are turning in favor of MHSH as a low-cost supplement to professional mental health care. Rigorous experimental evaluations indicate MHSH can be effective. Future research needs to identity the conditions under which MHSH initiatives both thrive and fail. Such knowledge can support a diffusion of effective MHSH initiatives that promote the well-being of mental health consumers and their family members. However, MHSH implementation will always remain an art that science can only help to refine.

References

Brown, L. D. (2009). Making it sane: Using life history narratives to explore theory in a mental health consumer-run organization. *Qualitative Health Research, 19*, 243–257.

Brown, L. D., Shepherd, M. D., Wituk, S. A., & Meissen, G. (2007). Goal achievement and the accountability of consumer-run organizations. *Journal of Behavioral Health Services and Research, 34*, 73–82.

Brown, L. D., Shepherd, M. D., Wituk, S. A., & Meissen, G. (2007). How settings change people: Applying behavior setting theory to consumer-run organizations. *Journal of Community Psychology, 35*, 399–416.

Burti, L., Amaddeo, F., Ambrosi, M., Bonetto, C., Cristofalo, D., Ruggeri, M., et al. (2005). Does additional care provided by a consumer self-help group improve psychiatric outcome? A study in an Italian community-based psychiatric service. *Community Mental Health Journal, 41*(6), 705–720.

Carling, P. J. (1995). *Return to community: Building support systems for people with psychiatric disabilities*. New York, NY: Guilford Press.

Chamberlin, J. (1990). The ex-patients' movement: Where we've been and where we're going. *Journal of Mind and Behavior, 11*, 323–336.

Chamberlin, J., Rogers, E. S., & Ellison, M. L. (1996). Self-help programs: A description of their characteristics and their members. *Psychiatric Rehabilitation Journal, 19*(3), 33–42.

Chien, W.-T., Norman, I., & Thompson, D. R. (2006). Perceived benefits and difficulties experienced in a mutual support group for family carers of people with schizophrenia. *Qualitative Health Research, 16*(7), 962–981.

Clay, S. (2005). About us: What we have in common. In S. Clay (Ed.), *On our own, together: Peer programs for people with mental illness*. Nashville, TN: Vanderbilt University Press.

Constantino, V., & Nelson, G. (1995). Changing relationships between self-help groups and mental health professionals: Shifting ideology and power. *Canadian Journal of Community Mental Health, 14*(2), 55–70.

Corrigan, P. W., Slopen, N., Gracia, G., Phelan, S., Keogh, C. B., & Keck, L. (2005). Some recovery processes in mutual-help groups for persons with mental illness; II: Qualitative analysis of participant interviews. *Community Mental Health Journal, 41*(6), 721–735.

Goldstrom, I. D., Campbell, J., Rogers, J. A., Lambert, D. B., Blacklow, B., Henderson, M. J., et al. (2006). National estimates for mental health mutual support groups, self-help organizations, and consumer-operated services. *Administration and Policy in Mental Health and Mental Health Services Research, 33*, 92–103.

Humphreys, K. (2004). *Circles of recovery: Self-help organizations for addictions*. Cambridge, UK: Cambridge University Press.

Kelly, T. B., Salmon, R., & Graziano, R. (2004). Mutual aid groups for older persons with a mental illness. In R. Salmon & R. Graziano (Eds.), *Group work and aging: Issues in practice, research, and education*. (pp. 111–126). Haworth Social Work Practice Press, Binghamton, NY.

Kimura, M., Mukaiyachi, I., & Ito, E. (2002). The House of Bethel and consumer-run businesses: An innovative approach to psychiatric rehabilitation. *Canadian Journal of Community Mental Health, 21*(2), 69–77.

Meissen, G. J., Gleason, D. F., & Embree, M. G. (1991). An assessment of the needs of mutual-help groups. *American Journal of Community Psychology, 19*, 427–442.

Milofsky, C. (1988). *Community organizations: Studies in resource mobilization and exchange*. New York: Oxford University Press.

Mohr, W. K. (2004). Surfacing the life phases of a mental health support group. *Qualitative Health Research, 14*, 61–77.

Mowbray, C. T., Greenfield, A., & Freddolino, P. P. (1992). An analysis of treatment services provided in group homes for adults labeled mentally ill. *The Journal of Nervous and Mental Disease, 180*, 551–559.

Mowbray, C. T., Robinson, E. A., & Holter, M. C. (2002). Consumer drop-in centers: Operations, services, and consumer involvement. *Health and Social Work, 27*, 248–261.

Nelson, G., Lord, J., & Ochocka, J. (2001). *Shifting the paradigm in community mental health: Towards empowerment and community*. Toronto, Canada: University of Toronto Press.

Nelson, G., Walsh-Bowers, R., & Hall, G. B. (1998). Housing for psychiatric survivors: Values, policy, and research. *Administration and Policy in Mental Health, 25*, 55–62.

Norcross, J. C. (2000). Here comes the self-help revolution in mental heath. *Psychotherapy: Theory, Research, Practice, Training, 37*(4), 370–377.

Powell, T. J., Hill, E. M., Warner, L., Yeaton, W., & Silk, K. R. (2000). Encouraging people with mood disorders to attend a self-help group. *Journal of Applied Social Psychology, 30*, 2270–2288.

Recovery International. (2009). History of Recovery International. Retrieved August 29, 2009, from http://www.recovery- inc.org/about/history.asp

Sabin, J. E., & Daniels, N. (2003). Managed care: Strengthening the consumer voice in managed care: VII. The Georgia peer specialist program. *Psychiatric Services, 54*(4), 497–498.

Salzer, M. S., & Shear, S. L. (2002). Identifying consumer-provider benefits in evaluations of consumer-delivered services. *Psychiatric Rehabilitation Journal, 25*(3), 281–288.

Segal, S. P., & Silverman, C. (2002). Determinants of client outcomes in self-help agencies. *Psychiatric Services, 53*, 304–309.

Sherman, S. R., Frenkel, E. R., & Newman, E. S. (1986). Community participation of mentally ill adults in foster family care. *Journal of Community Psychology, 14*, 120–133.

Sisson, R. W., & Mallams, J. H. (1981). The use of systematic encouragement and community access procedures to increase attendance at Alcoholic Anonymous and Al-Anon meetings. *American Journal of Drug and Alcohol Abuse, 8*, 371–376.

Smith, D. H. (2000). *Grassroots associations*. Thousand Oaks, CA: Sage.

Solomon, P. (2004). Peer support/peer provided services: Underlying processes, benefits, and critical ingredients. *Psychiatric Rehabilitation Journal, 27*, 392–401.

Swarbrick, M. (2007). Consumer-operated self-help centers. *Psychiatric Rehabilitation Journal, 31*, 76–79.

Veterans Health Administration. (2004). *VA Mental Health Strategic Plan*. Washington, DC: Office of Mental Health Services.

Wuthnow, R. (1994). *Sharing the journey: Support groups and America's new quest for community*. New York: Free Press.

Part I
Frameworks for Research and Practice

Chapter 2
Theoretical Foundations of Mental Health Self-Help

Louis D. Brown and Alicia Lucksted

Abstract This chapter reviews the theoretical perspectives commonly applied to mental health self-help (MHSH). First, *recovery* and *community integration* are multifaceted constructs often used to conceptualize the outcomes of participation in MHSH initiatives. Second, we present several perspectives on MHSH setting characteristics that influence individual outcomes, including *sense of community*, *behavior setting theory*, and *empowerment theory*. Third, we summarize theoretical perspectives providing insight into how individuals benefit from their interactions with self-help settings, including the *helper-therapy principle*, *experiential knowledge*, *social comparison theory*, and *social support theories*. Finally, the *Role Framework* provides a theoretical model that helps to integrate and extend these different perspectives in the literature.

There are a variety of theoretical frameworks that can be used to understand different aspects of MHSH settings, processes, and outcomes. Developing a rich theoretical understanding of MHSH can be helpful to MHSH leaders, potential members, mental health professionals, policy makers, and researchers. Theoretical frameworks provide insight into (1) how MHSH settings can be most effectively structured; (2) how mental health policy and professionals can effectively support MHSH; (3) who is likely to benefit from participation; and (4) how to design theoretically sound evaluations. To help readers develop a functional theoretical understanding of MHSH relevant to all chapters in this volume, this chapter reviews the most common theories and concepts applied to MHSH (see Table 2.1). To help integrate the various theoretical perspectives reviewed, we organized them into four categories: (1) conceptualizations of MHSH outcomes; (2) theories regarding how MHSH setting characteristics influence individual outcomes; (3) explication of interpersonal

---

L.D. Brown (✉)
Prevention Research Center, The Pennsylvania State University, 135 E, Nittany Ave, Suite 402, State College, PA 16801, USA
e-mail: ldb12@psu.edu

Table 2.1 Overview of perspectives used to understand MHSH

Theoretical perspective – Content addressed	Core insights
Recovery – MHSH Outcomes	MHSH can help people reach a point at which their knowledge and management of their illness, along with their skills and values enables them to live a meaningful, satisfying life.
Community integration – MHSH Outcomes	MHSH participation contributes to (1) physical integration by involving self-initiated interaction in the community; (2) social integration by enhancing social networks; (3) psychological integration by encouraging camaraderie and group collaboration.
Sense of community – MHSH settings	The interdependent, mutually supportive relationships at a MHSH initiative promote sense of community and commitment.
Behavior setting theory – MHSH settings	Overpopulated MHSH settings may have numerous capable leaders whereas underpopulated settings may encourage a larger proportion of members to undertake empowering leadership roles.
Empowerment theory – MHSH settings	MHSH promotes individual empowerment by emphasizing self-determination and coping strategies. Member control of organizational activities, governance, and administration provides organizational empowerment. Organizing advocacy and public education efforts enhances community empowerment.
Helper-therapy principle – How individuals benefit	Helping other MHSH participants can provides helpers with a sense of self-efficacy, equality in giving and taking, improved interpersonal skills, and positive regard from help recipients.
Experiential knowledge – How individuals benefit	MHSH participants may be more capable of extending empathy, emotional support, and relevant coping strategies because their similar experiences give them knowledge that is more accurate and a deeper appreciation of what a person is going through.
Social comparison theory – How individuals benefit	MHSH participation may normalize mental illness (lateral comparisons), provide accomplished role models who effectively manage mental illness (upward comparisons), and downward comparisons to those who are worse off, which may enhance self-esteem and appreciation of current capabilities.
Social support – How individuals benefit	From a stress-buffering perspective, MHSH provides participants with social resources in times of need. Long-term relationships also provide direct benefits (main effects), including a sense of stability, purpose, belonging, security, and self-worth.
Role Framework – Connects settings, participation, and outcomes	MHSH settings promote the development of help-seeker and help-provider roles, where participants (1) exchange emotional and informational resources, (2) obtain positive self-appraisals by helping others, (3) develop new skills to meet role expectations, and (4) adopt empowering help-provider role identities.

processes that lead to participation benefits; and (4) frameworks that help to connect settings, interpersonal processes, and outcomes.

Recovery and community integration help to conceptualize the goals and outcomes of MHSH. Behavior setting theory, empowerment theory, and sense of community describe how MHSH setting characteristics influence interpersonal processes and individual outcomes. The helper-therapy principle, experiential knowledge, social comparison theory, and social support theories help to explain how the interpersonal interactions within MHSH settings lead to individual outcomes. And finally, the Role Framework ties setting level characteristics, interpersonal processes, and individual outcomes together and helps integrate the other theoretical perspectives. The following sections explore each of these theories and concepts in more detail.

2.1 Conceptualization of MHSH Outcomes

2.1.1 Recovery

"Mental health recovery" has been described as both an outcome and as a process leading to that outcome (Bellack, 2006). As an outcome it refers to people with serious mental illnesses (SMI) reaching a point at which their knowledge and management of their illness, their skills and values, their use of helping modalities, and their personal stance toward their life in the context of their ongoing illness, together enable them to live a meaningful, satisfying life (Anthony, 1993). Recovery can be conceptualized as a combination of hope, self-responsibility, "getting on with life" beyond illness, and overcoming the challenge of disability (Deegan, 1988; Noordsy et al., 2002)

Participation in MHSH can be a powerful part of one's path toward recovery-as-outcome. MHSH is seen as helping people build capacity and learn skills to overcome stressors and recover wellness. MHSH can foster active coping and taking responsibility for the consequences of one's actions, and the shape of one's future and well-being. By developing new capacities, framing new goals, and ascribing new meaning to old experiences, participants can create new states of wellness with renewed hope for the future. These all contribute to a person's recovery. Thus, the concept of mental health recovery does not explain why or how MHSH benefits people. Instead, it highlights the larger picture that MHSH contributes to – helping people with mental illnesses improve and re-fashion their lives in an adaptive response to the challenges of mental illness.

2.1.2 Community Integration

The multidimensional construct of community integration provides a different framework for understanding the many different ways individuals can benefit from

MHSH participation. Being able to take part in the various facets of a community is both a right (according to the 1990 Americans with Disabilities Act and the 1999 Supreme Court Olmstead decision) and an avenue to psychological and social benefits that can result from taking advantage of opportunities in the community environment and feelings connected to the community. Wong and Solomon (2002) thoughtfully define the interrelated physical, social, and psychological components of community integration. "*Physical integration* refers to the extent to which an individual spends time, participates in activities, and uses goods and services in the community outside his/her home or facility in a self-initiated manner," (Wong & Solomon, 2002, p. 18). Whenever individuals participate in a MHSH initiative, they do all of these. Thus, physical community integration is inherent in the act of MHSH participation. The more someone replaces time spent in isolation with time spent involved in a MHSH initiative, the more physically integrated that person becomes into his/her community.

"*Social integration* has two subdimensions – an interactional dimension and a social network dimension. [The] interactional dimension refers to the extent to which an individual engages in social interactions with community members that are culturally normative both in quantity and quality, and that take place within normative contexts," (Wong & Solomon, 2002, p. 18). Again, MHSH participation inherently involves social interactions with community members. MHSH interactions are normative in the sense that participants voluntarily meet new people, share stories and discuss issues, solve problems, and take on leadership roles – activities common throughout community-based organizations. At the same time, MHSH interactions are also often non-normative in that participants interact only with other mental health consumers. This interaction may be helpful as participants share experiential knowledge in coping with mental illness (Borkman, 1999), typically creating an understanding, accepting, and supportive environment where participants have a great deal in common. Thus, MHSH facilitates social integration into the community of mental health consumers. However, viewed from the vantage of the wider geographic or societal community surrounding a given MHSH initiative, MHSH participation can also remain distant and separated from normative community interactions. Socializing *only* with other consumers or MHSH participants may limit a person's community integration to a narrow band.

"[The] *social network dimension* refers to the extent to which an individual's social network reflects adequate size and multiplicity of social roles, and the degree to which social relationships reflect positive support and reciprocity, as opposed to stress and dependency," (Wong & Solomon, 2002, p. 19). MHSH participation leads to the development of a new social network full of mutually supportive roles. The more involved participants become, the more their social network size and richness will grow. Dependency roles do not typically develop because MHSH participants act as both help providers and help seekers. The voluntary nature of MHSH roles and relationships allows people to disengage from relationships where stress outweighs the positive support received. Thus, MHSH participation can dramatically enhance participants' social integration.

2.1.3 Sense of Community/Psychological Integration

"*Psychological integration* refers to the extent to which an individual perceives membership in his/her community, expresses an emotional connection with neighbors, and believes in his/her ability to fulfill needs through neighbors, while exercising influence in the community," (Wong & Solomon, 2002, p. 19). This definition of psychological integration is very similar to the definition of psychological sense of community provided by McMillan and Chavis (1986). When interdependent, mutually supportive relationships form (at an MHSH initiative or otherwise), a sense of community develops. People become attached and committed to the setting. They further invest themselves into the initiative, contributing to it and receiving many benefits from it.

Forming a sense of community is important to MHSH settings because it promotes empowerment and catalyzes increased and sustained participation (Chavis & Wandersman, 1990; McMillan et al., 1995). Furthermore, a sense of belonging is a highly valued outcome of participation. A shared sense of community is catalyzed in many MHSH settings by the shared "experiential knowledge" that members in a self-help initiative possess (Borkman, 1999). In a beneficial spiral, the warm accepting atmosphere inherent to settings with a strong sense of community is rewarding in itself, and is critical to the development of roles and relationships where participants exchange and sustain mutual emotional support. By having a place where people trust and support each other, individuals gain confidence to take on new roles that are unfamiliar, exciting, and healthy. Settings rich with encouragement and acceptance allow people to take needed risks without the fear of social criticism. The trusting bonds enable communication around difficult issues and work as a healing mechanism (Gidron & Chesler, 1994).

Furthermore, developing a sense of community at a MHSH initiative can facilitate community attachment with other territorial (e.g., neighborhood) and relational (e.g., church) communities (Heller, 1989; McMillan & Chavis, 1986, Unger & Wandersman, 1985), thereby strengthening individual and the organizational resources and furthering community integration. Research suggests that MHSH participants are in fact involved in their communities, with over 90% taking part in at least one community activity outside of their MHSH initiative (Chamberlin, Rogers, & Ellison, 1996).

In summary, the physical, social, and psychological aspects of community integration are important outcomes that MHSH participation can promote, enhanced by the development of a sense of community. All fit with the larger conceptualization of recovery among people with serious mental illnesses. Several other setting characteristics are also important determinants of positive MHSH participation outcomes, including empowerment theory and behavior setting theory. The next section discusses these, beginning with behavior setting theory, which is useful in understanding how the MHSH setting characteristics of under- and overpopulation influence individual outcomes.

2.2 Setting Characteristic Theories

2.2.1 Behavior Setting Theory

A behavioral setting is a small social system defined by its standing pattern of behavior and occurring within particular temporal and spatial boundaries (Barker, 1968). Established patterns of behavior guide the interactions among the setting's various participants. MHSH initiatives are behavior settings that attempt to establish a mutually supportive pattern of behavior, where participants act as both help seekers and help providers, bounded temporally by their meeting hours and spatially by their meeting location.

For behavior settings to operate properly, the individual roles that make up the standing patterns of behavior need to be filled. Some MHSH settings may have one or two roles, such as group member and group leader. Others have more complex structures that require numerous roles, such as grant writer, budget manager, director, transportation provider, and board member. In behavior setting theory, participants are essential to fulfilling the functions of these roles, but individuals are considered relatively interchangeable because similar interactions occur regardless of who occupies each role in a setting. Assuming participants are equally effective in both help-seeker and help-provider roles, a MHSH setting will produce a similar pattern of mutually supportive exchanges regardless of who participates.

However, roles are not the same across even similar settings like MHSH. One critical factor in determining how individuals experience a given behavior setting is whether it is under- or overpopulated. An *under* populated behavior setting has more roles than members, making every member essential (Barker, 1968; Schoggen, 1989) and requiring that some members occupy more than one role. In this environment, there are many opportunities to develop new skills, and all available resources are used. For example, rather than screening out less adequate participants from leadership roles through "vetoing circuits," underpopulated settings develop "deviation-countering circuits" that help people learn the correct behavior and successfully perform the needed role. However, if the setting is too underpopulated, members may become overextended and burn out.

In contrast, *over* populated settings have more interested participants than roles available. Therefore, such settings develop dynamics that select only the members perceived to be most capable to fill leadership roles, excluding other less capable members. This process of exclusion within an overpopulated setting is called a "vetoing circuit." Both over- and underpopulation have important implications for individuals' experiences in that setting.

Research suggests that a strong leadership base is essential for effective MHSH operation (Kaufmann, Ward-Colasante, & Farmer, 1993). Overpopulated MHSH settings may be able to select only the strongest leaders and exclude weaker candidates. The competition can help MHSH settings cope with a surplus of potential leaders and to operate effectively by putting the most capable at the helm.

However, this exclusion of some members from leadership roles also may be problematic. Previous research indicates that involvement in organizational planning and decision making is an important predictor of participation benefits (Segal & Silverman, 2002). If there are a limited number of leadership roles, then overpopulated settings may confer less benefit on large proportions its participants. Instead, underpopulated settings may be more individually beneficial because all members are needed and encouraged to take on leadership roles. Furthermore, the idea that only some members are suitable for leadership contradicts the self-help ideals of minimal hierarchy and shared decision making (Riessman & Carroll, 1995).

Yet in any setting, participants gravitate to certain roles and avoid others depending on factors such as temperament, skill set, judgments of others, and opportunity. In overpopulated settings, involving everyone in planning and decision making can be slow and cumbersome. As groups grow, more participants are excluded from leadership roles since they are limited in number (Brown, Shepherd, Wituk, & Meissen, 2007). However, exclusion from leadership roles may not be particularly problematic, as participants can still benefit from the mutually supportive exchanges that occur in non-leadership roles (Brown, Shepherd, Merkle, Wituk, & Meissen, 2008). These challenges of balancing leadership and role differentiation with equality and effective operations are an important consideration for any MHSH initiative.

2.2.2 Empowerment Theory

Like behavior setting theory, empowerment theory provides insight into how setting characteristics contribute to outcomes – in this case, an empowering environment promotes individual empowerment and other benefits. Empowerment as a values framework posits that psychiatric consumers have the right to gain control over their lives, make informed decisions about how they will use mental health services rather than being passive recipients of others' treatment decisions, and take actions on their own behalf (Dickerson, 1998). As a process, empowerment involves a person developing skills and acquiring information that can enhance self-determination. Environments facilitate this process when they value consumers' recovery and readily offer opportunities to both develop skills and acquire valuable information. Further, empowerment is also an important outcome fostered by MHSH and positively related to indicators of physical and mental health (Israel, House, Schurman, Heaney, & Mero, 1989).

MHSH settings are uniquely empowering because they are consumer and family driven. Furthermore, MHSH is qualitatively different from professional mental health services in that MHSH participants not only receive help but provide it as well. Professionally delivered mental health services may provide excellent support, but even the most client-centered systems do not provide participants (clients) the benefits of helping others (see helper-therapy principle, next section). The emphasis of MHSH on building capacity to help oneself and others promotes empowerment (Trainor, Shepherd, Boydell, Leff, & Crawford, 1997).

Thus MHSH participation leads to empowerment at the individual, organizational, and community levels (Segal, Silverman, & Temkin, 1993). MHSH promotes individual empowerment by helping members obtain needed resources, develop skills needed to take initiative in directing their own lives, and to become socially engaged. This is reinforced at the group or organizational level, in that MHSH members control the activities that are pursued, their governance, and their administration. At the community level, many MHSH settings encourage participant involvement in social change and policy-making by organizing advocacy and public education efforts.

Thus, MHSH settings often manifest key characteristics of empowering community settings, including "(a) a belief system that inspires growth, is strengths-based, and is focused beyond the self; (b) an opportunity role structure that is pervasive, highly accessible, and multifunctional; (c) a support system that is encompassing, peer-based, and provides a sense of community; and (d) leadership that is inspiring, talented, shared, and committed to both setting and members" (Maton & Salem, 1995, p. 631). The sense of control and ownership that individuals can gain when participating in a MHSH initiative can transfer into a sense of personal and community level empowerment (Schulz, Israel, Zimmerman, & Checkoway, 1995; Zimmerman & Rappaport, 1988). Furthermore, involvement in empowering leadership roles is an important predictor of personal empowerment and social functioning (Segal & Silverman, 2002).

Empowerment, sense of community, and behavior setting theory all provide insight into how setting level characteristics influence individual outcomes. The next sections describe how interpersonal processes occurring within MHSH settings help create these setting characteristics and contribute to individual outcomes. Specifically, the helper-therapy principle, experiential knowledge, social comparison theory, and social support theories all help to explain how the interpersonal interactions that occur during MHSH participation are beneficial.

2.3 Interpersonal Processes Within MHSH Settings

2.3.1 The Helper-Therapy Principle

The helper-therapy principle states that the act of providing help can be more therapeutic than receiving help (Riessman, 1965). Research has demonstrated that the act of helping others can improve self-concept, increase energy levels, and improve physical health (Luks, 1991). MHSH initiatives provide many opportunities to help others in a mutually supportive environment. For example, self-help group participants help each other by providing emotional support, acceptance, and ideas about how to solve personal problems. Additionally, people in a MHSH leadership role can help others by accomplishing organizational tasks that are beneficial to everyone. Such helping roles are especially valuable to people with mental illnesses because psychiatric symptoms and the common consequences of severe mental illness (such as poverty and stigma) can reduce one's opportunities to make valuable contributions to others, such as through work, parenting, or civic leadership.

Skovholt (1974) theorized four benefits from helping others. One is an increased sense of competence or self-efficacy, which can occur when people successfully help others. For example, MHSH participants find that relating one's own experiences and coping strategies gives other participants helpful ideas. This reinforces a positive self-assessment of those experiences while also creating the rewarding experience of being valued by someone else. Second, Skovholt theorized that helping others promotes a sense of equality in one's giving and taking in relationships with others. This equality can help consumers become independent, self-supporting adults, who contribute as much as they consume. A third benefit of helping is that it can promote learning and the acquisition of personally useful knowledge. In a MHSH setting, people can apply their existing experience and knowledge in new ways, exercise problem-solving skills, expand their thinking about common challenges and improve their interpersonal skills through helping others. Fourth, the helper role often leads to appreciation and social approval from the person receiving help and other peers. This positive regard can provide the helper with a sense of importance, usefulness, and satisfaction.

2.3.2 *Experiential Knowledge*

Experiential knowledge refers to the insights, information, and skills that one develops through coping with life challenges. When people share a particular life challenge, experiential knowledge can help them relate to one another and provide appropriate support (Borkman, 1999). This shared experience is particularly powerful in an MHSH context because the stigma associated with mental illness often sets consumers apart from others. Experiences with psychiatric hospitalization, medications, hallucinations, suicidal ideation, and other symptoms are not only hard to fathom but often frightening. Friends, family, and even professional providers who have not had such experiences may therefore shy away from understanding these experiences, often by discouraging discussion of them and the feelings they provoke, changing the subject, or encouraging cheerfulness in spite of trauma (Coates & Winston, 1983; Dunkel-Schetter, 1984; Helgeson & Gottlieb, 2000). Such responses can frustrate and belittle people struggling to deal with mental illness.

Therefore, the *shared* experience with mental health problems among MHSH participants frequently acts as a key bonding point in the development of supportive relationships. This commonality can engender trust and a feeling of acceptance. Numerous studies have demonstrated the emotional benefits of sharing experiences with others who have faced similar hardships (Helgeson & Gottlieb, 2000), including validation, normalization of the experience, a reduction in social and emotional isolation, and a sense of belonging (Cowan & Cowan, 1986; Lieberman, 1993; Rosenberg, 1984; Toseland & Rossiter, 1989).

Additionally, people who have also "been there," are often better prepared to provide appropriate support to each other by virtue of the (often hard won) expertise and understanding that these experiences convey (Helgeson & Gottlieb, 2000). For example, mental health consumers may be more capable of extending empathy and emotional support to other mental health consumers because their similar experiences give them knowledge that is more accurate and a deeper appreciation of what a person is going through. By dealing with their own problems, MHSH participants also may have developed coping and problem-solving strategies that can be useful to others facing similar challenges (Borkman, 1999). Their experience in certain situations may have taught them certain information, coping strategies, or tips that can save others from having to learn through trial and error. Thus, the exchange of emotional and informational support in a MHSH setting, informed by experiential knowledge, can be invaluable.

2.3.3 Social Comparison Theory

In MHSH settings, participants' shared experiences enable several types of meaningful social comparison (Festinger, 1954). Lateral (peer) comparisons may serve to normalize and contextualize a person's experiences within the particular challenges shared by the group. For example, one reason that having a mental illness or caring for someone who does is often isolating is that others cannot relate to the challenge. Discussing hopes, fears, stories, and meanings in a MHSH setting, with peers going through related challenges, can help people realize they are not alone in their struggle nor abnormal in their reactions (Coates & Winston, 1983). Additionally, downward comparisons can be helpful. MHSH participants sometimes report that hearing other participants' more harrowing stories helps to put their challenges in perspective and increases their resolve (Lucksted, Stewart, & Forbes, 2008).

Secondly, MHSH leaders are often charismatic and accomplished people despite the serious challenges posed by their mental illness. Other members can make *upward* social comparisons to these people, viewing them as role models (Helgeson & Mickelson, 1995). Their success may help raise the expectations, dreams, and striving of MHSH participants. If such participants can also identify with these leaders, socially valued roles may become a new possibility in their minds, perhaps replacing assumptions of isolation and dependency. Such upward comparisons may inspire hope and the pursuit of new life-enhancing roles. However, social comparison theory also cautions that the benefits of upward comparisons can be compromised if the more-accomplished person is seen as a rare unattainable exception or too dissimilar from the upward-looking members (Suls, Martin, & Wheeler, 2002).

Every MHSH initiative has numerous members with a variety of capacities. Just as upward comparisons with the leaders are possible, *downward* comparisons with people in worse situations are also possible. Comparing one's self to those worse off may help people appreciate what they do have and provide a boost in self-esteem (Wills, 1981). Downward comparisons also sometimes help people persevere in their coping (Taylor, 1983), such as via thinking "if he can handle X then surely I should keep working on Y which is not as bad" (Lucksted et al., 2008). However, both upward and downward social comparisons are also potentially detrimental. Downward comparisons may lower expectations or contribute to demoralization, while upward comparisons may make people feel inferior (Helgeson & Gottlieb, 2000). How social comparisons play out in MHSH settings is poorly understood and further research is needed.

2.3.4 Social Support Theories

Social relationships are widely regarded as critical determinants of physical and mental health (Berkman, Glass, Brissette, & Seeman, 2000). Larger social networks among people with mental illness are linked to fewer psychiatric symptoms, improved quality of life, and higher self-esteem (Goldberg, Rollins, & Lehman, 2003). MHSH initiatives improve social networks by providing participants with the opportunity to participate in shared activities that they self-organize and within which they may develop relationships that transcend those specific activities (Hardiman & Segal, 2003). Furthermore, research suggests that making new friends is the most frequently cited benefit of MHSH participation (Mowbray & Tan, 1993). Relationships formed during MHSH participation can be not only richly rewarding and therapeutic in themselves but also valuable precursors to the development of relationships external to the MHSH initiative. Research by Trainor et al. (1997) supports the notion that MHSH can help participants build networks in the broader community, with 60% of MHSH participants indicating that contacts with non-consumers increased as a result of their MHSH involvement.

Social support, the perception that one is part of a caring network of people who are helpful during difficult times, (Cobb, 1976) is widely recognized as an important determinant of mental health and a powerful motivation for MHSH participation (Mowbray & Tan, 1993). However, *how* social support impacts mental health is extensively debated (Cohen, Gottlieb, & Underwood, 2000; Thoits, 1985). There are two prominent and competing models – the stress-buffering model and the main effects model. The *stress-buffering* perspective argues that social support mediates the relationship between stress and health. Enhanced coping ability made possible through social support can buffer the negative influence of stressful experiences on mental health, because the resources available from social support provide individuals with both confidence in their coping ability and real support in coping with imposed demands. By maintaining long-term relationships in a MHSH initiative, people are able to draw on these social resources in times of need.

In contrast, the *main effects* model of social support emphasizes the importance of social relationships in the direct production of positive affect and the reduction of psychological despair (Cohen et al., 2000; Thoits, 1985). Such relationships provide people with a sense of predictability, stability, purpose, belonging, security, and self-worth (Hammer, 1981; Thoits, 1983; Wills, 1985). MHSH initiatives also provide these direct positive effects, through enjoyable social interactions, positive settings for fostering further social relationships, and affirming exchanges about problems and challenges. Thus MHSH initiatives embody both the stress-buffering and the main effects models of how social support contributes to well-being.

The next section discusses the Role Framework, which uses a main effects model of social support to understand how relationships formed in MHSH initiatives are beneficial. The Role Framework also helps to draw connections between several of the other theories discussed, including sense of community, empowerment theory, behavior setting theory, the helper-therapy principle, and experiential knowledge.

2.4 The Role Framework

Several social science disciplines have used the concept of *roles* to understand human behavior, including sociology (Mead, 1934), psychology (Lewin, 1948), and anthropology (Linton, 1936). In this chapter, we use the phrase "the Role Framework" to denote a new integration of ideas from across these disciplines. Within the Role Framework, a role is defined as a set of behavioral expectations describing how one person is supposed to interact with others in a given environment (Brown, 2009a, 2009b; Brown et al., 2008). Numerous roles exist in MHSH settings. Two universally available roles are that of help seeker and help provider. These roles do not have strict expectations, but some general guidelines are clear. In help-seeker roles, participants may be expected to share problems, listen to feedback, decide for themselves which advice is useful, and develop plans to overcome personal challenges. Those in help-provider roles may be expected to provide empathy, share their own struggles with similar challenges, share problem-solving strategies that have worked, and accept others for who they are. MHSH participants typically occupy both help-seeker and help-provider roles on a regular basis, sometimes during a single conversation. Well-run MHSH initiatives maintain role structures that promote mutually supportive patterns of interaction and allow members to move easily between help seeker and help provider as their needs and the needs of others indicate.

Drawing from the previously discussed ideas of empowerment theory, sense of community, the helper-therapy principle, social support, and experiential knowledge, along with concepts from resource exchange theory (Foa & Foa, 1980) and identity theory (Burke, Owens, Serpe, & Thoits, 2003; Stryker & Burke, 2000), the Role Framework explains how people benefit from MHSH participation (Brown, 2009a, 2009b). More specifically, the role framework explains how the roles and relationships formed through MHSH initiatives can lead to new resources, positive self-appraisals, new skills, and new identities. Research exploring the Role Framework found it flexible enough to capture the personal experiences and outcomes described by 194 MHSH participants (Brown, 2009a). Another study, using prolonged observation and in-depth interviews, demonstrated that the Role Framework could accurately describe the change processes experienced by seven MHSH members from one MHSH initiative (Brown, 2009b). Therefore, although it is a new conceptualization of the beneficial processes involved in MHSH participation, we have initial evidence that it is a useful integration of numerous diverse relevant concepts. Figure 2.1 illustrates the Role Framework's six components: (a) person–environment interaction, (b) role and relationship development, (c) resource exchange, (d) self-appraisal, (e) skill development, and (f) identity transformation (Brown, 2009a). The subsections below describe each component, followed by an explanation of how theoretical concepts presented earlier in this chapter relate to the Role Framework.

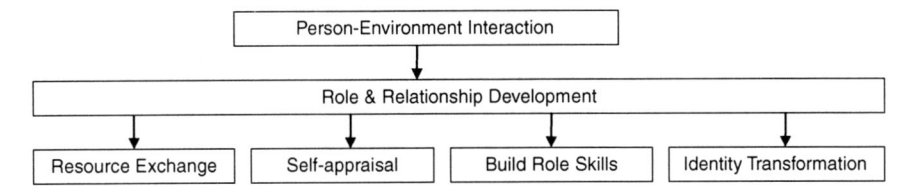

Fig. 2.1 Conceptual model of the Role Framework

2.4.1 Component One – Person–Environment Interaction

The first component of the Role Framework focuses how individual and environmental characteristics interact to shape the course of role and relationship development. Individual characteristics that are especially relevant to MHSH include having a mental illness or caring for someone who does and being interested in interacting with similar others. One particularly important environmental characteristic is that MHSH initiatives provide people who have mental illnesses a setting that emphasizes mutually supportive roles rather than the unidirectional help-recipient roles that operate when interacting with mental health professionals. As further discussed in the section, "*Relating the Role Framework to other theoretical perspectives*," environmental characteristics that influence person–environment interaction include the degree to which a MHSH initiative is empowering, has a sense of community, and is under- or overpopulated.

Identifying further individual and environmental characteristics that influence role and relationship development is a key research challenge facing MHSH. Improved understanding of how the environment influences the interpersonal interaction process could foster the development of even more effective MHSH environments that promote wellness-enhancing roles. Furthermore, understanding which individual characteristics influence the interaction process can help recruitment efforts target individuals who are most likely to benefit from participation and tailor skill-building programs within the setting.

2.4.2 Component Two – Role and Relationship Development

Whereas the first component focuses on characteristics of the person and environment (which influence role and relationship development), the second component focuses on describing the actual roles and relationships formed during MHSH participation. As touched on in the section on behavior setting theory, a myriad of roles can develop during MHSH participation, many of which are specific to a particular MHSH context. For example, a consumer-run drop-in center (see Chapter 7) may have an executive director, shift managers, and a board of directors. Listing the roles available in a setting and describing the expectations associated with each one can provide insight into the structure and pattern of interactions within that setting. In addition to the roles of help provider and help recipient, the self-governed nature of MHSH also promotes the development of empowering leadership roles among participants because the continued functioning of the initiative depends on multiple members taking on the responsibilities of leadership (Maton & Salem, 1995). These roles have important consequences for their occupants, which are described in the next four sections.

2.4.3 Component Three – Resource Exchange

The third component focuses on describing the resources that participants exchange in order to experience positive interactions and fulfill the expectations of the roles they occupy in a given MHSH setting. For example, participants in a help-seeker role are expected to receive resources whereas participants in a help-provider role are expected give resources. Because MHSH participants can switch quickly between the two roles or even occupy both during a single interaction (such as in a support group), the exchange of resources in MHSH can be complex and lively. Resources exchanged can include esteem, love, information, money, goods, and services (Foa & Foa, 1974). MHSH participants may exchange informational support such as coping strategies and love as a caring friend. MHSH members enacting leadership roles can give by completing organizational tasks that benefit everyone. In return, they may receive esteemed gratitude from the participants who benefit from their efforts.

2.4.4 Component Four – Self-Appraisal

Drawing from the ideas of identity theory, (Burke, 1991; Burke et al., 2003; Stryker, 1980) this component describes the process of self-appraisal and how it influences emotions and self-esteem. When people are successful in meeting role expectations, they appraise themselves positively for a job well done. For example, MHSH help-seekers who successfully reach out for and accept needed assistance may feel good that they are actively working to improve their lives. Additionally, meeting the expectations of help-provider roles may be particularly rewarding because the positive appraisals come from both the helper and those who they helped. Conversely, when people do not fulfill valued role expectations, they make negative self-appraisals and likely receive negative appraisals from others who value the role expectations.

Positive and negative appraisals cause positive and negative emotional responses (Burke, 2003). Self-appraisals similarly contribute to or detract from self-esteem (Cast & Burke, 2002; Thoits, 1985). Consequently, people are motivated to fulfill role expectations not only because they facilitate resource exchange but because of their direct influence on emotional well-being and self-esteem.

2.4.5 Component Five – Build Role Skills

When MHSH participants take on new roles, they may need to develop new skills in order to meet the new expectations. The fifth component focuses on understanding the skills that MHSH participants develop in order to meet expectations. For example, success in the help-provider role requires good listening skills; success in the help-seeker role requires the humility to ask for help and critical thinking skills to differentiate between good and bad advice. Leadership roles require participants to development decision-making abilities and other leadership skills. Skill development is one strategy people can use to meet the challenges and expectations of the roles they take on, and thus enable them to attain positive self-appraisals, positive emotions, and increased self-esteem.

2.4.6 Component Six – Identity Transformation

The sixth component focuses on understanding how the new role relationships developed within a MHSH setting transform the identities of participants. Roles are fundamental determinants of self-concept because each role an individual inhabits becomes a component of that person's identity if it is enacted on a regular basis. These identities then provide a framework that guides role-specific interactions the person has with others (Stryker & Burke, 2000). For example, people in the role of help providers may begin to see themselves as good listeners. Similarly, MHSH participants who take on leadership roles may begin to see themselves as leaders. Once these identity transformations take place, these MHSH participants may become more likely to move into help-provider or leadership roles in other community settings.

Identities shift as people embrace new role expectations and appraise their role performance. For example, a MHSH participant in a leadership role may expect to facilitate productive discussions during meetings. If the MHSH participant successfully meets expectations, she/he will think of him/herself as a good discussion leader and may expand his/her behavior and identity in this role. In contrast, failure to lead productive discussions will lead to negative self-appraisals, negative emotions, and reduced self-esteem. This can spark behavioral changes to bring one's actions more in line with the role – such as asking for coaching or other help in improving one's facilitation skills. However, if failures continue, the person may escape the role expectations by giving up their role and identity (here, as discussion leader). Thus, identity transformations are similar to skill development in that they are a strategy people can use to maintain congruence between expectations and behavior.

2.4.7 Relating the Role Framework to Other Theoretical Perspectives

Several previously discussed theoretical perspectives are directly related to the role framework, including sense of community, empowerment theory, behavior setting theory, the helper-therapy principle, experiential knowledge, social comparison theory, and social support theories. Within the person–environment component, sense of community operates as an important environmental characteristic of MHSH settings that promotes the development of mutually supportive relationships. Similarly, an empowering environment is critical for MHSH settings because it encourages participants to develop empowering leadership roles within the setting, thereby gaining greater control over their environment. When participants undertake empowering leadership roles they can experience empowering identity transformations and begin to see themselves as leaders capable of controlling their lives and making important contributions to the community. Within behavior setting theory, the concept of under- and overpopulation is a salient environmental characteristic for MHSH settings that influences role and relationship development by pulling participants into leadership roles (in the case of underpopulated settings) or excluding less qualified participants from leadership roles (in the case of overpopulated settings). Experiential knowledge relates to the role framework as an important individual characteristic that enhances person–environment interaction. The shared experience of coping with mental illness helps individuals understand and identify with one another. Experiential knowledge also relates to the resource exchange component because it serves as a valuable resource that participants share during mutually supportive interactions.

In the Role Framework, MHSH participants benefit from the helper-therapy principle when they take on helper roles. The four benefits of helping others described by Skovholt (sense of self-efficacy, equality in giving and taking, improved interpersonal skills, and positive regard from help recipients) directly relate to the consequences of role development described by the Role Framework. In the resource exchange component, people in mutually supportive helper roles develop a sense of equality in giving and taking. During the self-appraisal process, people in helper roles are likely to make positive self-appraisals because of the positive regard they receive from help recipients. Through helper roles, people can build new skills such as the interpersonal skills described by Skovholt. Developing a sense of self-efficacy is a type of identity transformation that occurs when people become confident they can meet the expectations associated with their helper role.

Among social support theories, both the stress-buffering model and the main effects model fit can be understood using the Role Framework. MHSH participants who maintain socially supportive friendship roles can buffer stressful experiences by drawing upon their social support resources in times of need. Similarly, participants can also benefit directly from their friendship roles when they fulfill role expectations for being a good friend and thereby obtain positive appraisals from both themselves and others. Successful friendship roles can also boost self-esteem and provide participants with purposeful identities as important people embedded in the social network of the MHSH initiative. Members of a MHSH social network also make upward, downward, and lateral social comparisons that can influence their self-appraisals and role expectations as a person with mental health problems.

2.4.8 Implications for MHSH Practice

Familiarity with the theoretical frameworks that provide insight into MHSH settings, interpersonal processes, and outcomes can help guide the development of effective MHSH initiatives. Understanding the outcomes associated with well-run MHSH initiatives and the processes by which people benefit can help MHSH leaders and allies explain the benefits to potential MHSH participants, and write more compelling funding applications to support MHSH initiatives. Furthermore, understanding the dynamics of MHSH settings and how they influence outcomes is essential for those aiming to develop and implement strategic efforts intended to enhance the effectiveness of the MHSH operations.

2.4.9 Implications for MHSH Researchers

Theoretical frameworks that explain the relations between MHSH settings, interpersonal processes, and outcomes are equally important for researchers. These frameworks can help guide the researcher into productive areas of inquiry, sharpening focus on insightful questions, appropriate analyses, and contextualized conclusions that help move the field forward. In particular, these theoretical perspectives can help researchers design rigorous studies that test the effectiveness of MHSH using outcome measures that are appropriate for the context while simultaneously examining relevant setting characteristics that may influence outcomes and mediating interpersonal processes that are critical to outcome attainment.

2.5 Conclusion

Although many MHSH initiatives developed without the use of formal theoretical frameworks, MHSH leaders and allies can nevertheless refine their efforts through careful reflection on how their actions lead to desired outcomes. This chapter reviewed some of the most common theories applied to MHSH and Table 2.1 provides a brief overview of each theoretical perspective. Readers can use these theoretical frameworks to enhance understanding of the different types of MHSH discussed in Chapters 4–10. Although all have some empirical support, none has undergone extensive or rigorous testing in a MHSH setting. It is likely that all are partially able to explain how people benefit from MHSH. However, we need future research and applied program development to improve our understanding of which theories demonstrate the most promise and explanatory power.

References

Anthony, W. A. (1993). Recovery from mental illness: The guiding vision of the mental health service system in the 1990s. *Psychosocial Rehabilitation Journal, 16,* 11–23.

Barker, R. G. (1968). *Ecological psychology.* Stanford, CA: Stanford University Press.

Bellack, A. S. (2006). Scientific and consumer models of recovery in schizophrenia: Concordance, contrasts, and implications. *Schizophrenia Bulletin, 32,* 432–442.

Berkman, L. F., Glass, T., Brissette, I., & Seeman, T. (2000). From social integration to health: Durkheim in the new millennium. *Social Science & Medicine, 51,* 843–857.

Borkman, T. J. (1999). *Understanding self-help/mutual aid: Experiential learning in the commons.* New Brunswick, NJ: Rutgers University Press.

Brown, L. D. (2009a). How people can benefit from mental health consumer-run organizations. *American Journal of Community Psychology, 43,* 177–188.

Brown, L. D. (2009b). Making it sane: Using life history narratives to explore theory in a mental health consumer-run organization. *Qualitative Health Research, 19,* 243–257.

Brown, L. D., Shepherd, M. D., Merkle, E. C., Wituk, S. A., & Meissen, G. (2008). Understanding how participation in a consumer-run organization relates to recovery. *American Journal of Community Psychology, 42,* 167–178.

Brown, L. D., Shepherd, M. D., Wituk, S. A., & Meissen, G. (2007). How settings change people: Applying behavior setting theory to consumer-run organizations. *Journal of Community Psychology, 35,* 399–416.

Burke, P. J. (1991). Identity processes and social stress. *American Sociological Review, 56*(6), 836–849.

Burke, P. J. (2003). Introduction. In P. J. Burke, T. J. Owens, R. Serpe & P. A. Thoits (Eds.), *Advances in identity theory and research* (pp. 1–7). New York: Kluwer/Plenum Publisher.

Burke, P. J., Owens, T. J., Serpe, R., & Thoits, P. A. (Eds.). (2003). *Advances in identity theory and research.* New York: Kluwer/Plenum Publisher.

Cast, A. D., & Burke, P. J. (2002). A theory of self-esteem. *Social Forces, 80,* 1041–1068.

Chamberlin, J., Rogers, E. S., & Ellison, M. L. (1996). Self-help programs: A description of their characteristics and their members. *Psychiatric Rehabilitation Journal, 19*(3), 33–42.

Chavis, D. M., & Wandersman, A. (1990). Sense of community in the urban environment: A catalyst for participation and community development. *American Journal of Community Psychology, 18,* 55–81.

Coates, D., & Winston, T. (1983). Counteracting the deviance of depression: Peer support groups for victims. *Journal of Social Issues, 39,* 169–194.

Cobb, S. (1976). Social support as moderator of life stress. *Psychosomatic Medicine, 38,* 300–314.

Cohen, S., Gottlieb, B. H., & Underwood, L. G. (2000). Social relationships and health. In S. Cohen, L. G. Underwood & B. H. Gottlieb (Eds.), *Social support measurement and intervention: A guide for health and social scientists* (pp. 3–28). Oxford: Oxford University Press.

Cowan, C. P., & Cowan, P. A. (1986). A preventive intervention for couples becoming parents. In C. Z. Boukydis (Ed.), *Research on support for parents and infants in the postnatal period.* New York: Ablex.

Deegan, P. E. (1988). Recovery: The lived experience of rehabilitation. *Psychosocial Rehabilitation Journal, 11*(4), 11–19.

Dickerson, F. B. (1998). Strategies that foster empowerment. *Cognitive and Behavioral Practice, 5,* 255–275.

Dunkel-Schetter, C. (1984). Social support and cancer: Findings based on patient interviews and their implications. *Journal of Social Issues, 40,* 77–98.

Festinger, L. (1954). A theory of social comparison processes. *Human Relations, 7,* 117–140.

Foa, U. G., & Foa, E. B. (1974). *Societal structures of the mind.* Springfield, IL: Thomas.

Foa, U. G., & Foa, E. B. (1980). Resource theory: Interpersonal behavior as exchange. In K. J. Gergen, M. S. Greenberg & R. H. Willis (Eds.), *Social exchange: Advances in theory and research* (pp. 77–94). New York: Plenum Press.

Gidron, B., & Chesler, M. (1994). Universal and particular attributes of self-help: A framework for international and intranational analysis. In F. Lavoie, T. Borkman & B. Gidron (Eds.), *Self-help and mutual aid groups: International and multicultural perspectives*. New York: The Haworth Press.

Goldberg, R. W., Rollins, A. L., & Lehman, A. F. (2003). Social network correlates among people with psychiatric disabilities. *Psychiatric Rehabilitation Journal, 26*, 393–402.

Hammer, M. (1981). Social supports, social networks, and schizophrenia. *Schizophrenia Bulletin, 7*, 45–57.

Hardiman, E. R., & Segal, S. P. (2003). Community membership and social networks in mental health self-help agencies. *Psychiatric Rehabilitation Journal, 27*, 25–33.

Helgeson, V. S., & Gottlieb, B. H. (2000). Support groups. In S. Cohen, L. G. Underwood & B. H. Gottlieb (Eds.), *Social support measurement and intervention: A guide for health and social scientists* (pp. 221–245). Oxford, : Oxford University Press.

Helgeson, V. S., & Mickelson, K. D. (1995). Motives for social comparison. *Personality and Social Psychology Bulletin, 21*, 1200–1209.

Heller, K. (1989). The return to community. *American Journal of Community Psychology, 17*, 1–15.

Israel, B. A., House, J. S., Schurman, S. J., Heaney, C. A., & Mero, R. P. (1989). The relation of personal resources, participation, influence, interpersonal relationships, and coping strategies to occupational stress, job strains and health: A multivariate analysis. *Work and Stress, 3*, 163–194.

Kaufmann, C. L., Ward-Colasante, C., & Farmer, J. (1993). Development and evaluation of drop-in centers operated by mental health consumers. *Hospital and Community Psychiatry, 44*, 675–678.

Lewin, K. (1948). *Resolving social conflicts*. New York: Harper and Brothers.

Lieberman, M. A. (1993). Self-help groups. In H. I. Kaplan & B. J. Sadock (Eds.), *Comprehensive group therapy*. Baltimore, MD: Williams & Wilkins.

Linton, R. (1936). *The study of man*. New York: D. Appleton-Century.

Lucksted, A., Stewart, B., & Forbes, C. (2008). Benefits and changes for family to family graduates. *American Journal of Community Psychology, 42*, 154–166.

Luks, A. (1991). *The helping power of doing good: The health and spiritual benefits of helping others*. New York: Fawcett Columbine.

Maton, K. I., & Salem, D. A. (1995). Organizational characteristics of empowering community settings: A multiple case study approach. *American Journal of Community Psychology, 23*, 631–656.

McMillan, B., Florin, P., Stevenson, J., Kerman, B., & Mitchell, R. E. (1995). Empowerment praxis in community coalitions. *American Journal of Community Psychology, 23*, 699–727.

McMillan, D. W., & Chavis, D. M. (1986). Sense of community: A definition and theory. *Journal of Community Psychology, 14*(6–23).

Mead, G. H. (1934). *Mind, self, and society*. Chicago, IL: University of Chicago Free Press.

Mowbray, C. T., & Tan, C. (1993). Consumer-operated drop-in centers: Evaluation of operations and impact. *Journal of Mental Health Administration, 20*, 8–19.

Noordsy, D., Torrey, W., Mueser, K., Mead, S., O'Keefe, C., & Fox, L. (2002). Recovery from severe mental illness: An interpersonal and functional outcome definition. *International Review of Psychiatry, 14*, 318–326.

Riessman, F. (1965). The "helper" therapy principle. *Social Work, 10*, 27–32.

Riessman, F., & Carroll, D. (1995). *Redefining self-help*. San Francisco: Jossey-Bass.

Rosenberg, P. P. (1984). Support groups: A special therapeutic entity. *Small Group Behavior, 15*, 173–186.

Schoggen, P. (1989). *Behavior settings: A revision and extension of Roger G. Barker's Ecological Psychology*. Stanford, CA: Stanford University Press.

Schulz, A. J., Israel, B. A., Zimmerman, M. A., & Checkoway, B. N. (1995). Empowerment as a multi-level construct: Perceived control at the individual, organizational and community levels. *Health Education Research, 10*, 309–327.

Segal, S. P., & Silverman, C. (2002). Determinants of client outcomes in self-help agencies. *Psychiatric Services, 53*, 304–309.

Segal, S. P., Silverman, C., & Temkin, T. (1993). Empowerment and self-help agency practice for people with mental disabilities. *Social Work, 38*, 705–712.

Skovholt, T. M. (1974). The client as helper: A means to promote psychological growth. *Counseling Psychologist, 4*, 58–64.

Stryker, S. (1980). *Symbolic interactionism: A social structural version.* Menlo Park, CA: Benjamin Cummings.

Stryker, S., & Burke, P. J. (2000). The past, present, and future of identity theory. *Social Psychology Quarterly, 63*, 284–297.

Suls, J., Martin, R., & Wheeler, L. (2002). Social comparison: Why, with whom and with what effect? *Current Directions in Psychological Science, 11*(5), 159–163.

Taylor, S. E. (1983). Adjustment to threatening events: A theory of cognitive adaptation. *American Psychologist, 38*(1161–1173).

Thoits, P. A. (1983). Multiple identities and psychological well-being. *American Sociological Review, 49*, 174–187.

Thoits, P. A. (1985). Social support and psychological well-being: Theoretical possibilities. In I. G. Sarason & B. R. Sarason (Eds.), *Social support: Theory, research, and applications* (pp. 51–72). Dordrecht: Martinus Nijhoff Publishers.

Thoits, P. A. (1986). Multiple identities: Examining gender and marital status differences in distress. *American Sociological Review, 51*, 259–272.

Toseland, R. W., & Rossiter, C. M. (1989). Group interventions to support family caregivers: A review and analysis. *Gerontologist, 29*, 438–448.

Trainor, J., Shepherd, M., Boydell, K. M., Leff, A., & Crawford, E. (1997). Beyond the service paradigm: The impact and implications of consumer/survivor initiatives. *Psychiatric Rehabilitation Journal, 21*, 132–140.

Unger, D. G., & Wandersman, A. (1985). The importance of neighbors: The social, cognitive, and affective components of neighboring. *American Journal of Community Psychology, 13*, 139–169.

Wills, T. A. (1981). Downward comparison principles in social psychology. *Psychological Bulletin, 90*, 245–271.

Wills, T. A. (1985). Supportive functions of interpersonal relationships. In S. Cohen & S. L. Syme (Eds.), *Social support and health* (pp. 61–82). New York: Academic.

Wong, Y. I., & Solomon, P. L. (2002). Community integration of persons with psychiatric disabilities in supportive independent housing: A conceptual model and methodological considerations. *Mental Health Services Research, 4*(1), 13–28.

Zimmerman, M. A., & Rappaport, J. (1988). Citizen participation, perceived control, and psychological empowerment. *American Journal of Community Psychology, 16*, 725–750.

Chapter 3
Participatory Action Research and Evaluation with Mental Health Self-Help Initiatives: A Theoretical Framework

Geoffrey Nelson, Rich Janzen, Joanna Ochocka, and John Trainor

Abstract In deciding whether or not to collaborate with one another in a research partnership, researchers and members of mental health self-help (MHSH) initiatives should address several questions. What values will underlie the partnership? How will power be shared? What will the focus of the research be? What type of knowledge will be sought? How will the knowledge be used? What roles will the different partners play? In this chapter, we present a theoretical framework that aims to clarify how researchers and mental health self-helpers might answer these questions as they co-construct a research project. The framework consists of six elements: (a) values, (b) participation and power-sharing, (c) social programming, (d) knowledge construction, (e) knowledge utilization, and (f) practice. For each element, we discuss the main issues; we illustrate these issues with examples from both our work and that of others; and we note lessons learned and provide recommendations for future research and evaluation with MHSH initiatives.

In this chapter, we propose a theoretical framework for participatory action research (PAR) and evaluation with mental health self-help (MHSH) initiatives. The framework borrows from and expands upon Shadish, Cook, and Leviton's (1991) theoretical formulation of program evaluation, our earlier conceptualizations of PAR and evaluation with MHSH initiatives (Nelson, Ochocka, Griffin, & Lord, 1998; Nelson, Ochocka, Janzen, Trainor, & Lauzon, 2004), and others' reactions to the approach that we have espoused (Isenberg, Loomis, Humphreys, & Maton, 2004). The purpose of this paper is to argue for the utility of this framework in guiding future PAR and evaluation with MHSH initiatives. In the following section, we discuss the six key elements of the theoretical framework: (a) values, (b) participation and power-sharing, (c) social programming, (d) knowledge construction, (e) knowledge utilization, and (f) practice. We conclude the chapter with recommendations for future research and evaluation.

G. Nelson (✉)
Department of Psychology, Wilfrid Laurier University, Waterloo, ON, Canada
e-mail: gnelson@wlu.ca

3.1 Elements of the Framework

3.1.1 Values

What values will underlie the partnership? Shadish et al. (1991) make a distinction between prescriptive and descriptive approaches to values in program evaluation. In a prescriptive approach, the evaluator seeks to determine if the program strives to promote a pre-determined set of values, whereas in a descriptive approach, the evaluator works to understand the values of program stakeholders. In most evaluation research, values are pushed to the background of the evaluation, while empirical data are in the foreground. Our approach to values is somewhat different. First, we assert that what is important is the congruence between the values of the research approach and the values of the program. Furthermore, we believe that the values underlying PAR fit well with the values of MHSH initiatives (Nelson et al., 1998), and that PAR should be the method of choice with these settings. We also believe that values should be front and center in any research with MHSH initiatives, as these alternative settings are strongly anchored in their values. Second, putting values into practice is challenging. Often there are value dilemmas within MHSH initiatives, as well as value conflicts with evaluators (Nelson, Janzen, Trainor, & Ochocka, 2008).

Value congruence between PAR and mental health self-help (MHSH) initiatives. PAR can be defined as a "research approach that involves active participation of stakeholders, those whose lives are affected by the issue being studied, in all phases of research for the purpose of producing useful results to make positive changes" (Nelson et al., 1998, p.12). The participatory quality of PAR calls for a highly collaborative process throughout the research, while the action component addresses the desires of stakeholders to use the research to create social change.

Both PAR and MHSH initiatives are guided by similar values (Nelson et al., 1998). One important value is that of consumer empowerment and power-sharing (Rappaport, 1981). Mental health consumers have a long history of marginalization, with little control over their involvement with mental health services or research. In contrast, in MHSH initiatives, consumers become agents of personal and social change, with real power, voice, choice, and control. Similarly, PAR emphasizes power-sharing and empowerment of marginalized people (Grant, Nelson, & Mitchell, 2008; Ochocka, Janzen, & Nelson, 2002). A second value is social inclusion. There still exists today pervasive exclusion and stigmatization of people with mental health problems (Hinshaw & Cicchetti, 2000). Both PAR and MHSH initiatives underscore the importance of supportive relationships and participation in valued social roles in the program and the wider community. Third, there is an emphasis on social change and social justice (Prilleltensky & Nelson, 2009). Most people with serious mental illness are unemployed and live in poverty with inadequate housing. PAR and many MHSH initiatives strive to create social change and improve consumer access to the valued resources of income, employment, education, and housing (Campbell, 2005). Finally, there is the value of continuous, mutual learning. PAR emphasizes an ongoing cycle of research, action, and reflective learning (Grant et al., 2008), while MHSH initiatives are based on the principle that members have the potential to learn and grow through receiving and providing support to one another and striving to create change (Isenberg et al., 2004).

Putting values into practice. In our research with MHSH initiatives, we have sought ways to concretize the values identified above (see Table 3.1). To share power and promote empowerment, we have used steering committees to guide the entire research process (e.g., developing the proposal, selecting the project sites, gathering the data) (Nelson, Lord, & Ochocka, 2001; Nelson et al., 2004). Our experiences with steering committees have been quite positive. In one study, a consumer chaired the bi-monthly meetings of this committee over the 7 years of the study. Consumers experienced a great deal of ownership over the research, and the researchers and consumers were able to develop shared goals for the project. In a study of self-helpers, Isenberg et al. (2004) found such experiences to be very important for establishing positive, collaborative relationships. For these reasons, we highly recommend the use of steering committees with consumer representation in future research.

Table 3.1 Values and strategies for implementing values in participatory action research and evaluation with mental health self-help initiatives

Values	Strategies for implementing values
Consumer empowerment and power-sharing	Provide opportunities for consumer participation in the research, including research steering committees and research teams
Social inclusion	Establish informal, positive working relationships among consumers and researchers on research steering committees and research teams
Social change and social justice	Hire and train consumer researchers; study social change activities and outcomes of mental health self-help initiatives
Continuous, mutual learning	Practice mutual reflection on the research process and research findings; share knowledge and experiences

The value of social inclusion entails the development of both authentic relationships and participation in valued social roles. We have implemented this value through both the research steering committee and a team of consumer researchers in two different studies. We enjoyed positive relationships with consumers in both of these projects. We believe that this is because we had a clear, written partnership agreement with the settings; we spent a great deal of time building informal relationships and learning about the settings; and we communicated openly, honestly, and regularly (Nelson et al., 2004; Ochocka et al., 2002). Isenberg et al. (2004) found that developing trusting, non-exploitive relationships is essential for collaborative research with MHSH initiatives.

We also experienced challenges in our relationships with the consumer researchers. Some of the researchers required a great deal of guidance and social support; two consumer researchers were hospitalized during the course of one the studies, including one who committed suicide shortly after being released from hospital; and we had to terminate the employment of two researchers for inadequate job performance. Mentoring and supporting the consumer researchers was a taxing job for us, especially during crisis periods. In spite of these challenges, we found many benefits to hiring the consumer researchers. The jobs benefited the consumers both financially and in terms of personal and professional development (Reeve, Cornell, D'Costa, Janzen, & Ochocka, 2002). Also, the consumer researchers were invaluable at recruiting participants and establishing rapport with them to do interviews for the project. Finally, consumers became co-mentors and co-supporters to each other as they collectively problem-solved challenges faced by the research team. While challenging, we recommend hiring and training consumer researchers, as this is important for promoting the value of social inclusion (Ochocka et al., 2002).

Hiring and training consumer researchers is also important for promoting the value of social justice and social change. In a multi-site study of MHSH initiatives in the United States, up to 40% of the grant went to the organizations for service enhancement, and the consumer groups had 51% control of decision-making power. Dr. Patrick Corrigan, one of the investigators for this study, noted that this financial and decision-making equality "gets us beyond good intention to true participation" (Isenberg et al., 2004, p. 132). Structural arrangements such as this are needed to promote greater equity between consumers and researchers in future research. We also believe that it is important to study the social change activities of MHSH initiatives. One of our studies was one of several projects funded under an initiative that was designed to examine the impacts of different types of community mental health programs on consumers (Dewa et al., 2002). Our steering committee decided to have an additional focus on the social change activities of the MHSH initiatives, since that is an important part of their raison d'être (Janzen, Nelson, Trainor, & Ochocka, 2006). More specifically, we examined the educational, advocacy, planning, and action research strategies that were designed to create systems-level changes in community attitudes, programs, and policies. These systems-level activities and outcomes were deemed as important as those activities and outcomes for individual members of the MHSH initiatives. We recommend that more research be devoted to examining the social change activities of MHSH initiatives.

The value of mutual learning was promoted through the steering committee, where all members had a chance to reflect upon the research process and findings. We learned a great deal about the MHSH initiatives and the experiential realities of consumers, and we, in turn, were able to educate and train consumers about research and demystify research concepts. The consumers learned about PAR and specific research strategies that we used. Similar themes about the importance of learning processes were reported in Isenberg et al.'s (2004) study of self-helpers. Creating spaces for shared dialogue is important for future research to promote this value of reciprocal learning.

3.1.2 Participation and Power-sharing

How will power be shared? Although not an original category of Shadish et al.'s (1991) formulation, we believe it is important to foreground participation and power-sharing in our framework because of its pre-eminence both in PAR and within MHSH initiatives. With regard to PAR, the active participation of stakeholders throughout the research process is its distinguishing feature (Nelson et al., 1998). But PAR recognizes the complexity that participation implies, especially in community settings where inequitable power differentials often exist among researchers, helping professionals, and community members (Israel, Schulz, Parker, & Becker, 1998). Drawing on critical theory, PAR acknowledges that research is conducted within a context that is fundamentally mediated by power relations that are social and historically constituted (Foley & Valenzuela, 2005). Therefore, no researchers are politically neutral. Rather research is a political exercise that can serve to further oppress or to liberate. While research has often reproduced elements within oppressive systems, whether these be based on class, race, gender, or ability (Kincheloe & McLaren, 2005), the aim of PAR is emancipatory, seeking to actively address power differences and to create a future that is not bound to the oppressive past (Kemmis & McTaggart, 2005; Mertens, 2003).

Such a stance resonates well with MHSH initiatives. Since the 1970s, MHSH initiatives have emerged that not only offer mutual support, but also have agendas for social and policy change (Chamberlin, 1978; Weitz, 1984). Many of these organizations view themselves as part of a broader social movement for the liberation of psychiatric survivors (Chamberlin, 1978, 1984; Everett, 1994). There is a long history of abuse in psychiatry (Deutsch, 1948; Whitaker, 2001), whether in its crude physical treatments (Collins, 1998) or forced incarceration (Szasz, 1974). MHSH initiatives therefore see their role as essential rudders for a mental health system that can run out of control. The active and equitable participation of consumers within MHSH initiatives is an integral component in achieving these goals. We suggest that such participation that emphasizes power-sharing can also be extended to MHSH initiative-based evaluations.

Engaging stakeholders and addressing relative power. Participatory approaches that emphasize multiple perspectives and a collaborative process of constructing knowledge are increasingly being applied to evaluation research (Bradley, Mayfield, Mehta, & Rukonge, 2002; Fine et al., 2003). There is growing awareness in the research community of the need to use methodologies that are appropriate for the unique circumstances of the settings being studied (Fisher & Ball, 2003). There is also an increasing recognition that evaluations need to be credible and relevant to stakeholders in order to be utilized (Patton, 2008).

It is our belief that these goals can be achieved using PAR. PAR is particularly well-suited to research *with* MHSH initiatives. Members of MHSH initiatives do not want to be "research subjects" but rather "active partners" in the research process (Rappaport, Seidman, Toro, McFadden, Reischl, Roberts, Salem, Stein, & Zimmerman, 1985). As member-driven organizations, MHSH initiatives are interested in participating in something that they believe is meaningful and will be useful for the organizations and its members (Nelson et al., 2004).

Yet, we believe that participation must also follow the traditions of democratic pluralism (Nelson et al., 2004). This tradition holds that the evaluation conversation should be broadened to include all perspectives and voices, and to do so in such a way that respects diversity of opinion (Ryan, Green, Lincoln, Mathison, & Mertens, 1998). Evaluators are therefore astute political managers who orchestrate the involvement of diverse interest groups (Weiss, 1983). Within evaluations that involve external stakeholders, democratic pluralism means that the experiential knowledge of consumers is valued equally to that of professional knowledge. It also means that intentional efforts are made to privilege the voice of consumers as the central stakeholder group – the group for whom the mental health system was created to serve.

From the beginning of one of our MHSH initiative studies, we worked closely with the Ontario Peer Development Initiative (OPDI), an umbrella organization for over 55 MHSH initiatives (called consumer/survivor initiatives or CSIs) in Ontario. When a call for proposals to evaluate these CSIs was announced, the researchers met with the Coordinator of the OPDI to consider applying for a grant. We began by holding a series of meetings with representatives of several CSIs and the OPDI Coordinator to collaboratively develop the proposal. Once funding was secured, the researchers and the OPDI Coordinator together developed criteria and selected four CSIs for participation in the research.

At this point we began to identify the range and optimal mix of stakeholders to sit on the project's steering committee (Cargo & Mercer, 2008; Ochocka et al., 2002). The committee was eventually composed of the Executive Directors of the four CSIs, the investigators and senior researchers who managed the project, an OPDI representative, and one CSI volunteer who chaired it since its inception. This steering committee was a forum where all decisions were made about the research activities, where knowledge and power were shared in all stages of the evaluation process, and where we achieved "a faithful representation" (Ryan et al., 1998, p. 117). As a committee we continually addressed power dynamics through an ongoing dialogue, by following the working principles that were collaboratively developed and by sharing research responsibilities.

Building evaluation capacity and empowerment. Power-sharing implies that the benefits of participation are shared. Within research these benefits are linked to capacity-building and empowerment, outcomes that enable people to gain mastery and control over their own lives (Rappaport, 1981). Despite certain differences, PAR and "empowerment evaluation" share a commitment toward the extensive participation of stakeholders (Fetterman, 2001). By giving more decision-making control to stakeholders, empowerment evaluation contends that stakeholders are more likely to benefit positively from the research process and to gain the capacity to conduct future evaluation on their own. PAR expands on this notion of power-sharing and empowerment to include the capacity of stakeholders in making social change (Grant et al., 2008) and to equip the marginalized to gain capacity for social action that is liberating (Fals-Borda & Rahman, 1991).

In our studies with CSIs, we attempted to share not only the work, but also the rewards of the research (Ochocka et al., 2002). This included co-presentations with consumers at conferences and co-authorship of some research publications (Reeve et al., 2002). In addition, the skills learned by consumer researchers were helpful in securing subsequent employment, as researchers and otherwise. Finally, the research enabled CSIs to better their systemic advocacy, including using evidence-based arguments to advocate directly to senior policy-makers for the expansion of CSIs.

3.1.3 Social Programming

What will the focus of the research be? According to Shadish et al. (1991), social programming refers to how programs are structured internally, how programs contribute to social change, and how programs are constrained by the external context. In this regard it is important to understand a program's theory of change and to evaluate the implementation and outcomes of a program. Typically the research questions in studies of mental health self-help groups and organizations center on the program processes and outcomes that are the key features of the program's theory of change.

Establishing program theory. Chen (2005) argues that in any evaluation of a social program that it is important to articulate the program's theory of change. That is, what are the processes or mechanisms that are believed to be or have been shown in previous research to be causally connected to changes in outcomes for individuals and communities? Different theoretical formulations of the mechanisms of change in mental health self-help groups and organizations have been developed, including the mechanisms of empowerment and social support (Brown, Shepherd, Merkle, Wituk, & Meissen, 2008), which link directly to the values of these settings that were noted in the previous section.

A useful way of clarifying a program's theory of change is through the use of a program logic model (Frechtling, 2007). A program logic model is a graphic illustration of what a program does and what it hopes to achieve, noting the rationale (or logic) between the two (Rush & Ogborne, 1991). If developed in a participatory way, program logic models are helpful in moving stakeholders toward a common understanding of a program's theory of change. They also aid in planning an appropriate evaluation design and in formulating data-gathering tools (McLaughlin & Jordan, 2004).

In our CSI study, we used program logic models to organize participating CSI's activities and outcomes (Nelson et al., 2004). Using a participatory process involving in-depth discussions with CSI staff and participants and reviewing program documents, we as researchers drafted one logic model for each of the four CSIs. Although each site was unique, we attempted to visually show the similarities among sites as well. We discussed and refined these program logic models during steering committee meetings throughout the early stages of the research study.

Finally, a synthesis logic model captured the similarities across sites (see Janzen et al., 2006 for a visual depiction).

The individual and synthesis logic models were useful in focusing our research. They featured two main levels of activity (individual and systems) with corresponding activity categories which where subsequently linked to short- and long-term outcomes. The individual-level activities were those that were meant to have an impact on and benefit individual consumers. For example, all CSIs had some combination of the following activity categories: internal member development, drop-ins, self-help groups, or one-to-one peer support. In this study we were interested in not only understanding individual-level outcomes over time, but also how these outcomes related to overall participation and the amount and type of participation in local CSIs. Using the program logic models as a basis, we were able to develop a common tool to help us track how our study participants were active in each participating CSI.

Systems-level activities, on the other hand, were those that attempted to impact the human service system, the broader community, and social policy. There were four main categories of activities: public education, political advocacy, community planning, and action research. All CSIs had some activities within each category. These categories were similar to the primary system-level components found in other studies (Nelson, 1994; Tefft, 1987). These four system-level categories formed the basis of a tool that was used to track system-level activities and outcomes during the study. As with the individual-level tracking tool, this tool was common and applicable across all sites, yet, flexible enough to identify the uniqueness of each site (see Janzen et al., 2006 to view the tool).

Evaluating program implementation and outcomes. Having developed a logic model that articulates the program's theory of change, the next steps in a program evaluation are to examine the implementation of program activities and the extent to which the expected outcomes of the program are achieved. Beginning with the evaluation of program activities, implementation has been defined as "what a program consists of when it is delivered in a particular setting" (Durlak & DuPre, 2008, p. 329).Implementation or process evaluation seeks to answer the following questions: Has the program been implemented as intended? What are the inputs, efforts, and access of the program? What is the quality of the program in terms of the experiences of different stakeholders? When the outcomes of a program are not successfully achieved, implementation evaluation helps to understand if this is due to a faulty theory or a program that was not well-implemented and thus provided a poor test of the program's theory of change (Patton, 2008).

In addition to evaluating implementation, it is also important to examine the outcomes of participation in MHSH initiatives. In developing a logic model, it is useful to distinguish between shorter- and longer-term outcomes. This is because some outcomes can be reasonably expected to occur in the short-term (e.g., increased social support), while other outcomes (e.g., obtaining employment or education) may take longer to develop. It is also important to define outcome goals in such a way that they are clear, specific, and measurable. Many MHSH initiatives have "empowerment" as an expected outcome, but empowerment needs to be defined in concrete terms.

Many of the social programs with whom we have worked in our role as evaluators do not operate from a clear theory of change. Therefore, we strongly recommend the use of logic models in future research with MHSH initiatives. Logic models can be beneficial in several ways. First, helping a program to articulate its theory of change through a collaborative process of developing a logic model can be very helpful for a program to understand what it is trying to achieve and how it should go about trying to achieve its goals. Second, logic models can also help to establish the evaluability of a program and guide the selection of tools to measure implementation and outcomes. Third, testing a program's theory of change can help to understand not just if self-help works, but why and how it works.

3.1.4 Knowledge Construction

What type of knowledge will be sought? Researchers and members of mental health self-help groups and organizations often have different ideas about what constitutes valid knowledge. Traditionally, researchers have typically sought to acquire knowledge through objective, controlled, quantitative research guided by the assumptions of the positivist or post-positivist paradigm, whereas self-helpers tend to rely on experiential knowledge gathered through qualitative methods (e.g., discussion, narratives), which reflect more of a social constructionist or naturalistic paradigm (Kennedy, Humphreys, & Borkman, 1994; Loveland, Weaver Randall, & Corrigan, 2005). Moreover, post-positivism is more concerned with knowledge about causal relationships, whereas social constructionism is more concerned with meaning and lived experience (Guba & Lincoln, 2005).

Also relevant to research with MHSH initiatives is the transformative paradigm. According to Mertens (2009)

> the transformative paradigm emerged in response to individuals who have been pushed to the societal margins throughout history and who are finding a means to bring their voices into the world of research. Their voices, shared with scholars who work as their partners to support the increase of social justice and human rights, are reflected in the shift to transformative beliefs to guide researchers and evaluators. (p. 3)

Valid knowledge in the transformative paradigm is that which unmasks unequal power relationships, challenges the societal status quo, and leads to a more equitable distribution of resources. Prilleltensky (2008) argues that transformative research should have psychopolitical validity, which entails a credible account of power and how to reduce unequal power relationships. Ultimately, the transformative paradigm is concerned with promoting social justice and eliminating unjust social conditions. Applied to people with mental health problems, the transformative approach aims to enhance consumer choice, control and power, promote social inclusion and eliminate stigma and discrimination, and increase access to valued resources, such as jobs and decent housing.

The different paradigms that we have identified above may appeal to different audiences in PAR with MHSH initiatives. An evaluation researcher may believe that a post-positivist paradigm yields the best knowledge about the causes and effects of self-help participation; a self-help group member may believe that a constructionist paradigm best captures knowledge about their experiences and the stories of fellow group members; and a psychiatric survivor activist may believe that a transformational paradigm is needed to gain knowledge about power inequities and transformational social change. Rather than view one paradigm as the *best* approach, we believe that it is important to consider the audience for the research and the questions that are important for the stakeholders to answer to determine what paradigm the research should operate from and which methods should be used. To overcome the limitations of exclusively relying one paradigm and one set of methods for knowledge creation, there has been a growing interest in mixed methods research, which combine quantitative and qualitative methods (Tashakkori & Teddlie, 2003). Greene (2008) has elaborated a variety of strategies for how different paradigms can work in concert with one another in mixed methods research. In the next sections, we discuss how both quantitative and qualitative methods can be used to obtain knowledge about implementation and outcomes.

Knowledge about implementation. There are three approaches to implementation or process evaluation that are based on the post-positivist paradigm. First, fidelity measures are used to determine the degree to which the program activities are faithfully implemented according to the program's theory of change. Johnsen, Teague, and Herr (2005) and Mowbray, Bybee, Holter, and Lewandowski (2006) developed fidelity measures of mental health MHSH initiatives. After identifying critical or common ingredients (e.g., consumer determination of policy, operations, and planning) of MHSH initiatives, the authors operationalized these ingredients so that they could be assessed by external observers. Johnsen et al. (2005) validated their measure by demonstrating that it differentiated traditional mental health services from MHSH initiatives. They also found that various dimensions of their fidelity measure differentiated consumer-run drop-in centers, peer support programs, and organizations that focused on education and advocacy.

A second post-positivist approach to implementation evaluation focuses on inputs (number of staff, staff–participant ratios, training), efforts (dosage, the amount or strength of the program intervention), and access (whether the program reached those it intended to reach). Corrigan (2006) found that participation in MHSH initiatives was positively associated with consumer recovery and empowerment. In our longitudinal study of the impacts of CSIs we used a bi-monthly tracking form to determine the frequency of consumer participation in different CSI activities. At a 3-year follow-up, we found that those CSI members with sustained and frequent participation experienced better outcomes than those who participated less frequently (Nelson, Ochocka, Janzen, Trainor, Goering, & Lomotey, 2007). We also used a different tracking form to assess the frequency of participation of CSI members in systems-level change activities (Janzen, Nelson, Hausfather, & Ochocka, 2007).

A third post-positivist approach assesses the quality of the program components. Consumers and staff can be asked about their experiences of different aspects of mental health self-help groups and organizations or the qualities of the group or organization can be observed. In our CSI study, we found that members' perceptions of the quality of their participation in the CSIs was a better predictor of outcomes than the actual amount of participation (Nelson & Lomotey, 2006). In another study of CSIs, Brown et al. (2008) found that experiences of organizational empowerment and social support in these settings were directly associated with consumer recovery. In an observational study of group interaction in GROW self-help groups, Roberts et al. (1999) found that members' giving support to others was associated improved functioning over time.

Qualitative research, based on social constructionist and transformative paradigms, can also be used for process evaluation (Patton, 2008). In our study of CSIs, members noted several helpful qualities of these settings: a safe and supportive environment and opportunities for participation and contribution both in the CSIs and in the larger community (Ochocka, Nelson, Janzen, & Trainor, 2006). Corrigan et al. (2005) found that GROW mental health self-help group members perceived peer support to be the most helpful quality of these groups. In another qualitative study of MHSH initiatives, Brown (2009a) found that work and recreational activities, peer relationships, and the positive atmosphere of the initiatives contributed to personal changes. This research is constructionist in its focus on consumer experiences, and it is transformative in that focuses on social inclusion, empowerment, and power-sharing among members of MHSH initiatives. Together, these quantitative and qualitative studies of program implementation point to some of the key qualities of MHSH initiatives and how these qualities are related to outcomes.

Evaluating program outcomes. There have been several recent reviews of the outcomes resulting from participation in MHSH initiatives (Nelson, Ochocka, Janzen, & Trainor, 2006; Pistrang, Barker, & Humphreys, 2008; Solomon 2004). Post-positivist approaches to outcome evaluation use experimental and quasi-experimental designs to determine if participation in these settings leads to causal changes in outcomes for consumers. The recent review by Pistrang et al. (2008) focused exclusively on controlled studies of self-help groups. While only 12 studies were found that met their inclusion criteria, these studies reported promising findings about the effectiveness of mental health self-help groups. Other recent controlled studies by Burti et al. (2005), Nelson et al. (2007), and Rowe et al. (2007), not included in the Pistrang et al. review, have also reported some positive outcomes.

Qualitative research based on a social constructionist paradigm has also been used to examine outcomes. While such research cannot pinpoint cause and effect, it does provide a more in-depth understanding of the changes experienced by consumers than can be obtained through quantitative research. In our research on CSIs, we found several positive outcomes (stable mental health, enhanced social support, and sustained work and participation in the community) in a longitudinal, qualitative study (Ochocka et al., 2006). Other recent qualitative studies of consumer narratives in MHSH initiatives by Brown (2009a, 2009b) and Weaver, Randall, and Salem (2005) have reported similar positive recovery outcomes.

3.1.5 Knowledge Utilization

How will the knowledge that is acquired be used? In PAR, it is important not just to generate knowledge, but to use that knowledge to create social change (Grant et al.,

2008). This is the action component of PAR. Similarly, Patton (2008) and others have emphasized the need for program evaluations to be "utilization-focused." This focus on action and utilization is part of a broader trend in the social and health sciences to pay more attention to what has been variously referred to as knowledge mobilization, transfer, translation, utilization, or exchange (Mitton, Adair, McKenzie, Patten, & Perry, 2007). Moreover, a focus on knowledge utilization is quite consistent with the needs of MHSH initiatives. Members of such groups often comment that they do not wish to partake in research that is not useful to them in some way. Mental health consumers are sometimes skeptical about the value of research for them based on previous negative experiences or views that research is too intrusive or burdensome (Isenberg et al., 2004).

Several different types of knowledge utilization have been identified in the evaluation literature (Patton, 2008). First, instrumental utilization entails the use of evaluation findings to affect changes in a program toward the goal of program improvement. Second, persuasive utilization refers to using evaluation findings as "political ammunition" to advocate for a specific purpose, such as increased program funding. Third, conceptual utilization is concerned with "altering (the) cognitive frameworks" of program managers or policy-makers (Cook & Shadish, 1986). While conceptual utilization may not lead directly to tangible changes in the short-term, it can serve to reframe policies or programs.

Dissemination and utilization. Constantino and Nelson (1995) interviewed hospital- and community-based mental health professionals and family and consumer self-help group members in a qualitative PAR study of current and preferred relationships between professionals and mental health self-helpers. The two main themes that came out of this research were professional ideology and practices and professional power and control. Self-helpers wanted more education and training of professionals about self-help and more collaboration and power-sharing between these two stakeholder groups. The authors observed instrumental utilization of the findings of this research, including the development of a self-help resource center by one of the mental health agencies, greater involvement of consumers and family members on the boards and committees of mental health agencies, and the creation of open forums to discuss how these different stakeholders could better collaborate with one another.

Our study of CSIs included an active dissemination process at the end of the study. The researchers and members of the CSIs disseminated the findings of the research across the province of Ontario so that other CSIs, mental health agencies, and other interested parties could learn about the research (Nelson, Ochocka, Lauzon, Towndrow, & Cheng, 2005). As part of the dissemination process, a professional film-maker, hired and guided by our Steering Committee, created a DVD "From Madhouse to Our House" that provided background on CSIs and the research process and findings. The primary purpose of the dissemination process was education and advocacy. The positive outcomes of CSIs that we found in the research not only educated stakeholders about the benefits of CSIs, but they also served to enhance the credibility of CSIs in the eyes of mental health service-providers and policy-makers. One policy-maker remarked to us that the findings of our research fit well with the current emphasis of evidence-based practice in the formulation of health policy and practice. In addition to this persuasive form of utilization, the findings of the study demonstrated the viability and utility of CSIs, as an alternative to the formal mental health system, thus serving the function of conceptual utilization. We recommend that PAR researchers and partners develop knowledge utilization plans and strategies to promote the different types of utilization. We further recommend that a dissemination policy be negotiated upfront among partners to lay out procedures that would ensure equitable participation and control in determining specific knowledge utilization strategies (Jacobson, Ochocka, Wise, Janzen, & the Taking Culture Seriously Partners, 2007).

3.1.6 Practice

What roles will the different partners play? According to Shadish et al. (1991), practice refers to tactics and strategies that evaluators follow in their work. While constrained by limited time, resources, and skills, evaluators attempt to conduct the most feasible evaluation that produces the most practical and useful information for program settings. One key consideration in this pursuit is the role that evaluation partners play. Within the context of MHSH initiatives, the two primary role clarifications revolve around the evaluator and MHSH members.

Clarifying the role of the evaluator. Traditionally, evaluators were social scientists interested in satisfying their own curiosity, were accountable only to their academic peers, and did not concern themselves with the utilization of evaluation findings, all to the exclusion of the interests and needs of other evaluation stakeholders (Shadish et al., 1991). Employing the expertise of a statistician (or other analytic know-how), the evaluator's primary role was to pronounce judgment on the merit and worth of a program (Scriven, 1980). Even among those evaluators who preached responsiveness to program settings, the locus of control often still rested in the hands of evaluators. In the words of Robert Stake, "For me, the inquiry belongs to the evaluator ... I do not see inquiry as a cooperative effort" (Abma & Stake, 2001, p. 9).

Historically, MHSH initiatives have been leery of this reliance on external professional experts. As with other alternative settings, MHSH initiatives de-emphasize mainstream professional services which are often viewed as bureaucratic and paternalistic (McCubbin & Cohen, 1996). Rather, they desire that members regain control over their recovery by stressing mutual aid and power-sharing among members (Chamberlin, 1990). This uneasy relationship with professionals extends to researchers. The regrettable history of disrespect, even abuse, in mental health research still lingers (Whitaker, 2001).

Evaluations within MHSH initiatives must contend with these issues of professionalism. Trust must be built between external evaluator and MHSH members, some of whom may have negative research experiences. Trust-building between researcher and community member may be time-consuming and effort intensive (Shoultz, Oneha, Magnussen, Hla, Bress-Suanders, Dela Cruz, & Douglas, 2006).

However, good intentions are not enough when engaging non-researchers into the research domain (Postma, 2008). We therefore suggest that evaluators entering a MHSH initiative intentionally clarify and adopt two primary evaluative roles. We believe that these roles are consistent with the ethos of both PAR and MHSH initiatives in valuing the contribution and control of MHSH evaluation participants.

The first primary role for evaluators within MHSH initiatives is that of *facilitator*. Such a role addresses the participatory component of PAR, in that it seeks to meaningfully engage those who have a stake in the evaluation. As a facilitator, the evaluator enables stakeholders to identify their common purpose and guiding principles, and nudges them toward achieving these aims. Evaluators as facilitators recognize that MHSH members are the experts (and the best judges) of their local context, and therefore in the best position to guide the evaluation process. In politically charged settings, the facilitative evaluator needs to contend with and address power differentials among people and groups. To do this, the evaluator ensures that all relevant stakeholder views are included, promotes extensive dialogue and understanding among stakeholders, and ensures adequate deliberation among all parties to reach valid conclusions (House, 2004). Fetterman expands on this facilitative role to include the notions of coach, critical friend, and knowledgeable colleague with evaluation expertise (Donaldson & Scriven, 2003). Regardless of label, this facilitative role implies that the evaluator does not simply hold research expertise, but demonstrates a high level of relational skills, all the while being open and clear about her/his own value-base.

The second role to be adopted by evaluators within MHSH initiatives is as a *co-agent of change*. This role addresses the action component of PAR. A co-agent of change recognizes that the hope of action is what draws many non-researchers into the research process (Postma, 2008). The evaluator affirms this motivation by using research as a platform to inspire and build relationships among people – not simply to produce new knowledge together—but to consider and debate how that new knowledge can best guide their collective future action. The evaluator recognizes the importance of existing change agents within the MHSH initiative, inviting them to join in the process of determining and implementing needed change. If successful, the action legacy therefore continues beyond the evaluation time-frame and long after the professional evaluator has gone home.

Clarifying the role of MHSH members. Our experience has taught us that adopting the two evaluator roles mentioned above increases the likelihood of receptivity (even enthusiasm) among MHSH initiatives to participate in evaluation. It is also important to clarify the roles that MHSH members can play within the evaluation. Again we offer two general options: that of evaluation "guiders" and of evaluation "co-researchers."

We have already made numerous references to the importance of the steering committee in guiding our research with MHSH initiatives. Whatever the exact mechanism to implement this guiding role, it remains integral in ensuring that MHSH members have input and control over all stages of the evaluation; from design, partnership agreements, tool development, data gathering, analysis, writing, dissemination, and future action. In effect evaluation guiders become the "MHSH conscience," ensuring that its agenda is being advanced and not harmed through evaluation. Indeed, MHSH advocates have warned about the potential of co-optation when working too closely with the formal mental health system (Chamberlin 1978; Everett, 1998). So too, MHSH evaluation guiders can warn of lurking research co-optation in which community partners become "strangers in their own communities" (Minkler, 2004, p. 691) even under the guise of community-friendly research. Moreover, MHSH members can keep professional researchers honest as they navigate their position on the insider–outsider continuum (Humphrey, 2007; Minkler, 2004).

While not all MHSH members have interest or time to participate in the details of evaluation implementation, clearly others do. As co-researchers MHSH members participate as full members of the research team. Their addition is both a matter of data quality (access to participants and insights into data analysis) and of social justice (the sharing of financial resources and capacity-building opportunities) (Ochocka et al., 2002). Consumer co-researchers will have their own challenges in negotiating their preferred insider–outsider stance (Humphrey, 2007). Still, we have found that creating a supportive research team environment is not only the training ground to enable the accomplishment of research tasks, but it also provides a safe forum to aid MHSH members in their reflexivity as researchers (Reeve et al., 2002).

3.2 Conclusion and Recommendations for Future Research

In this chapter, we proposed a theoretical framework for research and evaluation with MHSH initiatives that consists of six elements. These elements and related recommendations for future research can be found in Table 3.2. First, because of their shared value-base, PAR provides a good fit for research and evaluation with MHSH initiatives. However, it is important to have concrete strategies to implement the values of MHSH initiatives and PAR. Second, sharing knowledge, power, and control with members of MHSH initiatives makes evaluation research meaningful, credible, and relevant for all stakeholders and audiences (i.e., consumers, funders, researchers, policy-makers). MHSH initiatives provide a fascinating lens through which to explore the issues of PAR. People with mental illness are among the most devalued in terms of their ability to make knowledge claims, and carrying out projects with them as full partners is a direct way of confronting both objectifying research approaches and social stigma. The many examples provided in this chapter show clearly the value consumers bring to all aspects of research and evaluation.

Third, the social programming element of mental health self-help groups and organizations draws attention to the need for research and evaluation to focus on important processes and outcomes both for individuals and for communities. Program theories that emphasize transformative change are most compatible with MHSH initiatives because of their fundamentally different nature than mainstream mental health services (Mertens, 2009). Fourth, different research paradigms have emerged that are particularly applicable to MHSH initiatives. These different approaches to knowledge construction are related to the way that consumers are

Table 3.2 Elements of the theoretical framework and recommendations for future participatory action research and evaluation with mental health self-help initiatives

Elements	Recommendations for future research
Values	Establish values, principles, and strategies (e.g., steering committees, research teams) to guide research and evaluation projects; develop partnership agreements; study value clashes within these settings
Participation and power-sharing	Value consumers' experiential knowledge; provide opportunities for consumers to have "voice;" acknowledge and strive to reduce power differences; build evaluation capacity within the setting; share benefits of the research (e.g., publications, presentations) with consumers
Social programming	Use program logic models to clarify the program's theory of change; study program implementation and outcomes and the relationship between the two
Knowledge construction	Clarify the research questions to be addressed; decide what paradigm is the most appropriate to answer the research questions; uses quantitative and/or qualitative methods to answer the research questions regarding implementation and outcomes
Knowledge utilization	Develop plans and strategies to promote widespread and targeted dissemination of the findings; promote instrumental, persuasive, and/or conceptual utilization of the research findings
Practice	Clarify the roles of the researcher/evaluator, including facilitator and co-agent of change; clarify the roles of mental health self-help members, including guiders and co-researchers

thought of in mental health research. From being only passive subjects in traditional positivistic research, social constructionism recognizes that consumers have important things to say on their own behalf. The transformative approach of PAR opens up a new territory of consumer involvement, with consumers becoming partners in research for social and personal change. Fifth, a utilization-focused or action-oriented approach to research and evaluation is highly compatible with the ambitions of MHSH initiatives to create social change. Sixth, the approach to research and evaluation with MHSH initiatives that we have proposed requires new roles for both researchers and consumers. This approach requires a leap of faith on the part of researchers and consumers, but one that in our work has been richly rewarded.

References

Abma, R. A., & Stake, R. E. (2001). Stake's responsive evaluation: Core ideas and evolution. *New Directions in Evaluation, 92*, 7–22.
Bradley, J. E., Mayfield, M. V., Mehta, M. P., & Rukonge, A. (2002). Participatory evaluation of reproductive health care quality in developing countries. *Social Science and Medicine, 55*, 269–282.
Brown, L. D. (2009a). How people can benefit from mental health consumer-run organizations. *American Journal of Community Psychology, 43*, 177–188.
Brown, L. D. (2009b). Making it sane: Using narrative to explore theory in a mental health consumer-run organization. *Qualitative Health Research, 19*, 243–257.

Brown, L. D., Shepherd, M. D., Merkle, E. C., Wituk, S. A., & Meissen, G. (2008). Understanding how participation in consumer-run organizations relates to recovery. *American Journal of Community Psychology, 42*, 167–178.

Burti, L., Amaddeo, F., Ambrose, M., Bonetto, C., Cristofalo, D., Ruggeri, M., & Tansella, M. (2005). Does additional care provided by a consumer self-help group improve psychiatric outcomes? A study based in an Italian community-based psychiatric service. *Community Mental Health Journal, 41*, 705–720.

Campbell, J. (2005). The historical and philosophical development of peer-run support programs. In S. Clay, B. Schell, P. W. Corrigan, & R. O. Ralph (Eds.), *On our own, together: Peer program for people with mental illness* (pp. 17–64). Nashville, TN: Vanderbilt University Press.

Cargo, M., & Mercer, S. L. (2008). The value and challenges of participatory research: Strengthening its practice. *Annual Review of Public Health, 29*, 325–350.

Chamberlin, J. (1978). *On our own: Patient-controlled alternatives to the mental health system.* Toronto, ON: McGraw-Hill.

Chamberlin, J. (1984). Speaking for ourselves: An overview of the ex-psychiatric patients' movement. *Psychosocial Rehabilitation Journal, 8*(2), 56–63.

Chamberlin, J. (1990). The ex-psychiatric patients' movement: Where we've been and where we're going. *The Journal of Mind and Behavior, 11*, 323–336.

Chen, H.-T. (2005). *Practical program evaluation: Assessing and improving planning, implementation, and effectiveness.* Newbury Park, CA: Sage.

Collins, A. (1998). *In the sleep room: The story of the CIA brainwashing experiments in Canada.* Toronto, ON: Key Porter Books.

Constantino, V., & Nelson, G. (1995). Changing relationships between self-help groups and mental health professionals: Shifting ideology and power. *Canadian Journal of Community Mental Health, 14*(2), 55–70.

Cook, T. D., & Shadish, W. R. Jr. (1986). Program evaluation: The worldly science. *Annual Review of Program Evaluation, 37*, 193–232.

Corrigan, P. W. (2006). Impact of consumer-operated services on empowerment and recovery of people with psychiatric disabilities. *Psychiatric Services, 57*, 1493–1496.

Corrigan, P. W., Slopen, N., Gracia, G., Phelan, Keogh, C. B., & Keck, L. (2005). Some recovery processes in mutual-help groups for persons with mental illness; II: Qualitative analysis of participant interviews. *Community Mental Health Journal, 41*, 721–735.

Deutsch A. (1948). *The shame of the states.* New York: Harcourt Brace.

Dewa, C. S., Durbin, J., Wasylenki, D., Ochocka, J., Eastabrook, S., Boydell, K. M., & Goering, P. (2002). Considering a multisite study? How to take the leap and have a soft landing. *Journal of Community Psychology, 30*, 173–187.

Donaldson, S. I., & Scriven, M. (2003). Diverse visions for evaluation in the new millennium: Should we integrate or embrace diversity? In S. I. Donaldson & M. Scriven (Eds.), *Evaluating social programs: Visions for the new millennium* (pp. 3–16). Mahwah, NJ: Lawrence Erlbaum Associates.

Durlak, J. A., & DuPre, E. P. (2008). Implementation matters: A review of research on the influence of implementation on program outcomes and the factors affecting implementation. *American Journal of Community Psychology, 41*, 327–350.

Everett, B. (1994). Something is happening: The contemporary consumer and psychiatric survivor movement in historical context. *The Journal of Mind and Behavior, 15*, 55–70.

Everett, B. (1998). Participation or exploitation? Consumers and psychiatric survivors as partners in planning mental health services. *International Journal of Mental Health, 27*, 80–97.

Fals-Borda, O., & Rahman, M. A. (1991). *Action and knowledge: Breaking the monopoly with participatory action-research.* New York: The Apex Press.

Fetterman, D. M. (2001). *Foundations of empowerment evaluation.* Thousand Oaks, CA: Sage.

Fine, M., Torre, M. E., Boudin, K., Bowen, I., Clark, J., Hylton, D., Martinez, M., Missy, Roberts, R. A., Smart, P., & Upegui, D. (2003). Participatory action research: From within and beyond prison bars. In P. M. Camic, J. E. Rhodes, & L. Yardley, *Qualitative research in psychology* (pp. 173–198). Washington, DC: American Psychological Association.

Fisher, P. A., & Ball, T. J. (2003). Tribal participatory research: Mechanisms of a collaborative model. *American Journal of Community Psychology, 32*, 207–216.

Foley, D., & Valenzuela, A. (2005). Critical ethnography: The politics of collaboration. In N. Denzin & Y. S. Lincoln (Eds.), *The Sage handbook of qualitative research* (3rd ed., pp. 217–234). Thousand Oaks, CA: Sage.

Frechtling, J. A. (2007). *Logic modeling methods in program evaluation*. San Francisco: Jossey-Bass.

Grant, J., Nelson, G., & Mitchell, T. (2008). Negotiating the challenges of participatory action research: Relationships, power, participation, change, and credibility. In P. Reason & H. Bradbury (Eds.), *Handbook of action research* (2nd ed., pp. 589–607). Thousand Oaks, CA: Sage.

Greene, J. (2008). Is mixed methods social inquiry a distinctive methodology? *Journal of Mixed Methods Research, 2*, 7–22.

Guba, E. G., & Lincoln, Y. S. (2005). Paradigmatic controversies, contradictions, and emerging confluences. In N. Denzin & Y. S. Lincoln (Eds.), *The Sage handbook of qualitative research* (3rd ed., pp. 191–216). Thousand Oaks, CA: Sage.

House, E.R. (2004). The role of the evaluator in a political world. *Canadian Journal of Program Evaluation, 19*, 1–16.

Hinshaw, S.P., & Cicchetti, D. (2000). Stigma and mental disorder: Conceptions of illness, public attitudes, personal disclosure, and social policy. *Development and Psychopathology, 12*, 555–598.

Humphrey, C. (2007). Insider-outsider: Activating the hyphen. *Action Research, 5*(1), 11–26.

Isenberg, D., Loomis, C., Humphreys, K., & Maton, K. (2004). Self-help research: Issues of power sharing. In L. Jason, C. Keys, Y. Suarez-Balcazar, R. Taylor, M. Davis, J. Durlak, & D. Isenberg (Eds.), *Participatory community research: Theories and methods in action* (pp. 123–137). Washington, DC: American Psychological Association.

Israel, B.A., Schulz, A.J., Parker, E.A., & Becker, A.B. (1998). Review of community-based research: Assessing partnership approaches to improve public health. *Annual Review of Public Health, 19*, 173–202.

Jacobson, N., Ochocka, J., Wise J., Janzen, R., & the Taking Culture Seriously Partners (2007). Inspiring knowledge mobilization through a communications policy: The case of a Community University Research Alliance. *Progress in Community Health Partnerships: Research, Education and Action, 1*(1), 99–104.

Janzen, R., Nelson, G., Hausfather, N., & Ochocka, J. (2007). Capturing system level activities and impacts of mental health consumer-run organizations. *American Journal of Community Psychology, 39*, 287–299.

Janzen, R., Nelson, G., Trainor, J., & Ochocka, J. (2006). A longitudinal study of mental health consumer/survivor initiatives: Part IV – Benefits beyond the self? A quantitative and qualitative study of system-level activities and impacts. *Journal of Community Psychology, 34*, 285–303.

Johnsen, M., Teague, G., & Herr, E. M. (2005). Common ingredients as a fidelity measure for peer-run programs. In S. Clay, B. Schell, P. W. Corrigan, & R. O. Ralph (Eds.), *On our own, together: Peer program for people with mental illness* (pp. 213–238). Nashville, TN: Vanderbilt University Press.

Kemmis, S. & McTaggart, R. (2005). Participatory action research. In N.K. Denzin & Y.S. Lincoln (Eds.), *Handbook of qualitative research* (3rd ed., pp. 559–603).Thousand Oaks, CA: Sage.

Kennedy, M., Humphreys, K., & Borkman, T. (1994), The naturalistic paradigm as an approach to research with mutual-help groups. In T. J. Powell (Ed.), *Understanding self-help organizations* (pp. 172–189). Thousand Oaks, CA: Sage.

Kincheloe, J. L., & McLaren, P. (2005). Rethinking critical theory and qualitative research. In N. Denzin & Y. S. Lincoln (Eds.), *The Sage handbook of qualitative research* (3rd ed., pp. 303–342). Thousand Oaks, CA: Sage.

Loveland, D., Weaver Randall, K., & Corrigan, P.W. (2005). Research methods for exploring and assessing recovery. In R. O. Ralph & P. W. Corrigan (Eds.), *Recovery in mental illness: Broadening our understanding of wellness* (pp. 19–59). Washington, DC: American Psychological Association.

Mertens, D.M. (2003). Mixed methods and the politics of human research: The transformative-emancipatory perspective. In A. Tashakkori & C. Teddlie (Eds.), *Handbook of mixed methods in social & behavioral research* (pp. 209–240). Thousand Oaks, CA: Sage.

Mertens, D.M. (2009). *Transformative research and evaluation.* New York: The Guilford Press.

McCubbin, M., & Cohen, D. (1996). Extremely unbalanced: Interest divergence and power disparities between clients and psychiatry. *International Journal of Law and Psychiatry, 19,* 1–25.

McLaughlin, J.A., & Jordan, G.B. (2004). Using logic models. In J. S. Wholey, H. P. Hatry, & K. E. Newcomer (Eds.), *Handbook of practical program evaluation* (pp. 7–32). Thousand Oaks, CA: Sage.

Mitten, C., Adair, C. E., McKenzie, E., Patten, S. B., & Perry, B. W. (2007). Knowledge transfer and exchange: Review and synthesis of the literature. *Milbank Quarterly, 85,* 729–768.

Mowbray, C. T., Bybee, D., Holter, M. C., & Lewandoswki, L. (2006). Validation of a fidelity rating instrument for consumer-operated services. *American Journal of Evaluation, 27,* 9–27.

Nelson, G. (1994). The development of a mental health coalition: A case study. *American Journal of Community Psychology, 22,* 229–255.

Nelson, G., Janzen, R., Trainor, J., & Ochocka, J. (2008). Putting values into practice: Public policy and the future of mental health consumer-run organizations. *American Journal of Community Psychology, 42,* 192–201.

Nelson, G., & Lomotey, J. (2006). Quantity and quality of participation and outcomes of participation in mental health consumer/survivor initiatives. *Journal of Mental Health, 15,* 1–12.

Nelson, G., Lord, J., & Ochocka, J. (2001) *Shifting the paradigm in community mental health: Towards empowerment and community.* Toronto, ON: University of Toronto Press.

Nelson, G., Ochocka, J., Janzen, R., Trainor, J., Goering, P., & Lomotey, J. (2007). A longitudinal study of mental health consumer/survivor initiatives: Part V – Outcomes at three-year follow-up. *Journal of Community Psychology, 35,* 655–665.

Nelson, G., Ochocka, J., Lauzon, S., Towndrow, J., & Cheng, R. (2005). Disseminating the findings of a longitudinal study of mental health Consumer/Survivor Initiatives in Ontario. *The Community Psychologist, 38*(2), 41–43.

Nelson, G., Lord, J., & Ochocka, J. (2001) *Shifting the paradigm in community mental health: Towards empowerment and community.* Toronto, ON: University of Toronto Press.

Nelson, G., Ochocka, J., Griffin, K., & Lord, J. (1998). Nothing about me, without me: Participatory action research with self-help/mutual aid organizations for psychiatric consumer/survivors. *American Journal of Community Psychology, 26,* 881–912.

Nelson, G., Ochocka, J., Janzen, R., & Trainor, J. (2006). A longitudinal study of mental health consumer/survivor initiatives: Part I – Literature review and overview of the study. *Journal of Community Psychology, 34,* 247–260.

Nelson, G., Ochocka, J., Janzen, R., Trainor, J., & Lauzon, S. (2004). A comprehensive evaluation approach for mental health consumer-run organizations: Values, conceptualization, design, and action. *Canadian Journal of Program Evaluation, 19*(3), 29–53.

Ochocka, J., Janzen, R., & Nelson, G. (2002). Sharing power and knowledge: Professional and mental health consumer/survivor researchers working together in a participatory action research project. *Psychiatric Rehabilitation Journal, 25,* 379–387.

Ochocka, J., Nelson, G., Janzen, R., & Trainor, J. (2006). A longitudinal study of mental health consumer/survivor initiatives: Part III – A qualitative study of impacts of participation on new members. *Journal of Community Psychology, 34,* 273–283.

Patton, M. Q. (2008). *Utilization-focused evaluation* (4th ed.). Thousand Oaks, CA: Sage.

Pistrang, N., Barker, C., & Humphries, K. (2008). Mutual help groups for mental health problems: A review of effectiveness studies. *American Journal of Community Psychology, 42,* 110–121.

Prilleltensky, I. (2008). The role of power in wellness, oppression, and liberation: The promise of psychopolitical validity. *Journal of Community Psychology, 36*, 116–136.

Prilleltensky, I., & Nelson, G. (2009). Community psychology: Advancing social justice. In D. Fox, I. Prilleltensky, & S. Austin (Eds.), *Critical psychology: An introduction* (2nd ed., pp. 126–143). Thousand Oaks, CA: Sage.

Postma, J. (2008). Balancing power among academic and community partners: The case of El Proyecto Bienestar. *Journal of Empirical Research on Human Research Ethics, 3*(2), 17–32.

Rappaport, J. (1981). In praise of paradox: A social policy of empowerment over prevention. *American Journal of Community Psychology, 9*, 1–25.

Rappaport, J., Seidman, E., Toro, P. A., McFadden, L. S., Reischl, T. M., Roberts, L. J., Salem, D. A., Stein, C. H., & Zimmerman, M. A. (1985). Finishing the unfinished business: Collaborative research with a mutual help organization. *Social Policy, 16*, 12–24.

Reeve, P., Cornell, S., D'Costa, B., Janzen, R., & Ochocka, J. (2002). From our perspective: Consumer researchers speak about their experience in a community mental health research project. *Psychiatric Rehabilitation Journal, 25*, 403–408.

Roberts, L. J., Salem, D. A., Rappaport, J., Toro, P. A., Luke, D. A., & Seidman, E. (1999). Giving and receiving help: Interpersonal transactions in mutual-help meetings and psychosocial adjustment of members. *American Journal of Community Psychology, 27*, 841–868.

Rowe, M., Bellamy, C., Baranoski, M., Wieland, M., O'Connell, M. J., Benedict, P., Davidson, L., Buchanan, J., & Sells, D. (2007). A peer-support group intervention to reduce substance use and criminality among persons with severe mental illness. *Psychiatric Services, 58*, 955–961.

Rush, B., & Ogborne, A. (1991). Program logic models: Expanding their role and structure for program planning and evaluation. *Canadian Journal of Program Evaluation, 6*, 95–106.

Ryan, K., Green, J., Lincoln, Y., Mathison, S., & Mertens, D. (1998). Advantages and challenges of using inclusive evaluation approaches in evaluation practice. *American Journal of Program Evaluation, 19*, 101–122.

Shadish, W. R., Cook, T. D., & Leviton, L. C. (1991). *Foundations of program evaluation: Theories of practice*. Newbury Park, CA: Sage.

Shoultz, J., Oneha, M. F., Magnussen, L., Hla, M. M., Bress-Suanders, Z., Dela Cruz, M. D., & Douglas, M. (2006). Finding solutions to challenges faced in community-based participatory research between academic and community organizations. *Journal of Interprofessional Care, 20*, 133–144.

Solomon, P. (2004). Peer support/peer provided services: Underlying processes, benefits, and critical ingredients. *Psychiatric Rehabilitation Journal, 27*, 392–401.

Scriven, M. (1980). *The logic of evaluation*. Inverness, CA: Edgpress.

Szasz, T. (Ed.). (1974). *The age of madness*. New York: Jason Aronson.

Tashakkori, A., & Teddlie, C. (Eds.). (2003). *Handbook of mixed methods in social and behavioral research*. Thousand Oaks, CA: Sage.

Tefft, B. (1987). Advocacy coalitions as a vehicle for mental health system reform. In E.M. Bennett (Ed.), *Social intervention: Theory and practice* (pp. 155–185). Lewiston, New York: The Edwin Mellen Press.

Weaver Randall, K., & Salem, D. A. (2005). Mutual-help groups and recovery: The influence of settings on participants' experience of recovery. In R. O. Ralph & P. W. Corrigan (Eds.), *Recovery in mental illness: Broadening our understanding of wellness* (pp. 173–205). Washington, DC: American Psychological Association.

Weiss, C. (1983). The stakeholder approach to evaluation: Origins and promise. In A. S. Bryk (Ed.), *Stakeholder-based evaluation* (Vol. 17, pp. 3–14). San Francisco, CA: Jossey-Bass.

Weitz, D. (1984). "On Our Own": A self-help model. In D. P. Lumsden (Ed.), *Community mental health action: Primary prevention programming in Canada* (pp. 312–320). Ottawa, ON: Canadian Public Health Association.

Whitaker, R. (2001). *Mad in America: Bad science, bad medicine, and the enduring mistreatment of the mentally ill*. Cambridge, MA: Perseus.

Part II
MHSH Groups

Chapter 4
The Contributions of Mutual Help Groups for Mental Health Problems to Psychological Well-Being: A Systematic Review

Nancy Pistrang, Chris Barker, and Keith Humphreys

Abstract This chapter systematically reviews empirical studies on whether participating in mutual help groups for mental health problems leads to improved psychological and social functioning. It first outlines how mutual help groups fit into the broader picture of mental health self-help initiatives, and discusses some issues involved in conducting effectiveness research on mutual help groups (i.e., how to determine whether they are beneficial to their members). The methods and results of the review are then presented. To be included, studies had to satisfy four sets of criteria, covering: (1) characteristics of the group, (2) target problems, (3) outcome measures, and (4) research design. The 12 studies meeting these criteria provide limited but promising evidence that mutual help groups benefit people with three types of problems: chronic mental illness, depression/anxiety, and bereavement. Seven studies reported positive changes for those attending support groups. The strongest findings come from two randomized trials showing that the outcomes of mutual help groups were equivalent to those of substantially more costly professional interventions. Five of the 12 studies found no differences in mental health outcomes between mutual help group members and non-members; no studies showed evidence of negative effects. There was no indication that mutual help groups were differentially effective for certain types of problems. The studies varied in terms of design quality and reporting of results. More high-quality outcome research is needed to evaluate the effectiveness of mutual help groups across the spectrum of mental health problems.

N. Pistrang (✉)
Department of Clinical, Educational and Health Psychology, University College London, London, UK
e-mail: n.pistrang@ucl.ac.uk

4.1 Introduction

Mental health self-help brings many images to mind. Perhaps shelves of books on how to improve one's life, or interactive self-paced therapy programs on CD-ROMs or on the Internet. Perhaps national organizations such as Alcoholics Anonymous or GROW, or the local chapters of these organizations, with a small group of people meeting together in a church basement to discuss a common concern. Perhaps online support groups, in which people can use Internet message boards or forums to exchange support and help, without restriction of time or place. Or organizations founded and run by mental health service users ("consumer/survivor initiatives") that aim to provide advocacy, work, or housing. Or what might be described as meta-self-help organizations, the clearing houses that aim to encourage and support self-help groups and to disseminate information about them: the self-help clearing houses in New Jersey, Toronto, or Nottingham, or SHARE (the Self Help and Recovery Exchange) in Los Angeles are prominent examples. All of these entities, activities, and organizations can justly claim the label "mental health self-help."

Mental health self-help therefore is clearly an umbrella term that covers a bewildering variety of approaches. The present chapter will concentrate on one small but important corner of the territory, namely that of the effectiveness of member-led mutual help groups. However, we will first briefly address the broader area of interpersonal self-help modalities, i.e., small groups or larger organizations, which involve people giving and receiving help from each other. Individually focused modalities, such as self-help books (bibliotherapy) and computerized forms of individual therapies, lie outside of the scope of the present volume, but have been thoroughly reviewed elsewhere (den Boer, Wiersma, & van den Bosch, 2004).

Interpersonal forms of self-help (often termed "mutual help" or "mutual aid") may manifest themselves in different ways, but all have a common core: people are enabled to take charge of their own lives, and to deal with their problems with the support of others like them, without professional input. It is usually non-stigmatizing and non-pathologizing, and the person with the problem stays in control of what happens to them.

One of the first writers to discuss the phenomenon of mutual aid was the remarkable Russian anarchist thinker Petr Kropotkin. His book *Mutual Aid: A Factor of Evolution* (Kropotkin, 1902) argued from an evolutionary standpoint for the existence of mutual aid processes, thereby mitigating the popular image of the Darwinian natural universe as being invariably "red in tooth and claw." Kropotkin marshaled examples of how mutual aid processes may be biologically adaptive as well as socially desirable, and makes a strong argument for furthering this form of social organization.

Interestingly, mutual aid appeals to thinkers on both the left and the right of the political spectrum. From the right, conservative thinkers are sympathetic to the ethos of individualistic self-improvement and of communities solving problems without the input of government hired professionals. From the left, progressive thinkers like Kropotkin are sympathetic to the cooperative, communitarian sense of solidarity: people joining together to improve their own lot and to challenge social injustice – processes analogous to the mutual aid processes that occur in labor unions.

4.1.1 Dimensions of Mental Health Self-Help Groups and Organizations

Clearly, mental health self-help initiatives differ along many different dimensions. The most important ones are described below.

4.1.1.1 Target Problem

The problem that the group or organization addresses is obviously its most important feature, one usually reflected in its name (e.g., Schizophrenics Anonymous, Bipolar Disorder Support Association). There are self-help groups and organizations for most conceivable human problems, within and outside of mental health. Within mental health, partly for historical reasons, groups and organizations for people with substance abuse problems tend to be treated separately from those focusing on other mental health problems, although there are groups and organizations that cover "dual diagnoses," i.e., for those experiencing both substance abuse and other mental health problems.

4.1.1.2 Aims

Some groups and organizations exist purely to give advice and emotional support, whereas others focus on more practical issues, such as housing or employment. Others focus on advocacy; others take a more political stance and focus on changing social policy or legislation. These aims are not mutually exclusive: many groups and organizations work in several areas simultaneously.

4.1.1.3 Guiding Philosophy

Many groups and organizations have an explicit philosophical basis, often articulated by its founder(s). The most important distinction is between those groups that follow the "12-step" approach and those that do not. The 12 steps were originally articulated in the context of Alcoholics Anonymous (1939), and involve first admitting that you are powerless over alcohol and then placing yourself in the care of a "higher power." Groups with Anonymous in their title tend to use this framework. An alternative philosophical framework is that of Recovery, Inc., a mutual help organization for individuals with psychiatric problems, which maintains that symptoms can be controlled using "Will Training." This is markedly different from the 12-step philosophy, which emphasizes the limits of members' self-control rather than how to enhance it.

4.1.1.4 Membership

Most groups and organizations are aimed directly at people who are experiencing the target problem, but there is also the important category of "one-step removed groups" (a different type of step than that in 12-step groups), in other words groups for the families or carers of the people experiencing the target problem. Although not experiencing a mental health problem themselves, members of one-step removed groups are united by the concerns of caregiving.

4.1.1.5 National or Local Organization

Mutual help groups are often organized as chapters of a larger umbrella organization. The national organization provides the overall structure and, in some but not all cases, funding. For example, it may maintain a website or a local directory and referral system, and it may also carry out political or research work. However, some purely local groups also exist, formed spontaneously by a group of people in the community with a common concern.

4.1.1.6 Modality of Communication

Groups and organizations vary in the extent to which they emphasize face-to-face communication, as opposed to the telephone or the Internet. Some organizations now operate entirely over the Internet, allowing them to become more international in scope, whereas others maintain a more traditional basis in their local communities. Organizations also vary in the extent to which they involve group interaction or one-to-one communication, an example of the latter being "buddy" systems which provide peer support.

Subsequent chapters in this volume will examine several of these different forms of groups or organizations. The present chapter will focus on mutual help groups (rather than multifaceted organizations), targeted at people directly experiencing a mental health problem. (It will not include groups for friends and family members. For a discussion of these, See Chapter 6, this volume.)

4.1.2 Mutual Help Groups

The last 20 years have seen a burgeoning of mutual help groups for people with mental health problems. Although, historically, these groups began in the addictions area (Alcoholics Anonymous being the prototypical example), there are long-established mutual help groups for the full gamut of mental health problems. This is, of course, in addition to groups catering to a plethora of physical disorders (Davison, Pennebaker, & Dickerson, 2000).

Approximately one in six of the US adult population has participated in a mutual help group (but not necessarily for mental health problems) at some point in their lives (Jacobs & Goodman, 1989; Kessler, Mickelson, & Zhao, 1997), as has a smaller, but still significant proportion of Canadians (Gottlieb & Peters, 1991). Goldstrom et al. (2006) estimated that there were over 3,000 mental health mutual help groups in the USA, and that over 40,000 people attended their last meetings. There are no comparable surveys outside of North America, but there are indications that mutual help groups have a significant presence in other industrialized countries (Borkman, 1999; Munn-Giddings, & Borkman, 2005; Schäfer et al., 2005; Trojan, 1989).

A mutual help group can be formally defined as a group of people sharing a problem, who meet regularly to exchange information and to give and receive psychological support (Chinman, Kloos, O'Connell, & Davidson, 2002; Levy, 2000). Groups are run principally by the members themselves, rather than by professionals, even though professionals may have provided extensive assistance during the groups' founding years. Traditionally, groups meet face-to-face, but Internet-based groups have expanded rapidly in recent years (Eysenbach, Powell, Englesakis, Rizo, & Stern, 2004). Mutual help groups are described in the literature under a variety of labels, including, for example, "mutual aid" and "mutual support" groups, as well as the broader terms "self-help groups" and "support groups." The latter two terms encompass a wide variety of activities, many of which fall outside the definition of a mutual help group (e.g., structured bibliotherapy interventions or professionally-led support groups), causing considerable confusion in the literature.

From a theoretical point of view, mutual help groups can be conceptualized as drawing on the potential benefits of socially supportive interactions (Helgeson & Gottlieb, 2000). Specifically, they utilize support from people who have gone through similar difficulties and participants therefore can easily empathize with each other. This type of peer support may compensate for deficiencies in people's natural support networks. In addition, group members possess "experiential knowledge" (Borkman, 1990), in contrast to the professional knowledge of service providers. A number of benefits would be expected from such supportive interactions, including feeling more understood and less isolated, an increased sense of empowerment and self-efficacy, and acquiring more effective ways of coping with one's difficulties (Helgeson & Gottlieb, 2000). Therefore, it is important to study how effective mutual help groups are, and conditions that enhance their effectiveness.

4.1.3 What Constitutes Evidence of Effectiveness?

The present review was driven by the question "What is the evidence that participating in a mutual help group brings about positive changes for people with mental health problems?" This raises the thorny issues of what kind of changes to focus upon and what type of evidence to consider in determining whether such changes occur. A large literature of surveys, qualitative studies, and first-person accounts attests to the subjective benefits of mutual help groups (see, for example, Borkman, 1999; Davidson, 2003; Humphreys, 2000; Levy, 2000). These studies often give a vivid picture of the types of changes that members experience in terms of identity, life narrative reconstruction, spiritual development, and sense of feeling cared about, but they are not designed to yield evidence about causal relationships between group involvement and more traditional "psychiatric outcomes" such as reduction of symptoms and hospitalizations. Randomized controlled trials present different tradeoffs. On the one hand, they are powerful tools for evaluating causality and measuring quantitative, standardized indicators of mental health. But the high level of researcher standardization and control inherent in a clinical trial can distort the informal, peer-driven processes essential to mutual help organizations (Humphreys & Rappaport, 1994).

Our own position is a pluralist one: we believe that multiple sources of evidence are important and valuable for addressing this issue (Barker & Pistrang, 2005; Humphreys & Rappaport, 1994). However, for the purposes of this review, we adopt a more specific focus, namely, that which Humphreys (2004) has labeled the "treatment-evaluation" perspective. In other words, we will examine the evidence that bears on whether mutual help groups "work," in terms of providing the kinds of outcomes at which a professionally led intervention would aim. Some readers may question the wisdom of such a focus, since it runs the danger of implying that mutual help is simply another professionally organized treatment. This is emphatically not our position: we actively celebrate the many features of mutual help groups that set them apart from professional interventions. However, as Humphreys (2004) has argued, it is still essential to examine the evidence on outcomes from a treatment-evaluation point of view, i.e., to determine the extent to which groups help their members directly with the problems that brought most of them into the group in the first place. This is important in order to assist consumers who may be considering investing their time and energy in a mutual help group and also to demonstrate that an evidence base exists for interventions that are organized from a grass-roots rather than a professional level. We fully acknowledge, however, that the treatment-evaluation perspective adopted here addresses only part of the range of potential benefits from mutual help.

Following Kyrouz, Humphreys, and Loomis (2002), the current review is therefore limited to quantitative studies employing either group-comparison or longitudinal designs. These designs allow some degree of causal inference to be drawn about changes resulting from group membership for people with mental health problems. In terms of outcome measurement, the review examines studies that address improvement in psychological or social functioning. This review differs from related reviews in terms of the range of interventions and the types of target problems that are covered (see Table 4.1).

Most prior reviews have focused on a broader range of interventions such as self-help, in general, (den Boer et al., 2004; Lewis et al., 2003) or social support interventions (Hogan, Linden, & Najarian, 2002), many of which are professionally led. Moreover, the distinction between professionally and member-led groups often is not made, making it difficult to know what is being evaluated. Two reviews (Eysenbach et al., 2004; Ybarra & Eaton, 2005) have focused specifically on online support groups and other online interventions. In terms of target problem, several have included both physical and mental health problems (e.g., Hogan et al., 2002; Levy, 2000), whereas others have focused on specific types of mental health problems (e.g., severe mental illness in Davidson et al., 1999 and mood and anxiety disorders in den Boer et al., 2004). The most closely related review (Kyrouz et al., 2002) is an intentionally, informal narrative review, aimed at a general audience,

Table 4.1 Recent reviews that include studies of mutual help groups for mental health problems

Review	Population or type of problem	Type of intervention	Method of review	Main difference from current review
Barlow et al. (1999)	Physical and mental health	Self-help and professionally facilitated support groups	Meta-analysis	Focused mostly on professionally led groups
Davidson et al. (1999)	Severe mental illness	Mutual support groups; consumer-run services; consumers as providers	Narrative review	Focused on severe mental illness
den Boer et al. (2004)	Chronic mood and anxiety disorders	Self-help, including bibliotherapy and self-help groups	Meta-analysis	Narrower spectrum of mental health problems; limited to RCTs; mostly focused on bibliotherapy
Eysenbach et al. (2004)	Physical and mental health	Electronic (online) peer support	Systematic review	Focused on electronic support
Hogan et al. (2002)	Physical and mental health	Social support interventions including peer support groups	Systematic review	Focused on interventions aiming to improve social support
Kyrouz et al. (2002)	Physical and mental health	Self-help mutual aid groups	Narrative review	Less formal review intended for non-professional audience
Lewis et al. (2003)	Mental health problems	Self-help in general including books, CD-ROMs, self-help groups, etc.	Systematic review	Focused on self-help materials
Levy (2000)	Physical and mental health	Self-help groups	Selective narrative review	Focused more on methodological and public policy issues rather than effectiveness
Ybarra & Eaton (2005)	Mental health problems	Self-directed and therapist-led online therapies including online support groups	Systematic review	Focused on Internet interventions

covering mutual help groups for a broad range of psychological and physical health problems. The present chapter builds on Kyrouz et al. (2002) by using systematic search strategies and inclusion criteria to focus on mental health problems and examining in detail each study's outcome and methodological approach. It represents material from our recent journal article (Pistrang, Barker, & Humphreys, 2008).

4.2 Method

4.2.1 Inclusion and Exclusion Criteria

To be included in the review, studies had to satisfy four sets of criteria. These addressed: (1) characteristics of the group, (2) target problem, (3) outcome measures, and (4) research design.

4.2.1.1 Characteristics of the Group

Studies were included if the group being evaluated met all of the following criteria: (1) it aimed to provide support by and for people with a common problem; (2) it was primarily run by its members or facilitated by someone with the same problem (i.e., at most, outside professionals provided occasional consultation); (3) the content of the sessions was determined by members (e.g., the group was not built around a structured self-help intervention such as a series of prescribed cognitive-behavioral techniques; and (4) members met either face-to-face or via the Internet. Groups meeting these criteria could be described under a variety of labels (e.g., self-help group, support group, mutual help group, or mutual aid group). Studies were excluded if the group was only one aspect of a larger mutual help or consumer-run organization which meant that the effects of group membership could not be isolated.

4.2.1.2 Target Problems

Studies were included if the group membership comprised adults with mental health problems. This criterion was broadly interpreted to include specific problems such as depression or anxiety, as well as more vaguely defined problems such as "chronic mental illness." Bereavement was included as these groups partly focus on reducing depression. Substance misuse and addictions were excluded because this is a distinct specialism with its own large, mutual help literature (recently reviewed by Humphreys, 2004), the only exception being groups specifically designed for people with both chronic mental illness and a substance use disorder. Groups for caregivers (e.g., relatives of people with Alzheimer's disease or of people with serious mental illness) were also excluded as they focus on reducing caregivers' stress or burden rather than on specific mental health problems.

4.2.1.3 Outcome Measures

Studies were included only if they reported at least one mental health outcome measure, assessing either (1) psychological symptoms, (2) rates of hospitalization, (3) adherence to psychiatric medication, or (4) social functioning.

4.2.1.4 Research Design

It was anticipated that randomized controlled trials would be rare because most of the literature has focused on existing, community-based support groups (to which randomized assignment is usually impossible). Therefore, in line with other, related reviews (Davidson, et al., 1999; Kyrouz et al., 2002), the inclusion criterion was that the study used either a comparison group (randomized or non-randomized) or a prospective longitudinal design comparing data from two or more time points.

4.2.2 Search Strategy

Three procedures were used to identify all relevant studies published prior to our cut-off date of May 2006. First, we used existing reviews of the literature in this and related areas: mutual aid/self-help groups (Kyrouz et al., 2002; Levy, 2000), peer support in severe mental illness (Davidson et al., 1999), social support interventions (Hogan et al., 2002), self-help interventions (den Boer et al., 2004; Lewis et al., 2003), and online support groups (Eysenbach et al., 2004). Second, the PsychInfo database from 1989 to May 2006 was searched using the terms "mutual support," "mutual aid," "mutual help," "online support," and "internet support." Searches using the broader terms "support group" and "self-help group" yielded a greatly over-inclusive set of studies, even when further delimited by using mental health terms such as anx*, depress*, and psych* (the asterisk is a standard wildcard convention used to encompass variant terms such as depression, depressed, depressive, etc.). As several recent reviews covered these areas we limited our search to the 2003 to May 2006 database for these terms, but also searched the additional databases of Medline (which focuses on biomedicine and the life sciences), Cinahl (which focuses on nursing-orientated research), and EMBASE (which focuses on biomedical and pharmacological research). Third, potential papers were identified from reference lists, manual searches of several key journals, and recommendations by experts in the field. Only English-language papers published in peer-reviewed journals were considered for the review.

Judgments about the eligibility of studies for the review were made initially by a research assistant and then by the first author. When eligibility was not clear-cut, the first two authors read and discussed the paper and came to a decision; if any doubt remained, the third author was consulted. Of the studies focusing on mental health problems (criterion 2), the majority of exclusions were made on the grounds of characteristics of the group (criterion 1, e.g., they were professionally led), or design (criterion 4). Studies that met the design criterion almost always met the criterion for outcome measures (criterion 3).

4.2.3 Examples of Excluded Studies

Several studies came close to meeting the inclusion criteria, but were eventually excluded. Some did not fully meet the criteria concerning characteristics of the group or provided insufficient information for making a judgment. For example, Rathner, Bönsch, Maurer, Walter, and Söllner (1993) report on a group for bulimic women which appeared to be based around a structured self-help intervention designed by professionals. In a few other studies, the outcome measure was not considered to be assessing a mental health variable as defined above. For example, in Dunham et al.'s (1998) otherwise excellent study of computer-mediated support for young single mothers, utilized parenting stress as the only pre–post outcome measure.

In some other studies, the effects of the mutual help groups could not be disentangled from that of a larger intervention. For example, in Vachon, Lyall, Rogers, Freeman-Letofsky, and Freeman's (1980) frequently cited study of a "widow-to-widow" program, the intervention comprised one-to-one as well as group support. Similarly, in Segal and Silverman's (2002) study of self-help agencies, mutual support groups were only one of many activities, and in Burti et al.'s (2005) well-designed Italian study, the self-help group was embedded in a multifaceted "Psychosocial Center."

4.3 Results

Twelve studies met the inclusion criteria for the review. Table 4.2 summarizes the characteristics of the mutual help groups under investigation and Table 4.3 summarizes the methodological characteristics of the studies.

Four of the studies used randomized controlled designs to evaluate mutual help groups set up for the purpose of the study. The other eight used quasi-experimental or prospective longitudinal designs to evaluate pre-existing groups, seven of which were part of national self-help organizations and one Internet-based. All 12 studies included standardized outcome measures, mostly assessing

Table 4.2. Summary characteristics of the mutual help groups

Feature	Number of studies
Target problem:	
Chronic mental illness	3
Depression/anxiety	4
Bereavement	5
Modality:	
Face-to-face	11
Internet	1
Status:	
Pre-existing group	8
Group set up for the study	4

4 The Contributions of Mutual Help Groups for Mental Health Problems

Table 4.3 Methodological characteristics of the studies

Feature	Number of studies
Design:	
Randomized controlled trial	4
Non-randomized controlled trial	3
Prospective longitudinal	4
Cross-sectional	1
Type of comparison group:	
Established psychological therapy	2
Wait-list control	1
No-intervention control	4
Community (probability) sample	1
No comparison group	4
Type of outcome measure:[a]	
Psychological symptoms	10
Social functioning	5
Use of psychiatric medication	4
Number of measurement occasions:	
One	1
Two	5
Three	3
Four	3

[a]Totals add up to more than 12 because some studies used more than one type of outcome measure

psychological symptoms. Nearly all studies used more than one outcome measure; there was a heavy reliance on self-report measures with only three studies supplementing these with independent interviewers' ratings. Sample sizes were moderate to large, ranging from 61 upwards; most studies had a hundred or more participants. In ten studies, the sample comprised a high proportion (70% or over) of women. All studies except one were North American.

The standard of reporting of findings was variable. In particular, the majority of studies did not provide sufficient information (i.e., cell means and standard deviations) to compute Cohen's d, the standard measure for effect sizes in meta-analytic reviews. However, two of the best-designed studies were also very thorough in their reporting of results.

Details of the individual studies are summarized in Table 4.4. Below we highlight the main findings for each of the three clusters of studies according to target problem.

4.3.1 Groups for Chronic Mental Illness

Three studies examined groups for general psychiatric problems or chronic mental illness, one of which was specifically targeted at individuals with a concurrent substance use disorder. Two used prospective longitudinal (uncontrolled) designs and one used a cross-sectional design. All three studies report some evidence for

Table 4.4 Description of individual studies

Author (date)	Target problem	Nature of group	Design	Assessment points[a]	Sample size	Outcome measures[b]	Results
Groups for chronic mental illness:							
Galanter (1988)	General psychiatric disorders	National self-help organization for people with psychiatric problems ("Recovery")	Cross-sectional comparison of recent members, longstanding members and community controls	Single time point in on-going groups	155 recent members, 201 longstanding members, 195 controls	General Well-Being Schedule; Neurotic Distress Scale; mental health treatment (including use of psychiatric medication)	Longstanding members higher on well-being, lower on neurotic distress and receiving less mental health treatment than recent members. Longstanding members similar to controls on well-being
Magura et al. (2002)	Chronic mental illness plus substance use disorder	12-step groups ("Double Trouble in Recovery")	Prospective longitudinal	Baseline plus 1 year	240	Adherence to psychiatric medication	Consistent attendance associated with better adherence after controlling for baseline variables
Roberts et al. (1999)	Serious mental illness	National mutual help organization for people experiencing mental illness ("GROW")	Prospective longitudinal	Baseline plus 6–13 months later	98	SCL-90; SAS; interviewer-rated adjustment	Improvement over time on all three outcome measures

Table 4.4 (continued)

Author (date)	Target problem	Nature of group	Design	Assessment points[a]	Sample size	Outcome measures[b]	Results
Groups for depression and anxiety:							
Bright et al. (1999)	Depression	10-session, weekly mutual support group	Randomized 2 × 2 design: mutual support group vs. group cognitive-behavioral therapy, peer- vs. professional-led	Pre and post	98	BDI; Hamilton; Hopkins Symptom Checklist; Automatic Thoughts Questionnaire	Improvement on all measures: mutual support group equivalent to CBT group; peer-led groups equivalent to professional-led groups
Cheung & Sun (2000)	Depression and anxiety	Support groups, meeting monthly, in a mutual aid organization in Hong Kong	Prospective longitudinal	3 time points: pre-group, 6 months, and 12 months	65	GHQ, STAI, CES-D, self-efficacy, social support	No changes over time
Houston et al. (2002)	Depression	Internet-based depression support groups	Prospective longitudinal	Baseline, 6 and 12 months	103	CES-D	Overall 34% resolved their depressive symptoms; more frequent users more likely to have resolution

Table 4.4 (continued)

Author (date)	Target problem	Nature of group	Design	Assessment points[a]	Sample size	Outcome measures[b]	Results
Powell et al. (2001)[c]	Mood disorders (mostly unipolar depression)	Manic-depressive and depressive association groups	Partially randomized assignment to support groups and to no-intervention control	Pre, 6 months and 1 year	144	Daily functioning; management of illness	No effects for being assigned self-help group sponsor, but group involvement predicted improved illness management
Groups for bereavement							
Caserta & Lund (1993)[c,d]	Bereavement (death of spouse)	Short-term (8 weekly sessions) and long-term (10 additional monthly sessions) self-help groups	Randomized assignment to short-term or long-term self-help group or to a no-intervention control	Pre, post-short-term groups, post-long-term groups, plus follow-up	295	Geriatric Depression Scale; Texas Revised Inventory of Grief	No main effects for group attendance. Among those with initially low interpersonal and coping skills, group attendance predicted less depression and grief

Table 4.4 (continued)

Author (date)	Target problem	Nature of group	Design	Assessment points[a]	Sample size	Outcome measures[b]	Results
Lieberman & Videka-Sherman (1986)	Bereavement (death of spouse)	National self-help organization for widows and widowers ("THEOS")	Comparisons of members with different levels of involvement and with "non-members" (attended <3 meetings) and with normative bereaved sample	Baseline plus 1 year	394 members, 108 non-members	Hopkins Symptom Checklist; self-esteem; well-being; life satisfaction; mastery; use of psychotropic medication	Members showed more improvement than normative sample on most measures; more improvement than non-members on only 2 measures. More involved members showed more positive change
Marmar et al. (1988)	Bereavement (death of husband)	12-session, weekly mutual help group	Random assignment to mutual help group or brief dynamic psychotherapy	Pre and post, plus 4 month and 1 year follow-up	61	SCL-90; BDI; BPRS; IES; clinician-rated stress; SAS; GAS	Improvement on most measures. Mutual help group equivalent to brief psychotherapy
Tudiver et al. (1992)	Bereavement (death of wife)	9-session, weekly mutual help group	Randomized assignment to group or wait-list control	Pre, post (2 months), 8 months, 14 months	113	GHQ-28; BDI; STAI; SAS	No main effects for group membership; whole sample showed improvement over time on psychological but not social variables

Table 4.4 (continued)

Author (date)	Target problem	Nature of group	Design	Assessment points[a]	Sample size	Outcome measures[b]	Results
Videka-Sherman & Lieberman (1985)	Bereavement (death of child)	National self-help organization for bereaved parents ("Compassionate Friends")	Comparison of non-members and members at varying participation levels	Baseline plus 1 year	97 non-members; 289 members at various levels of participation	Hopkins Symptom Checklist; self-esteem; life satisfaction; mastery; use of psychotropic medication; social role functioning	No effect for group membership; whole sample showed little improvement over time (small changes on only two measures)

[a]"Baseline" refers to a first measurement in an on-going group. "Pre" refers to a measurement taken before the start of the group

[b]Abbreviations of measures: BDI = Beck Depression Inventory; BPRS = Brief Psychiatric Rating Scale; CES-D = Center for Epidemiological Studies Depression Scale; GAS = Global Assessment Scale; GHQ = General Health Questionnaire; Hamilton = Hamilton Rating Scale for Depression; IES = Impact of Event Scale; SAS = Social Adjustment Scale; SCL-90 = Symptom Checklist-90; STAI = State-Trait Anxiety Inventory

[c]Powell et al. (2001) and Caserta & Lund (1993) did not report cell means and it was unclear whether the sample as a whole changed over time

[d]Half the groups in the Caserta & Lund study were facilitated by peers and half by professionals. The analysis does not distinguish between these

the effectiveness of mutual help groups although their designs do not allow firm conclusions to be drawn.

In a well-designed longitudinal study of groups for people with serious mental illness, Roberts et al. (1999) found improvement over a 1-year-period on measures of psychological symptoms and social adjustment. A particular strength of the study was that it examined associations between interpersonal transactions during meetings (using observer ratings) and the outcome variables. One interesting finding was that giving help was associated with improved functioning, but receiving help was associated with improved functioning only for those members who reported higher group integration.

Magura, Laudet, Mahmood, Rosenblum, and Knight (2002) studied 12-step groups for people with both chronic mental illness and substance use disorder. The outcome variable of interest was adherence to psychiatric medication. Consistent attendance at meetings was associated with better adherence when independent predictors of adherence (such as severity of psychiatric symptoms) were controlled. However, the degree of overall change in adherence was not examined.

Using a cross-sectional design to study groups for people with psychiatric problems, Galanter (1988) compared longstanding members, recent members, and community controls on a number of mental health outcome variables. Longstanding group members reported higher well-being (comparable to that of community controls), lower neurotic distress, and less use of psychiatric medication, compared to recent members. Because the "longstanding" members had been in the groups for many years and had become group leaders, they were probably a highly select group, which could mean these results overstate or understate the benefits of participation (cf. Klaw, Horst, & Humphreys, 2006). A number of other findings concerning improvements since joining the groups were reported (e.g., a reduction in neurotic distress) but these were based on members' retrospective reports rather than longitudinal data.

4.3.2 Groups for Depression and Anxiety

Three studies examined groups for depression, and one for depression and anxiety. Two provide evidence for effectiveness and two do not. The strongest evidence comes from Bright, Baker, and Neimeyer's (1999) well-designed, randomized study comparing the relative efficacy of group cognitive-behavioral therapy (CBT) and mutual help groups for depression, both professionally and non-professionally (peer) led. Self-report measures as well as ratings by an independent clinician were used to assess pre–post change. Participants improved on all measures, the outcomes of the mutual help groups being equivalent to those of the CBT groups, and peer leaders were as effective as professional therapists. This study did not include a formal cost-effectiveness analysis, but it goes without saying that the training and employment of professionals is substantially more costly than "helping" provided by peer volunteers. In other words, this finding of equal effectiveness demonstrates superior cost-effectiveness for the peer-led groups.

In the only study of Internet support groups, Houston, Cooper, and Ford (2002) used a longitudinal design to assess depressive symptoms over time. One-third of members showed a resolution of depressive symptoms with more frequent users more likely to improve (after adjusting for a number of other variables). The investigators were concerned that use of an online support group might have the unfortunate consequence of a decrease in face-to-face social support but they found that social support scores did not change over time.

Powell and colleagues (Powell, Hill, Warner, Yeaton, & Silk 2000; Powell, Yeaton, Hill, & Silk, 2001) used a "partially randomized" design (the study began with a quasi-experimental design and later became fully randomized) to study self-help groups for adults hospitalized for unipolar or bipolar depression. The experimental condition involved providing a "sponsor" (an experienced group member) to introduce participants to the group. An intent-to-treat analysis showed that the intervention increased the likelihood of group attendance nearly threefold (Powell et al., 2000). At 1-year follow-up, the team evaluated impact on two outcomes: Daily functioning and management of illness. Experimental participants did not have significantly higher scores than controls on either outcome measure (Powell et al., 2001). However, self-rated level of involvement in the group predicted improved management of illness. Unfortunately, the project team did not employ a two-stage, sample selection, data analytic model (see Humphreys, Phibbs, & Moos, 1996) which could have determined whether the negative results for the experimental condition reflected lack of an effect of self-help group participation per se or the fact that many individuals who were assigned a sponsor never attended any meetings.

Cheung and Sun (2000) studied groups for people with anxiety and depression in Hong Kong. Unusually, all participants had received 12 sessions of group cognitive-behavioral therapy before joining a mutual aid group. The prospective longitudinal design had three measurement points. At the time of joining the mutual aid group, participants had mean scores on mental health outcome variables within the clinical range (it is unclear how much change resulted from the previous group therapy) and there was no overall change over the 1-year-period of the study. The authors also examined self-efficacy as a potential mediator of outcome. Changes in self-efficacy were associated with changes in mental health, but whether this shared variance is a true mediational effect or a case where two measures tap quite similar aspects of psychological adjustment is not clear.

4.3.3 *Groups for Bereavement*

Five studies examined groups for bereavement (loss of a spouse or a child), three of which used randomized designs. One study provides strong evidence and one somewhat weaker evidence for effectiveness; the remaining three show no effects. Strong evidence is provided by Marmar, Horowitz, Weiss, Wilner, and Kaltreider's (1988) randomized study comparing a 12-week, peer-led mutual help group with brief individual psychodynamic psychotherapy for unresolved grief reactions in bereaved women. Participants in both conditions showed a reduction in stress-specific and general symptoms as well as improvement in social functioning (based on both self-report measures and independent clinician ratings). The outcomes of the mutual help group were equivalent to those of the psychotherapy intervention. Again, it is worth noting that even in the absence of a formal cost-effectiveness analysis, equivalent findings for effectiveness here suggest superior cost-effectiveness for the mutual help condition.

Some evidence for effectiveness is also provided by Lieberman and Videka-Sherman's (1986) study examining changes in mental health status among members of a self-help organization for widows and widowers. The study used a quasi-experimental design, over a 1-year time period, to compare participants with different levels of involvement in the groups and also to compare members with a normative bereaved sample. Members showed more improvement than the normative sample. There were few differences between members and "non-members" (individuals who had attended a maximum of two meetings). However, when level of involvement in the groups was examined, those members who participated more actively and formed social linkages within the groups were found to show more positive change. Interestingly, those members who had received additional professional help (e.g., psychotherapy) did not improve more than other members.

Three other studies found no differences between members and non-members. Tudiver, Hilditch, Permaul, and McKendree's (1992) randomized controlled trial of the efficacy of mutual help groups for recently bereaved men found no evidence of the intervention being superior to a waiting-list control. Caserta and Lund (1993) also used a randomized design to compare groups for bereaved older adults with a no-intervention control condition, in terms of the outcome variables of depression and grief. No main effects for group membership were found although the analysis and presentation of the data make it difficult to fully understand the findings (e.g., cell means are not presented). However, there was some indication that, for members with lower interpersonal and coping skills, greater meeting attendance was associated with reduced depression and grief.

Finally, in Videka-Sherman and Lieberman's (1985) quasi-experimental study of a national self-help organization for parents whose child had died, there were no differences in mental health or social functioning between members and non-members over a 1-year-period. Sadly, there were few signs of recovery for any of these parents regardless of whether they were members of the organization or their level of involvement within it (the one exception being some change in attitudes for highly involved members). There were also no differences between those who reported receiving professional help and those who did not. This study differs from the previously discussed "no difference" findings of other studies in that no intervention seemed to alleviate the high levels of distress in this population. However, parents did report subjective benefits from group membership such as feeling more confident, more in control, and freer to express feelings, but these data were based on retrospective accounts rather than longitudinal comparisons.

4.4 Discussion

The 12 studies reviewed here clustered into three areas – chronic mental illness, depression/anxiety, and bereavement – and our conclusions are therefore restricted to those areas. Overall, they provide limited but promising evidence that mutual help groups are beneficial for people with these types of problems. Seven of the 12 studies reported some positive changes in mental health for group members. The strongest findings come from two randomized studies showing that the outcomes of mutual help groups were equivalent to those of established, more costly, professionally provided psychological interventions. Five of the 12 studies found no differences in mental health outcomes between mutual help group members and non-members; no studies showed any evidence of negative effects. There was no indication that mutual help groups were beneficial for certain types of problems, but not others.

Despite the large and growing literature on mutual help groups only a handful of studies met our criteria for inclusion. Many studies that are frequently cited in the literature as providing evidence for the effectiveness of mutual help groups were excluded from our review because they did not fulfill the criteria concerning either characteristics of the group under study, outcome measures, or research design. Even those that met the criteria were of variable quality in terms of design and reporting of results.

4.4.1 Methodological Issues

We have tried in this review to take a middle line between two different methodological positions. On the one hand, traditional evidence-based medicine regards the randomized controlled trial (RCT) as the gold standard in research design. On the other hand, RCTs can be a poor methodological choice for evaluating mutual help groups if researchers operate the group themselves and take control of participation, in effect changing it from a peer-led to a professionally controlled intervention (Humphreys & Rappaport, 1994). Although RCTs are rare in the mutual help literature, our review included some good examples in which the autonomy of group members seemed to have been preserved. The review also included examples of carefully conducted quasi-experimental and longitudinal designs.

This review has been restricted to studies utilizing mental health outcome measures such as those common in professional treatment evaluations. Although important to study, such outcomes do not capture the full range of benefits of mutual help groups. Levy (2000) has argued that the outcomes important to group members may not be those that are assessed by symptom-oriented measures. First-person accounts, surveys, and qualitative studies have indicated that relevant outcomes include, for example, reduced isolation, increased confidence, changes in identity, and a sense of empowerment (Borkman, 1999; Munn-Giddings & Borkman, 2005; Rappaport, 1993). Although some of the studies in the current review found that participants reported such benefits, measurements of these variables were not incorporated into the longitudinal or quasi-experimental designs.

Another issue concerns the heterogeneity of the groups under study. Not only were there differences in target problems, but also differences in the nature of the groups. For example, some groups were set up as part of a research study whereas others were naturally occurring. These two types of groups likely differed on several dimensions (e.g., degree of structure and training of peer facilitators) although there were no apparent differences in outcome between them. Due to the small number of studies in the review and their heterogeneous nature, it was not possible to identify factors that could explain the variability in reported outcomes.

Finally, in any study aiming to demonstrate the effect of group membership, the definition of "membership" is problematic (Levy, 2000). This is particularly the case for naturally occurring groups, which may run over long periods of time with a fluctuating attendance at group meetings. Differences in attendance and level of participation may account for differences in outcome, a phenomenon analogous to the "dose-response" relationship in pharmacology. Several studies in the current review reported a correlation between higher levels of participation or involvement (operationalized in various ways) and positive outcomes (Caserta & Lund, 1993; Houston et al., 2002; Lieberman & Videka-Sherman, 1986; Magura et al., 2002). These findings are consistent with the hypothesis that greater involvement may lead to more positive change but they might also be taken to reflect differential attrition (i.e., the more severely troubled participants drop out). It is worth noting, however, that in a study of an alcohol-focused self-help group (Klaw et al., 2006), people with more serious problems were *more* rather than less likely to become long-term group members. Thus, selective attrition can lead to understatement as well as overstatement of the effects of mutual help groups.

4.4.2 Recommendations for Future Research

Many of the studies included in our review did not adequately report their results. Cell means and standard deviations were often absent making it impossible to calculate effect sizes (and therefore conduct a meta-analysis) and to estimate the clinical significance (as opposed to the statistical significance) of the findings. Information on the number of participants joining or declining and the pattern of attrition was also rarely provided. The CONSORT statement (Consolidated Standards of Reporting Trials), which has been widely disseminated (e.g., Moher, Schulz, & Altman, 2001), provides guidelines for the reporting of randomized trials. These can be adapted for research using other types of designs and we recommend that investigators consult them for guidance.

The characteristics of the groups being studied also need to be clearly described by investigators so that judgments can be made about whether these meet the definition of a mutual help group. This is particularly important because the terms "support group" and "self-help group" subsume a range of different types of groups. Published reports are sometimes disappointingly ambiguous about the degree to which putative mutual help groups are member-led and whether they are built around a structured self-help program (such as a cognitive-behavioral therapy package). In addition, empirical studies need to address a wider range of groups in terms of target problems. The studies in our review examined groups for three general problem areas: chronic mental illness, depression/anxiety, and bereavement. Further research is needed to evaluate the effectiveness of mutual help groups for other common mental health problems such as phobias and eating disorders.

Regarding outcome measures, we recommend that investigators include some standardized mental health outcome measures and, where possible, some assessment of costs. Although symptom reduction and cost-effectiveness are clearly not the only legitimate criteria of benefit, it is still important to assess this domain of outcomes if research findings in this field are to be used to inform public health and social policy decisions. In addition, investigators could draw on both the theoretical literature and qualitative studies to assess outcomes that have particular relevance to mutual help. For example, ratings of empowerment could be incorporated into a longitudinal or quasi-experimental design. When investigators have included such variables, they have tended to rely on participants' retrospective reports, which provide less convincing evidence.

With respect to research design, more studies should use longitudinal designs with comparison groups in order to provide more clearly interpretable data about the effectiveness of mutual help groups. Whether such studies are randomized should depend not on an a priori judgment but on the purpose of the study and whether randomization will or will not conflict with the peer control inherent in mutual help groups. Last, we note that whereas researchers often design studies of professional treatment "versus" mutual help groups, studies of combined forms would better match the reality that many individuals access both forms of help (Kessler et al., 1997).

In the current review, we have addressed the broad question of whether mutual help groups are "effective" for people suffering from mental health problems. Clearly, more fine-grained questions also need to be answered concerning who benefits (and who does not) and how any benefits or changes come about. The studies included in this review mostly concentrated on global outcome comparisons but some did examine potential mediating variables. One promising lead is the finding across several studies that individuals who make greater social links with other group members tend to benefit more. Future research is needed to examine this in more detail so that the possible causal processes can be disentangled.

Another promising direction is the examination of how group process variables, such as levels of self-disclosure and of giving and receiving help, relate to outcomes (Roberts et al., 1999). Research focusing on such process variables might take several forms including behavioral observations of the type conducted by Roberts et al. as well as in-depth qualitative studies investigating members' experiences of participation and change. Previous qualitative studies also point to possible mediating variables that could be incorporated into quantitative studies of effectiveness. For example, mutual help group members frequently describe a process of identity change (e.g., Rappaport, 1993; Solomon, Pistrang, & Barker, 2001).

Whether identity changes mediate changes in psychological symptoms is a question to be investigated in future research.

Davidson et al. (1999), in reviewing the effectiveness of mutual help for individuals with severe mental illness, observed that the literature showed "promising trends" but that "conclusions ... will remain tentative, however, until there are more systematic, prospective studies completed with comparison groups" (p. 171). Despite the increasing interest in mutual help groups, in particular the popularity of online groups, the picture has improved only marginally. There is clearly still a pressing need for high-quality outcome research evaluating mutual help groups for the full range of mental health problems. The outcome data from the studies we have reviewed here are promising but not definitive. We have traveled some distance along Humphreys and Rappaport's (1994) "one journey" toward a better understanding of the effectiveness of mutual help groups, but still have, in the words of Robert Frost, miles to go before we sleep.

References

Alcoholics Anonymous (1939). *The story of how many thousands of men and women have recovered from alcoholism*. New York: AA World Services.

Barker, C., & Pistrang, N. (2005). Quality criteria under methodological pluralism: Implications for doing and evaluating research. *American Journal of Community Psychology, 35*, 201–212.

Borkman, T. J. (1990). Experiential, professional, and lay frames of reference. In T.J. Powell (Ed.), *Working with self-help* (pp. 3–30). Silver Spring, MD: NASW Press.

Borkman, T. J. (1999). *Understanding self-help/mutual aid: Experiential learning in the commons*. New Brunswick, NJ: Rutgers University Press.

Burti, L., Amaddeo, F., Ambrosi, M., Bonetto, C., Cristofalo, D., Ruggeri, M., & Tansella, M. (2005). Does additional care provided by a consumer self-help group improve psychiatric outcome? A study in an Italian community-based psychiatric service. *Community Mental Health Journal, 41*, 705–720.

Bright, J. I., Baker, K. D., & Neimeyer, R. A. (1999). Professional and paraprofessional group treatments for depression: A comparison of cognitive-behavioral and mutual support interventions. *Journal of Consulting and Clinical Psychology, 67*, 491–501.

Caserta, M. S., & Lund, D. A. (1993). Intrapersonal resources and the effectiveness of self-help groups for bereaved older adults. *The Gerontologist, 33*, 619–629.

Cheung, S. -K., & Sun, S. Y. K. (2000). Effects of self-efficacy and social support on the mental health conditions of mutual-aid organization members. *Social Behavior and Personality, 28*, 413–422.

Chinman, M., Kloos, B., O'Connell, M., & Davidson, L. (2002). Service providers' views of psychiatric mutual support groups. *Journal of Community Psychology, 30*, 349–366.

Davidson, L. (2003). *Living outside mental illness: Qualitative studies of recovery in schizophrenia*. New York: New York University Press.

Davidson, L., Chinman, M., Kloos, B., Weingarten, R., Stayner, D., & Tebes, J. K. (1999). Peer support among individuals with severe mental illness: A review of the evidence. *Clinical Psychology: Science and Practice, 6*, 165–187.

Davison, K. P., Pennebaker, J. W., & Dickerson, S. S. (2000). Who talks? The social psychology of illness support groups. *American Psychologist, 55*, 205–217.

den Boer, P. C. A. M., Wiersma, D., & van den Bosch, R. J. (2004). Why is self-help neglected in the treatment of emotional disorders? A meta-analysis. *Psychological Medicine, 34*, 971.

Dunham, P. J., Hurshman, A., Litwin, E., Gusella, J., Ellsworth, C., & Dodd, P. W. D. (1998). Computer-mediated social support: single young mothers as a model system. *American Journal of Community Psychology, 26*, 281–306.

Eysenbach, G., Powell, J., Englesakis, M., Rizo, C., & Stern, A. (2004). Health related virtual communities and electronic support groups: Systematic review of the effects of online peer to peer interaction. *British Medical Journal, 328*, 1166–1170.

Galanter, M. (1988). Zealous self-help groups as adjuncts to psychiatric treatment: A study of Recovery, Inc. *American Journal of Psychiatry, 145*, 1248–1253.

Goldstrom, I. D., Campbell, J., Rogers, J. A., Lambert, D. B., Blacklow, B., Henderson, M. J., & Manderscheid, R. W. (2006). National estimates for mental health mutual support groups, self-help organizations, and consumer-operated services. *Administration and Policy in Mental Health and Mental Health Services Research, 33*, 92–103.

Gottlieb B. H., & Peters, L.A. (1991).A national demographic portrait of mutual aid participants in Canada. *American Journal of Community Psychology, 19*, 651–666.

Helgeson, V. S., & Gottlieb, B. H. (2000). Support groups. In S. Cohen, L. G. Underwood, & B. H. Gottlieb (Eds.), *Social support measurement, and intervention: A guide for health and social scientists* (pp. 221–245). New York: Oxford University Press.

Hogan, B. E., Linden, B. E., & Najarian, B. (2002). Social support interventions: Do they work? *Clinical Psychology Review, 22*, 381–440.

Houston, T. K., Cooper, L. A., & Ford, D. E. (2002). Internet support groups for depression: A 1-year prospective cohort study. *American Journal of Psychiatry, 159*, 2062–2068.

Humphreys, K. (2000). Community narratives and personal stories in Alcoholics Anonymous. *Journal of Community Psychology, 28*, 495–506.

Humphreys, K. (2004). *Circles of recovery: Self-help organizations for addictions*. Cambridge: Cambridge University Press.

Humphreys, K., Phibbs, C. S., & Moos, R. H. (1996). Addressing self-selection effects in evaluations of mutual help groups and professional mental health services: An introduction to two-stage sample selection models. *Evaluation and Program Planning, 19*, 301–308.

Humphreys, K., & Rappaport, J. (1994). Researching self-help/mutual aid groups and organizations: Many roads, one journey. *Applied and Preventive Psychology, 3*, 217–231.

Jacobs, M. K. & Goodman, G. (1989). Psychology and self-help groups: Predictions on a partnership. *American Psychologist, 44*, 536–545.

Kessler, R. C., Mickelson, K. D., & Zhao, S. (1997). Patterns and correlates of self-help group membership in the United States. *Social Policy, 27*, 27–46.

Klaw, E., Horst, D., & Humphreys, K. (2006). Inquirers, triers, and buyers of an alcohol harm reduction self-help organization. *Addiction Research and Theory, 14*, 527–535.

Kropotkin, P. (1902). *Mutual aid: A factor of evolution*. Boston, MA: Reprinted by Extending Horizon Books.

Kyrouz, E. M., Humphreys, K., & Loomis, C. (2002). A review of research on the effectiveness of self-help mutual aid groups. In B. J. White & E. J. Madara (Eds.), *American self-help clearinghouse self-help group sourcebook* (7th ed., pp. 71–85). Cedar Knolls, NJ: American Self-Help Group Clearinghouse.

Levy, L. H. (2000). Self-help groups. In J. Rappaport & E. Seidman (Eds.), *Handbook of community psychology* (pp. 591–613). New York: Kluwer.

Lewis, G., Anderson, L., Araya, R., Elgie, R., Harrison, G., Proudfoot, J., Schmidt, U., Sharp, D., Weightman, A., & Williams, C. (2003). *Self-help interventions for mental health problems*. London: Report to the Department of Health R&D programme.

Lieberman, M. A., & Videka-Sherman, L. (1986). The impact of self-help groups on the mental health of widows and widowers. *American Journal of Orthopsychiatry, 56*, 435–449.

Magura, S., Laudet, A. B., Mahmood, D., Rosenblum, A., & Knight, E. (2002). Adherence to medication regimens and participation in dual-focus self-help groups. *Psychiatric Services, 53*, 310–316.

Marmar, C. R., Horowitz, M. J., Weiss, D. S., Wilner, N. R., & Kaltreider, N. B. (1988). A controlled trial of brief psychotherapy and mutual-help group treatment of conjugal bereavement. *American Journal of Psychiatry, 145*, 203–209.

Moher, D., Schulz, K. F., & Altman, D. G. (2001). The CONSORT statement: revised recommendations for improving the quality of reports of parallel-group randomized trials. *Journal of the American Medical Association, 285*, 1987–1991.

Munn-Giddings, C., & Borkman, T. (2005). Self help/mutual aid as a psychosocial phenomenon. In S. Ramon & J. E. Williams (Eds.), *Mental health at the crossroads. The promise of the psychosocial approach.* Aldershot: Ashgate Publishing.

Pistrang, N., Barker, C., & Humphreys, K. (2008). Mutual help groups for mental health problems: A review of effectiveness studies. *American Journal of Community Psychology, 42*, 110–121.

Powell, T. J., Hill, E. M., Warner, L., Yeaton, W. H., & Silk, K. R. (2000). Encouraging people with mood disorders to attend a self-help group. *Journal of Applied Social Psychology, 30*, 2270–2288.

Powell, T. J., Yeaton, W. H., Hill, E. M., & Silk, K. R. (2001). Predictors of psychosocial outcomes for patients with mood disorders: The effects of self-help group participation. *Psychiatric Rehabilitation Journal, 25*, 3–11.

Rappaport, J. (1993). Narrative studies, personal stories, and identity transformation in the mutual help context. *Journal of Applied Behavioral Science, 29*, 239–256.

Rathner, G., Bönsch, C., Maurer, G., Walter, M. H., & Söllner, W. (1993). The impact of a "guided self-help group" on bulimic women: a prospective 15 month study of attenders and non-attenders. *Journal of Psychosomatic Research, 37*, 389–396.

Roberts, L. J., Salem, D. A., Rappaport, J., Toro, P. A., Luke, D. A., & Seidman, E. (1999). Giving and receiving help: Interpersonal transactions in mutual-help meetings and psychosocial adjustment of members. *American Journal of Community Psychology, 27*, 841–868.

Schäfer, A., Meyer, F., Matzat, J., Knickenberg, R. J., Bleichner, F., Merkle, W., et al. (2005). Utilization of and experience with self-help groups among patients with mental disorders in Germany. *International Journal of Self Help and Self Care, 4*, 5–19.

Segal, S. P., & Silverman, C. (2002). Determinants of client outcomes in self-help agencies. *Psychiatric Services, 53*, 304–309.

Solomon, M., Pistrang, N., & Barker, C. (2001). The benefits of mutual support groups for parents of children with disabilities. *American Journal of Community Psychology, 29*, 113–132.

Trojan, A. (1989). Benefits of self-help groups: a survey of 232 members from 65 disease related groups. *Social Science and Medicine, 29*, 225–232.

Tudiver, F., Hilditch, J., Permaul, J. A., & McKendree, D. J. (1992). Does mutual help facilitate newly bereaved widowers? Report of a randomized controlled trial. *Evaluation and the Health Professions, 15*, 147–162.

Vachon, M. L. S., Lyall, W. A. L., Rogers, J., Freeman-Letofsky, K., & Freeman, S. J. J. (1980). A controlled study of self-help intervention for widows. *American Journal of Psychiatry, 137*, 1380–1384.

Videka-Sherman, L., & Lieberman, M. A. (1985). The effects of self-help and psychotherapy intervention on child loss. *American Journal of Orthopsychiatry, 55*, 70–82.

Ybarra, M. L. & Eaton, W. W. (2005). Internet-based mental health interventions. *Mental Health Services Research, 7*, 75–87.

Chapter 5
Online Self-Help/Mutual Aid Groups in Mental Health Practice

J. Finn and T. Steele

Abstract An ever-expanding number of online self-help mutual aid groups are available to provide information and support over the Internet for a wide variety of social and mental health issues. They offer advantages to consumers since they are not bound to time, place, or social presence. Research supports their benefits in areas of health, mental health, addictions, stigmatized identities, trauma and violence recovery, and grief support. Harm may also come from participation in these groups due to disinhibited communication, privacy concerns, and misinformation. Mental health practitioners need to be knowledgeable about these groups as both sources of additional support and potential stressors for consumers. Future development of online support through social networking sites and virtual communities will become new resources for consumers.

5.1 Online Self-Help /Mutual Aid Groups in Mental Health Practice

Today, a wide variety of online groups and communities focus on almost every aspect of social life, including political and religious organization, recreation and hobbies, arts and culture, health, romance, and self-help/mutual aid. The focus of this chapter is on online self-help/mutual aid groups (OSHMAGs). We define OSHMAGs, describe their extent of use and common characteristics, present the advantages and disadvantages of OSHMAGs, discuss their implications for mental health practitioners, and present potential future directions for development of online support.

OSHMAGs are defined as groups that meet via the Internet, whose purpose is to provide information, support, and mutual aid to its members about a specific area

---

J. Finn (✉)
Social Work Program, University of Washington, Tacoma, WA, USA
e-mail: finnj@u.washington.edu

of personal concern. Although there are several different ways in which members of OSHMAGs communicate with each other, such as voice over Internet protocol (VoIP), voice and video chat, as well as Virtual Reality (VR) settings, this chapter's primary focus is on OSHMAGs which use text-based Computer Mediated Communication (CMC). Text-based OSHMAGs meet either in synchronous (simultaneous interaction, e.g., chat-based) or asynchronous (delayed interaction, e.g., email-based) mode. The vast majority of OSHMAGs are email-based (Meier, 2004) and use a Usenet model in which members access a Web site to post and read messages. Other groups function through a Listserv, in which members subscribe to a "list" and then receive all emails posted to the group.

It is also important to note that for the purposes of this chapter, we refer to interaction between individuals who are physically present in the same tangible location as "physical space." Although not applicable to the discussion of text-based OSHMAGs, the term "face-to-face" (FtF) implies the ability to gain information for facial and other nonverbal expressions; new technology research is emerging that shows that although there are differences, live video chat can also considered FtF (Anderson & Rainie, 2006; Bos, Gergle, Olson, & Olson, 2001).

5.1.1 Extent of Use of OSHMAGs

Self-help groups have been described as an essential human resource and a permanent social utility (Katz, 1992). Barak, Boniel-Nissim, and Suler (2008) note that OSHMAGs have become a mass social phenomenon that is estimated to number hundreds of thousands of groups worldwide. There is no comprehensive directory of online support groups and there are a variety of ways to access groups. A 2001 PEW survey found that 84% of Internet users had contacted an online group (Horrigan, 2001). Although, information changes at a rapid pace on the Internet and the number and type of OSHMAGs is proliferating rapidly through a variety of formats, the following provides some idea of what is available. Google groups (www.groups.google.com) lists approximately 1300 OSHMAGs, with 500 in the Health subarea and 800 in other subareas. Similarly, Yahoo Groups (www.Yahoo.dir.group.yahoo.com) lists almost 18,000 OSHMAGs in the "diseases and conditions" subsection, almost 5,000 groups in the "addictions and recovery" subsection and over 1,000 groups in "abuse survivors." OSHMAGs can also be found using *Harley Hahn's Master List of Usenet Groups* (http://www.harley.com/usenet/) in which support groups are located in the health subsection. For example, a search on "Depression" found 14 groups related to depression support. *PsychCentral* (http://forums.psychcentral.com/) offers mental health-related OSHMAGs called "forums" that are moderated by professionals or highly experienced group members. In December, 2008, the Depression forum on *PsychCentral* reported almost 65,000 postings. Groups that function through a Listserv can be found at *L Soft List Search* (http://www.listserv.net/lists/list_q.html). A 2008 search for "Support Group" found 99 mental health listservs covering a wide variety of health and mental health issues.

5.1.2 Characteristics of OSHMAGs

There is an OSHMAG for almost every imaginable issue for which people seek support. These include several types of OSHMAGs: personal change (e.g., addictions and weight loss), "friends of" (e.g., spouses of sexual abuse survivors and non-offending parent(s) of sexually abused children), medical condition support (e.g., cancer survivors and diabetes), and "stigmatized identity" (e.g., non-conforming gender identity and sexual orientation). Table 5.1 summarizes characteristics of OSHMAGs. Even though OSHMAGs meet primarily online, group dynamics are both similar to and different from groups that meet in physical space (Maloney-Krichmar & Preece, 2002). In general, their goals are very similar, (Barak et al., 2008). They are based on principles of empowerment, inclusion, nonhierarchical decision making, shared responsibility, and a holistic approach to people's cultural, economic, and social needs. The values of these groups include cooperative self-organization, non-bureaucratic mutual helping methods, and social support (Segal, Silverman, & Temkin, 1993). Members are viewed as having much to contribute to the helping of others as well as themselves. They differ primarily in lack of physical space contact, use of written rather than verbal exchange, and in the size of membership, with some OSHMAGs having hundreds and even thousands of participating members.

Table 5.1 A comparison of In-Person and Online mutual aid/self-help groups

Characteristic	Physical space group	OSHMAG
Purpose	Self-help/mutual aid through empathy, problem solving, self-disclosure, universality, multiple models, and empowerment.	Self-help/mutual aid through empathy, problem solving, self-disclosure, universality, multiple models, and empowerment.
Access	Limited to specific time and place. Limited access for those with communication, transportation, speech and hearing difficulties and care-giving responsibilities. High anxiety for those with interpersonal difficulties.	Asynchronous groups meet any time from any location with computer and Internet access. No barriers related to speech or hearing. Lower anxiety for those with interpersonal difficulties. Chat-based groups may be limited to a specific time or may be open whenever two or more people wish to chat.
Leadership	Nonprofessional leadership from members. May have professional adviser.	Nonprofessional leadership from members. May have professional adviser. Leader may prevent some comments from being posted.
Membership	Relatively small number from local geographic area. High similarity among members.	Diverse membership from global community. May range from a small number to several thousand members.

Table 5.1 (continued)

Characteristic	Physical space group	OSHMAG
Boundary	Generally open to all interested people. May be open-ended or time-limited. Members may know each other outside of group.	Generally open to all interested people. May be open-ended or time-limited. Few members will know each other outside of group.
Communication	Face-to-face, synchronous. Social status norms related to age, race, sex, income may influence and constrain member behavior. All participants' communications are observed.	Asynchronous or synchronous depending on method of online communication. Anonymous communication lowers social status differences and increases self-disclosure, adherence to group norms and hyperpersonal communication. A person may "participate" by reading messages but not contributing to the group (lurk).
Information exchange	Resource, experience sharing – verbally or print.	Digital: resource, experience sharing via multimedia e.g., text, hyperlinks, digital pictures, video, music.
Misinformation	Group members immediately challenge misinformation.	Members challenge misinformation, but correction may take longer due to asynchronous format. Misinformation may remain in the group as long as the message remains posted online.
Privacy	Group norms focus on privacy and confidentiality. Physical identity is known. There is no transcript of communications.	Group norms focus on privacy and confidentiality. Physical identity is not known. A written record of a person's exact words is maintained and could be forwarded to others.

The majority of OSHMAGs are informal with leadership based on experience and expertise with the group rather than on formal education and training. Many informal groups, in fact, have no designated leader. Membership is not fee based, and the group is started and maintained by individuals seeking support (see, for example, groups at http://yahoo.groups.com). Some OSHMAGs, however, are formally supported by an organization and charge a fee for participation. For example, a health organization may sponsor moderated discussion groups on their Web site (e.g., Group Health Cooperative) that are staffed by mental health professionals (Ralston et al., 2007). In addition, some OSHMAGs are part of an Internet Service Provider (ISP) and the groups are only available to those who subscribe to that ISP (for example, groups at www.aol.com), or groups can be provided by an Internet Content Host (ICH) which charges a membership fee to access a Web site with a single OSHMAG topic (e.g., weight loss). Informal organizations also have different netiquette (communication rules) than formal OSHMAGs, whose sponsoring organization sets the rules that the group members must follow. Participation in informal OSHMAGs is governed by the will of the group; if an individual is not following proper netiquette they can be made "invisible" (they may be able to contribute, but what they contribute is not visible) by other members or they can be banned, by members contacting the ICH, with a formal request and evidence of inappropriate behavior. While there are philosophical and structural similarities between physical space and OSHMAGs, as is discussed below, OSHMAGs also differ from physical space groups in ways that are both therapeutic and potentially harmful.

It should be noted that self-help groups, whether meeting online or in physical space, differ substantially from a therapy group, although a support group may provide many therapeutic processes (Barak et al., 2008). Several core differences are noted. First, unlike a therapy group, self-help groups often have no pre-planned, targeted treatment protocol that is conducted or delivered. Second, the purpose of support groups is primarily to offer relief, improved feelings, and social support. Third, support groups may operate without a leader or manager, whereas therapy groups always have trained professionals who lead them. Fourth, a support group is usually an open forum in which participants can join or leave at anytime, whereas a therapy group is seldom open. Fifth, support groups typically last without specific time limits, whereas therapy groups are usually time-limited. While therapy and self-help groups differ in structure and intent, there are many similarities in providing conditions that have been shown to be therapeutic, as discussed below.

5.1.3 Advantages and Benefits of OSHMAGs

OSHMAGs use therapeutic principles found in physical space self-help groups. Both types of groups provide assistance to members through a variety of helping mechanisms that include the following: empathy; a sense of universality; mutual problem solving; modeling; sharing information, ideas, facts, and resources; engaging in dialogue to reveal multiple perspectives; discussing "taboo" subjects; experiencing mutual support; overcoming alienation and isolation; engaging in catharsis; taking on the role of helper; developing inspiration and hope; and developing social networks. (Archibald, 2007; Lieberman, 1976; Yalom, 1985).

The theoretical and practical advantages of OSHMAGs for providing help and support have been examined (Barak et al., 2008; Ferguson, 1996; Finn & Lavitt, 1994). An OSHMAG can provide support for members when physical space groups are not available or in conjunction with a formal group that meets in physical space. Participation barriers related to time and distance are nearly eliminated. These advantages are especially important to those whose work schedule, illness, disability, care-giving responsibilities, or geographic isolation makes it difficult or impossible to attend a physical space group. In addition, OSHMAGs offer a greater degree of anonymity than physical space groups. Using pseudonyms, members may choose to communicate without cues related to age, sex, race, and physical appearance. For many members with severe physical or mental disabilities this is a tremendously empowering experience (Barak et al., 2008; Braithwaite, Waldron & Finn, 1999).

The nature of relatively anonymous and asynchronous communication creates conditions that intensify both the benefits and potential harm on OSHMAGs. Walther (1997) describes *hyperpersonal* or *disinhibited* interaction in online groups in which online communication intensifies characteristics of "normal" interaction and tends to be viewed as highly desirable by participants. Hyperpersonal communication develops in part because of the limited nonverbal, historical, and contextual information available in mediated contexts. In this environment, message senders are able to carefully manage the presentation of self. Lacking an external reality against which perceptions might be checked, message recipients can develop idealized perceptions of their fellow members. The asynchronous nature of mediated communication and the limited cues available (primarily the often carefully crafted written messages of fellow members) can create a kind of feedback loop that intensifies and magnifies the interpersonal experiences of participants. As a result, when compared to physical space support, mediated support may be more focused and emotionally intense. Group identity and members' sense of obligation may be heightened. Relationships may become intimate more quickly (Kurtz, 1997). Thus hyperpersonal communication may result in OSHMAGs with greater self-disclosure, higher empathy, higher cohesion, and stronger peer pressure for change. These are characteristics associated with effective support groups.

Anonymity allows some members, especially in groups dealing with stigmatized issues such as disfiguring or contagious medical conditions, sexual orientation, and mental illness to more easily and safely begin to explore sensitive issues and find support for a positive self-identity. Members of OSHMAGs report that they are more likely to engage in self-disclosure than in physical space groups, a condition associated with therapeutic processes (Kummervold et al., 2002). In addition, research suggests that when members participate from the privacy of their homes rather than in a physical space setting, they are likely to be more open and receptive to altering their habitual biases and stereotypes when interacting with diverse groups (McKenna, Green & Gleason, 2002).

Additionally, members with physical communication disabilities, interpersonal difficulties, or social anxiety find sharing information in a written, anonymous form a safe way to begin to explore personal issues and are more likely to engage on an equal footing in online groups (McKenna & Seidman, 2005). The use of journals, stories, and poetry, often found on OSHMAGs, has been an effective tool for promoting self-awareness, self-esteem, and recovery (Dinsmore, 1991). The asynchronous nature of some OSHMAGs allows members to develop and respond to messages at their own speed and to send coherent and complete personal communications. For persons with disabilities who experience partial or complete loss of the ability to communicate orally, who have difficulty with auditory functions, and individuals with learning disabilities (e.g., dyslexia), the computer functions as an adaptive tool; programs can read text aloud or transform spoken words in to text.

The use of adaptive technology, in a group setting, provides a platform of inclusion and can provide an empowering experience (Nelson, 1995).

OSHMAGs' lack of distance barriers creates the possibility for a greater number of participants to contribute information and share perspectives drawn from a worldwide community. The large number of members may help to promote a sense of universality that decreases feelings of alienation. The group, then, becomes a communal, safe, and non-judgmental virtual location for individuals who may feel isolated and different (Wright & Bell, 2003). As with physical space groups, discussion among members of an OSHMAG relates to the whole person and is not limited to seeking or giving support for the topic of the OSHMAG. Kristen Eichhorn's research of posts on OSHMAG for eating disorders found that 44.2% were not explicitly giving support and 46.1% were not explicitly seeking support (Eichhorn, 2008). Issues of family, relationships, work, and recreation related to a person's broader life were also discussed. Finally, online groups also provide a learning opportunity for new members, friends, relatives, and professionals. A person may "lurk" (read messages but not participate in the discussion) in order to assess the group interaction, learn the group culture, and vicariously participate. For participants, lurking, in some cases, has led to eventual participation in the group and/or to seeking physical space services (Finn and Lavitt, 1994). "Lurking," however, has its negative connotations in some OSHMAGs since it can be taken as someone's attempt to "spy" on the group (Marvin, 1995). A practitioner or researcher who lurks must take precautions to avoid being intrusive or disturbing the group process and must be aware of ethical standards related to informed consent (O'Boyle, 2002; Riegelsberger, Sasse, & McCarthy, 2003).

Finally, OSHMAGs have a growing body of empirical research that supports positive outcomes for participants. Empirical research has documented that OSHMAGs offer support related to a wide variety of specific issues such as siblings of children with special needs (Tichon & Shapiro, 2003), adults with ovarian or prostate cancer (Sullivan, 2003), those with multiple sclerosis (Weis et al., 2003), child care (Worotynec, 2000), diabetes (van Dam et al., 2005), breast cancer (Radin, 2006), food allergy (Coulson & Knibb, 2007), hysterectomy (Bunde, Suls, Martin, & Barnett, 2007), women in midlife transition dealing with menopause (Bresnahan & Murray-Johnson, 2002), and multiple sclerosis (Weis et al., 2003), among others. A number of outcome studies have documented that OSHMAGs are beneficial to members (Barak et al., 2008; Braithwaite et al., 1999, Finn & Lavitt, 1994). For example, Kernsmith and Kernsmith (2008) found that a group for recovering sex offenders showed improvement based on changes in the number of fantasies or cognitive distortions present in the posts over time. Murray and Fox (2006) found that the majority of respondents in a self-harm OSHMAG viewed the discussion group as having positive effects, with many respondents reducing the frequency and severity of their self-harming behavior as a consequence of group membership. Barak & Dolev-Cohen's (2006) study of an OSHMAG for suicidal and severely distressed adolescents found that although the level of participants' distress did not change over time, on the average, it was significantly correlated with activity level, with a higher the number of posts and replies associated with lower levels of distress. Eysenbach, Powell, Englesakis, Ruizo and Stern (2004) in their review of OSHMAGs in the health and mental health areas, however, found little support for the effectiveness of OSHMAGs and concluded that very few studies assessed the outcomes of peer-to-peer communities. Based on a limited sample of six studies, they concluded that most studies did not show change in measures of depression or social support nor was there evidence to support concerns over virtual communities harming people. Further research is needed to document the impact of OSHMAGs on behavior change, social support, self-esteem, mental health, and life satisfaction.

5.1.4 Disadvantages and Potential Harm of OSHMAGs

Research has also identified potential disadvantages of OSHMAGs. Little is known about the extent to which members experience harm through negative, hostile, or malicious encounters. It has been found that in some instances online communication is disinhibited or hyperpersonal since members are anonymous and do not experience the social cues that normally constrain behavior (Spears, Postmes, Lea & Wolbert, 2002; Suler, 2004; Walther, 1997). Communication may include a "flame" in which a member castigates, curses, and personally attacks another member. Some groups are monitored and some have ground rules about the type of interactions permitted, and some groups have a moderator who screens messages before they are posted; however, many groups do not.

Participation in an OSHMAG may open a person to online or real-world harassment. Private information is available through online background databases or simply may be on public records searchable through the Internet, allowing someone to acquire personal information simply by knowing a person's legal name. (Tavani & Grodzinsky, 2002). Because OSHMAGs' members share personal feelings and information about their lives, OSHMAGs' members must be vigilant about not posting or sharing personal information, especially not a legal name. OSHMAGs with moderators tend to monitor for personal or identifying information and may delete such messages (Ralston et al., 2007). Cyber-harassment, such as unwanted contact through email, chat, or text messages, or someone posting personal information on other OSHMAGs can also lead to the phone calls or to stalking and harassment in physical space. Cyber-harassment may produce feelings of lack of control, humiliation, or degradation as well as anxiety and depression in some people from not knowing who or when someone might contact them (Southworth, Finn, Dawson, Fraser & Tucker, 2007). Cyber-harassment is illegal, though many times it is difficult to prosecute because the perpetrators are usually anonymous or known only by their nickname. Harm may also come to members because OSHMAGs are vulnerable to "cyber-terrorism" (Finn & Banach, 2000). The majority of OSHMAGs are not moderated so anyone can post a message. If one (or several) members join the group and then post racist and sexist messages, for example, the rest of the group may start arguing with the poster(s), and thus lose track of the original purpose of the group. Eventually, members leave the group because it no longer meets their needs. Waldron, Lavitt, and Kelley (2000) described two online self-help groups for people with emotional issues and sexual abuse recovery that disbanded as a result of receiving a barrage of sexually explicit advertising and messages.

While not as malicious as cyber-terrorism, *Munchausen by Internet* (i.e., help seeking for imaginary or made-up problems to gain attention) may also disrupt group process. Feldman (2000) describes scenarios in which a person may use an OSHMAG to obtain reinforcement and sympathy for a fictitious illness. Feldman believes that these members have a negative impact on other OSHMAG members by creating a division between those who believe the tale and those who do not, possibly resulting in having some members leave the group. In addition, the interaction may distract the group from its purpose by forcing it to focus on the poser.

Misinformation is another potential disadvantage of online groups. Members may receive misinformation and not have it corrected by other members until a later date due to the time delay in asynchronous communications. The limited research in this area has found that instances of misinformation do occur, although other group members generally correct them (Finn & Lavitt, 1994). Misinformation can be especially harmful when it is purposefully provided. Similar to cyber-terrorism, one way this occurs is when a "member" posts a message that includes a link to a Web site. The Web site may at first appear to be a resource, but on closer inspection is filled with misinformation, hostile rhetoric, or pornography. While such tactics are merely an annoyance to some members, they can be extremely disturbing to those already in emotional distress. It is important to note, however, that research suggests that in most cases the information provided by lay people in online support groups is not erroneous or harmful (Hwang et al., 2007).

Internationally, both popular Internet and print media attempt to warn consumers about the potential danger and harm of OSHMAGs. For example, Dr Miriam Stoppard, M.D, D.Sc, FRCP, DCL (2008), who blogs for The Mirror, a popular tabloid in the United Kingdom, posted a piece titled *How Safe Are Internet Health Forums*? in which she discusses the vulnerability of consumers when they are seeking information or help through an OSHMAG. Divya Vasisht (2003), a journalist with The Times of India, published a piece titled, *E-medicine Is Just What the Doctor Didn't Order*, in which she discusses the fact that consumers are using their computer mouse before they see their doctor and at times instead of seeing a doctor. In an article published by Reader's Digest (2006), *Thrills That Kill: Kids Are Taking Risks in Dangerous New Ways*, Mary Fischer tells the stories and gives warnings about OSHMAGs encouraging dangerous behaviors.

Finally, researchers have also raised concerns that Internet use may be "addictive" (Young, 1998), psychologically harmful, or may take time away from other more personal forms of social contact (Lebow, 1998; Turkle, 1995). A longitudinal study of families who were given computers and Internet access suggested that greater Internet use was associated with declines in communication with other family members, declines in the size of one's social circle, and increases in depression and loneliness (Kraut et al, 2002). The authors hypothesized that the results are due to substitution of higher quality primary relationships for more superficial ties. The study focused primarily on the use of email and the Web, and did not address a population that chose to use online support groups. More recent studies, however, failed to replicate these results, finding that Internet use was generally associated with positive effects on communication, social involvement, and well-being (Howard et al., 2001; Kraut et al., 2002; Moody, 2001). Further research is needed to document the extent to which participation in OSHMAGs' supplements or substitutes for physical space relationships.

5.1.5 Extreme Communities

Some online groups or "extreme communities" (Bell, 2007) provide a forum for those who hold views that support members in attitudes and behavior that may be considered harmful by the professional community. For example, pro-anorexia ("pro-ana") or pro-bulimia ("pro-mia") OSHMAGs were found to promote anorexia or bulimia as a "lifestyle choice" rather than a psychological disorder and to normalize participants' thoughts and behaviors through the sharing of a secret identity and the creation of a cohesive group. Group members may share ultra-thin pictures of themselves or celebrities as well as tips about diet drugs and how to avoid parental or medical controls over their eating behavior (Davies & Lipsey, 2003; Gavin, Rodham, & Poyer, 2008; Tierney, 2006). Similarly, Bell et al. (2006) found a social network of a likely psychotic group of individuals who formed a cohesive online community. In this case, the OSHMAG is used to collectively gather and reference online material in support of their beliefs. Participants may reject any medical explanation of their illness; rather, they argue that they are better off with the destructive behavior or some even claim that their condition is caused by external forces such as technology "thought control weapons." Similarly, some pro-cutting OSHMAGs see self-mutilation as a legitimate method for release of pain.

Some extreme communities promote behavior that may further damage physical health or mental health; other sites promote suicide as one legitimate option among many possible personal choices. Concern has been raised about groups that promote suicide or provide a venue for individuals who do not wish to die alone. Groups may encourage passive individuals to take their own lives through group conformity effects (Rajagopal, 2004) and may provide information on effective methods that may lead to an increase in completed suicides (Becker & Schmidt., 2004; Prior, 2004). Biddle et al. (2008) found that "pro-suicide" was at the top of search results, meaning they have high viewership. [Pro-suicide "extreme sites" should not be confused with advocates of "death with dignity" for terminally ill individuals (www.deathwithdignity.org/)]. Alao et al. (2006) found that "pro-suicide" groups may actively discourage individuals to seek psychiatric help. Additionally, pro-drug OSHMAGs discuss ways of obtaining and using both illegal and legal drugs (Murguía, Tackett-Gibson, & Lessem, 2007). Groups that support behaviors related to eating disorders, suicide, and drug use share many aspects of OSHMAGs since these groups meet online and members develop a sense of "community," engage in mutual support and problems solving, and create norms that support group goals.

Several countries, including Great Britain and Australia, have enacted laws aimed at restricting OSHMAGs that advocate for members to harm themselves or others. In addition, laws prevent groups from distributing illegal material. Examples of OSHMAGs that could be considered illegal are those that advocate for suicide, hate and violence, drugs and illegal medical advice, pedophilia, and sex slavery. Internet laws in the United States vary from state to state. These laws differ from Internet filtering done by China, Japan, and North Korea, which restricts access to sites. Rather, these laws target ISP or ICH owners of the technology and hardware where OSHMAGs' data and software is stored. Under some circumstances prosecution of members or those who start the OSHMAGs is allowed (Biddle, Donovan, Hawton, Kapur, & Gunnell, 2008; Loundy, n.d.).

Groups that offer support in recovery for issues in the same arena as "extreme sites" must be careful to differentiate themselves from the extreme sites. For example, pro-ana OSHMAGs support the actions of individuals to continue their anorexic behavior, whereas a recovery-based OSHMAGs give support to individuals who wish discontinue anorexic behavior. The use of "pro" is best understood as supporting the option to engage in the behavior versus "pro-recovery" as supporting the *individual* to stop self-harming behavior. A clear distinction between these groups is difficult based on their name alone. Education is needed for both mental health professionals and consumers about the nature of these groups.

5.1.6 Mental Health Practitioners and OSHMAGs

Given the growing number of consumers who use the Internet for health and mental health-related information and the extensive use of OSHMAGs, it is imperative that mental health practitioners become familiar with these resources. Table 5.2 outlines

Table 5.2 Checklist for mental health practitioners

☑ As part of the assessment process for all clients, ask about online activities including OSHMAGs, chat rooms, blogs, and social networking sites. Evaluate the usefulness and appropriateness of these resources.
☑ Search for groups using trusted sources such as psychcentral.com, International Society for Mental Health Online (ISHMO.org), or recommendations from colleagues and your personal experience.
☑ Determine the purpose and membership requirements of the group.
☑ Visit the group and read a sample of messages to understand the language, culture and focus of the group.
☑ Determine whether the group is moderated or not. Explain the difference to consumers.
☑ Determine the extent to which the group is anonymous.
☑ Discuss with consumers possible negative aspects of groups such as disinhibited communication, privacy concerns, and misinformation.
☑ Review basic "netiquette" with consumers.
☑ Explain a specific group's norms e.g., using a warning and blank space before "triggering" material is presented.
☑ As part of treatment, ask about any positive or negative experiences encountered in online groups.

a checklist that mental health practitioners might consider when connecting people to online groups. A fundamental decision is whether to refer consumers to an OSHMAG. The research supports OSHMAGs as a valuable means of increasing people's general well-being and social support, but is less clear about OSHMAGs' value in producing specific therapeutic change (Barak et al., 2008). Barak et al argue that OSHMAGs are not a substitute for therapy but rather a supplement to traditional treatment. This may be done prior to treatment as part of wait-list support, during treatment as a supplement to concurrent services, and/or following treatment as supportive follow-up services (Finn, 1995). The evidence is also clear, however, that OSHMAGs may include harmful interactions and misinformation. Referral to an OSHMAG must be predicated on insuring that a consumer is well informed about the benefits and potential harm in OSHMAGs and upon a practitioner's thorough understanding of the quality of the information and interactions of the specific OSHMAG to which a referral is made. This requires that practitioners understand the culture of online communities in general. Practitioners should investigate a specific group before a referral is made; this can be accomplished by personally observing the specific group, asking other colleagues for suggestions, or using a trusted OSHMAG directory. For example, Psychcentral (http://psychcentral.com/resources/) provides links to many online resources, including OSHMAGs. Additionally, they must be similarly knowledgeable about OSHMAGs in order to advise a consumer *not* to participate in an OSHMAG when necessary. Mental health professionals must support the development of information sites that describe and evaluate the purpose of OSHMAGs related to mental health issues.

OSHMAG users may become material that is discussed in physical space sessions since it is increasingly likely that a practitioner will encounter consumers who participate in OSHMAGs and bring their online experiences to treatment. This may include challenges to authority when a consumer finds information or advice in OSHMAGs that contradicts a practitioner's diagnosis or treatment plan. Consumers may also bring negative or painful interactions in OSHMAGs for discussion in therapy sessions. They may develop relationships in online groups that negatively impact marital and family relationships. OSHMAG participants may seek a practitioner's advice about whether to join or continue in an OSHMAG. Dealing with these issues requires that practitioners relate to issues concerning online communities.

Leadership is another important issue for mental health practitioners to consider. Most OSHMAGs are not led or moderated by mental health professionals. A minority of OSHMAGs do, however, provide professional input. Given the shortage of mental health services and trained group workers, practitioners and mental health organizations may want to consider development of partnerships with OSHMAGs in order to provide moderated, safe, and professionally informed online communities.

There is very little formal education about online practice in the curriculum of educational programs for mental health professionals (Murphy, McFadden, & Mitchell, 2008; Finn, 2002). In order to stay current with the online experiences of consumers, mental health professionals must be aware of the strengths and limitations of OSHMAGs and be influential in the development and shaping of the targets, applications, and evaluation of these new services. Professionals must also, however, be aware that OSHMAGs are consumer-driven and members may view input by professionals as disempowering and unwanted if presented in a way that violates group norms (Brown, Shepherd, Wituk, & Meissen (2007). In addition, mental health professional education can help form students' attitudes about OSHMAGs by providing information about the growth and extent of OSHMAGs, the types of OSHMAGs that consumers might currently encounter, strengths and weakness of this modality, and the emerging research on OSHMAG outcomes. In order to help students understand OSHMAGs, educators might include curriculum to allow students to observe ("lurk") in an online support group and discuss the extent to which it is "therapeutic"; learn ethics of online ethnographic research; hold class debates on the efficacy and ethics of referral to OSHMAGs; create research assignments that include content analysis of OSHMAG messages; examine the attitudes and practices of local social agency practitioners with regard to OSHMAGs; and review outcome studies and encourage outcomes research by students in Masters and PhD programs.

5.2 Future Directions

New directions in online self-help are already beginning. The majority of studies on OSHMAGs focus on text-mediated communication. In recent years, the advent of faster Internet connections, cheap video-cam Internet communications, and development of social networking sites (SNS) such as *MySpace* (www.myspace.com) and *Facebook* (www.facebook.com) may alter the format for OSHMAG participation. Research is needed to determine the impact that visual cues will have on group participation and process. The rapid development of social networking sites also warrants investigation into their use as a supportive community. Although OSHMAGs do form out of contacts on Social Networking Sites (SNS), it is important to recognize how OSHMAGs differ from SNS. Social Networking Sites such as MySpace and Facebook are usually an extension of an individual's physical space social network (Boyd & Ellison, 2007), whereas members of OSHMAGs may develop deep connections between members who may not naturally extend into an individual's social network in physical space. Research is needed to understand the quality and types of social support provided by social networking sites that do not focus on a specific problem issue, but rather provide more holistic social engagement that includes support around specific issues. The extent to which social networking sites promote the development of "extreme communities" also warrants investigation.

Another new development, which has both practical and therapeutic interest to mental health providers, is the use of graphically rich multi-user online role-playing sites that have become popular with millions of subscribers. These sites allow players to chose and visually design their own characters (avatars) and become immersed in a virtual reality-like environment. For example, Freddolino and Blaschke (2008) describe *Support for Healing*, a virtual island in *Second Life* (http://secondlife.com) where avatars can go for relief from life's problems. Island resources are free on a 24-h basis to any avatar in *Second Life*. Support groups for depression, anxiety, psychosis, chronic pain and illness, women's issues, weight loss, and others are available. Aside from support groups, the *Support for Healing* island also provides avatars with quiet areas for meditation and relaxation in beautifully crafted landscapes with running streams, blue skies, and colorful flowers. These sites provide a vastly different experience to previously studied methods of communication. Preliminary research suggests that they may have unique psychological features (Bailenson & Yee, 2005). Additional research is needed to examine both the user experience and the outcomes of participation in these sites for mental health consumers.

Future OSHMAG research is also needed to judge the increasing effect of a virtually connected society in which relationships, group affiliations, and individuals themselves are connected with the mobile 24/7 connection to the Internet through cell phones, netbooks, and other mobile communication devices. These devices will provide people with support on an as needed basis or even as an event is happening. The development and impact of "just-in-time" support through communication utilities such as Twitter (www.twitter.com), capitalizing on SMS (small messaging service) that supports exchange of quick, frequent messages, is a new area for mental health services, practice, and research.

5.3 Conclusion

Computer-mediated communications are altering social relationships and changing the psychology and sociology of the communication process itself (Vallee, 1982). This is extending to helping relationships as well. The Internet will likely play an increasing role in the organizational strategies of human service agencies as more people and human service organizations come online. (Finn & Schoech, 2008). The potential for OSHMAGs to provide help and support in an era of limited professional resources is enormous. Given the hundreds of thousands of people already involved in OSHMAGs, it is our obligation to evaluate processes and outcomes of these groups and to educate professionals and consumers about their benefits and potential harm. If further research continues to validate the usefulness of OSHMAGs, it will be important to promote their development through referral and clearing house activities, to understand and facilitate the organizational structures that maintain them, and to teach consumers how to best access and utilize them. Current research suggests that OSHMAGs provide support for specific life issues as well as growth and development in the meaning and quality of life. OSHMAGs are likely to take on even greater importance as the use of computer communications enters ever-widening areas of social life.

The impact of computers on human services has been pervasive. Information technology has allowed users to communicate and share information since the early 1970s (Wooley, 1994). By the early 1980s the French computer scientist, Jacque Vallee, predicted that information technology could create a "Grapevine Society" in which everyone had access to information and mutual support through computer communications (Vallee, 1982). He predicted that perhaps the most widespread and profound change from the computer revolution will come about through the use of the computer as a communication tool. At present, the era of "Grapevine Society" is firmly rooted in the developing world and offers great potential to provide helping resources on a global basis. Current OSHMAGs and future "virtual communities" will provide holistic, empowerment-based resources for mutual support and assistance. Mental health professionals will need to participate in the proliferation, evaluation, and improvement of these resources through education, research, and collaborative practice.

Concluding, it is also important to note the issues that affect all interactions on the Internet and thus influence OSHMAGs as well. These issues are important considerations but go beyond the scope of this chapter. They include the following: the Internet being predominantly English-based and therefore excludes, marginalizes, or disconnects some segments of the world community (Zhou, Burgoon, Zhang, & Nunamaker, 2004); national and cultural differences in communication (Grace-Farfaglia, Dekkers, Sundararajan, Peters, & Park, 2006); the socioeconomic and geographical "digital divide" in Internet use in general and in online medical services specifically (Chang et al., 2004; Coiera & Clarke, 2004); age-specific differences in Internet access and group dynamics (Sum, Mathews, Pourghasem, & Hughes, 2008; Vastag, 2001); laws and issues surrounding minors on the Internet (Berson, 2003; Greenfield & Yan, 2006); advances in telecommunication, specifically wireless technologies, enabling "mhealth" (mobile health systems) to reconstruct how health and mental health services are provided (Istepanian, Laxminarayan & Pattichis, 2006) and how mobile/virtual work is impacting the health and mental health profession (Eisenbach, 2000, Andriessen & Vartiainen, 2006);and the impact that the Internet and OSHMAGs may have on the health and mental health profession (Eisenbach, 2000).

References

Alao A. O., Soderberg, M., Pohl, E. L., & Alao A. L. (2006). Cybersuicide: review of the role of the internet on suicide. *Cyberpsychology & Behavior: The Impact of the Internet, Multimedia and Virtual Reality on Behavior and Society, 9*(4), 489–493. doi:10.1089/ cpb.2006. 9.489

Anderson, J. Q., & Rainie, L. (2006). The future of the Internet II. Pew Internet & American Life Project. Retrieved December 30, 2008, from http://www.pewinternet.org/pdfs/PIP_Future_of_Internet_2006.pdf.

Andriessen, J. E., & Vartiainen, M. (2006). *Mobile Virtual Work*. New York: Springer.

Archibald, M. E. (2007). *The evolution of self-help: How a health movement became an institution.* New York: Palgrave Macmillan.

Bailenson, J. N., & Yee, N. (2005). Digital chameleons: Automatic assimilation of nonverbal gestures in immersive virtual environments. *Psychological Science, 16*(10), 814–819. doi:10.1111/j.1467-9280.2005.01619.x

Barak, A., & Dolev-Cohen, M. (2006). Does activity level in online support groups for distressed adolescents determine emotional relief? *Counselling & Psychotherapy Research. 6*(3), 186–190. doi:10.1080/14733140600848203

Barak, A., Boniel-Nissim, M., & Suler, J. (2008). Fostering empowerment in online support groups. *Computers in Human Behavior, 24*(5), 1867–1883. doi:10.1016/j.chb.2008.02.004

Becker, K., & Schmidt, M. (2004). Internet chat rooms and suicide. *Journal of the American Academy of Child and Adolescent Psychiatry, 43*(3), 246–247. doi:10.1097/01.chi.0000106848.88132.c5

Bell, V. (2007). Online information, extreme communities and Internet therapy: Is the Internet good for our mental health? *Journal of Mental Health, 16*(4), 445–457. doi:10.1080/09638230701482378

Bell, V., Maiden, C., Muñoz-Solomando, A., & Reddy, V. (2006). "Mind control experiences" on the Internet: Implications for the psychiatric diagnosis of delusions. *Psychopathology, 39*(2), 87–91. doi:10.1159/000090598

Berson, I. R. (2003). Grooming Cybervictims: The psychosocial effects of online exploitation for youth. *Journal of School Violence, 2*(1), 5–18. doi:10.1300/J202v02n01_02.

Biddle, L., Donovan, J., Hawton, K., Kapur, N., & Gunnell, D. (2008). Suicide and the Internet. *BMJ: British Medical Journal, 336* (7648), 800. doi:10.1136 bmj.39525.442674.AD

Boreman, L. D., Brock, L. E., Hess, R., & Pasquale, F. L. (1982). *Helping people to help themselves: Self-help and prevention*. New York: Haworth Press.

Bos, N,. Gergle, D., Olson, J. S., & Olson,G. M. (2001). Being there versus seeing there: trust via video, *CHI '01 extended abstracts on Human factors in computing systems*. doi:10.1145/634067.634240

Boyd, D. M., & Ellison, N. B. (2007). Social Network Sites: Definition, History, and Scholarship. *Journal of Computer-Mediated Communication, 13*(1), article 11. Retrieved December 24, 2008, from http://jcmc.indiana.edu/vol13/issue1/boyd.ellison.html.

Braithwaite, D. O., Waldron, V. R., & Finn, J. (1999). Communication of social support in computer-mediated groups for people with disabilities. *Health Communication, 11*(2), 123–151. doi:10.1207/s15327027hc1102_2

Brown, L. D., Shepherd, M. D., Wituk, S. A., & Meissen, G. (2007). Goal achievement and the accountability of consumer-run organizations. *Journal of Behavioral Health Services and Research, 34*, 73–82.

Chang, B. L., Bakken, S., Brown, S. S., Houston, T. K., Kreps, G. L., & Kukafka, R., et al. (2004). Bridging the digital divide: Reaching vulnerable populations. *Journal – American Medical Informatics Association, 11*, 448–457. doi:10.1197/jamia.M1535

Coiera E., & Clarke R. (2004). E-Consent: The design and implementation of consumer consent mechanisms in an electronic environment. *Journal of the American Medical Informatics Association : JAMIA, 11*(2). doi:10.1197/jamia.M1480

Coulson, N. S., & Knibb, R. C. (2007). Coping with food allergy: Exploring the role of the online support group. *CyberPsychology and Behavior, 10*, 145–148.

Davies, P., & Lipsey, Z. (2003). Ana's gone surfing. *The Psychologist, 16*, 424–425.

Dinsmore, C. (1991). *From surviving to thriving: Incest, feminism and recovery*. Albany, NY: State University of New York Press.

Eichhorn, K. (2008). Soliciting and providing social support over the Internet: An Investigation of online eating disorder support groups. *Journal of Computer Mediated Communication, 14*(1), 67–68. Retrieved December 19, 2008, from http://www3.interscience.wiley.com.offcampus.lib.washington.edu/cgi-bin/fulltext/121527996/PDFSTART. doi:10.1111/j.1083-6101.2008.01431.x

Eysenbach, G., Powell, J., Englesakis, M., Ruizo, C., & Stern, A. (2004). Health related virtual communities and electronic support groups: systematic review of the effects of online peer to peer interactions. *British Medical Journal, 328*(7449), 1166–1172. doi:10.1136/bmj.328.7449.1166

Eysenbach, G. (2000). Consumer health informatics. *British Medical Journal, 320*(7251), 1713–1716. doi:10.1136/bmj.320.7251.1713

Freddolino, P.,& Blaschkem C. M. (2008). Therapeutic applications of online gaming. *Journal of Technology and Human Services, 26* (2–4), 423–446.

Feldman M. D. (2000). Munchausen by Internet: detecting factitious illness and crisis on the Internet. *Southern Medical Journal, 93*, 669–672. doi:10.1080/ 15228830802099998

Ferguson, T. (1996). *Health online*. Reading, MA: Addison-Wesley.

Finn, J., & Schoech, D. (2008). Internet-delivered therapeutic interventions in human services: Methods, issues, and evaluation. 3 volume issue of *Journal of Technology and Human Services*, 26 (2–4). Philadelphia, PA: Haworth Press.

Finn, J. (2002). MSW Student Perception of the Ethics and Efficacy of Online Therapy. *Journal of Social Work Education, 38*(3), 403–420. Retrieved December 30, 2008, from http://eric.ed.gov/ERICWebPortal/recordDetail?accno=EJ657601.

Finn, J., & Banach, M. (2000). Victimization Online: The downside of seeking services for women on the Internet. *Cyberpsychology and Behavior, 3*(2), 776–785. doi:10.1089/10949310050191764

Finn, J. (1995). Computer-based self-help groups: A new resource to supplement support groups. *Social Work with Groups, 18*(1), 109–117. doi:10.1300/J009v18n01_11

Finn, J., & Lavitt, M. (1994). Computer-based self-help groups for sexual abuse survivors. *Social Work with Groups, 17*(1/2), 21–45. doi:10.1300/J009v17n01_03

Fischer, M. A. (2006, February). *Reader's Digest*. Retrieved December 30, 2008, from http://www.rd.com/living-healthy/choking-games-and-thrills-that-kill/article19581.html.

Gavin, J., Rodham, K., & Poyer, H. (2008). The presentation of "pro-anorexia" in online group interactions. *Qualitative Health Research, 18*(3), 325–333. doi:10.1177/1049732307311640

Grace-Farfaglia, P., Dekkers, A., Sundararajan, B., Peters, L., & Park, S.-H. (2006). Multinational web uses and gratifications: measuring the social impact of online community participation across national boundaries. *Electronic Commerce Research, 6* (1), 75–101. doi:10.1007/s10660-006-5989-6

Greenfield P., & Yan Z. (2006). Children, adolescents, and the internet: A new field of inquiry in developmental psychology. *Developmental Psychology, 42*(3), 391–394. doi:10.1037/0012-1649.42.3.391

Horrigan, J. (2001). *Online communities: Networks that nurture long-distance relationships and local ties*. Washington DC: Pew Internet & American Life Project. Retrieved February 8, 2008 from: www.pewInternet.org/PPF/r/47/report_display.asp.

Howard, P., Rainie, L., & Jones, S. (2001). Days and nights on the internet: The impact of a diffusing technology. *American Behavioral Scientist, 45*(3), 383–404. doi:10.1177/0002764201045003003

Hwang, K. O., Farheen, K., Johnson, C. W., Thomas, E. J., Barnes, A. S., & Bernstam, E. V. (2007). Quality of weight loss advice on Internet forums. *American Journal of Medicine, 120*, 604–609. doi:10.1016/j.amjmed.2007.04.017

Istepanian, R. S. H., Laxminarayan, S., & Pattichis, C. S. (2006). *M-health: Emerging mobile health systems*. New York: Springer.

Katz, A. H. (1992). *Self help: Concepts and applications*. Philadelphia, PA: Charles Press.

Kernsmith, P. D., & Kernsmith, R. M. (2008). A safe place for predators: Online treatment of recovering sex offenders. *Journal of Technology in Human Services, 26* (2/4), 223–238. doi:10.1080/15228830802096598

Kraut, R., Patterson., M., Lundmark, V., Kiesler, S., Mukhopadhyay, T., & Scherlis, W. (1998). Internet paradox: A social technology that reduces social involvement and psychological well-being? *American Psychologist, 53*, 1017–1031. doi:10.1037/0003-066X.53.9.1017

Kummervold, P. E., Gammon, D., Bergvik, S., Johnsen, J. K., Hasvold, T., & Rosenvinge, J. H. (2002). Social support in a wired world. Use of online mental health forums in Norway. *Nordic Journal of Psychiatry, 65*, 56–59. doi:10.1080/08039480252803945

Kurtz, L. F. (1997). *Self-help and support groups: A handbook for practitioners.* Thousand Oaks, CA: Sage.

Lebow, J. (1998). Not just talk, maybe some risk: The therapeutic potentials and pitfalls of computer-mediated conversation. *Journal of Marital and Family Therapy, 24,* 203-206. doi:10.1111/j.1752-0606.1998.tb01076.x

Lieberman, M.A. (1976). Change induction in small groups. *Annual Review of Psychology,* 27, 217-250.

Loundy, D. (n.d.). Internet governance through self-help remedies. Retrieved December 21, 2008, from http://www.loundy.com/CPSR-Self-Help.html.

Maloney-Krichmar, D., & Preece, J. (2002). The meaning of an online health community in the lives of its members: Roles, relationships and group dynamics social implications of information and communication technology. *2002 International Symposium on Technology and Society* ISTAS'02, 20-27. Retrieved December 30, 2008, from http://www.ifsm.umbc.edu/~preece/Papers/02_The_meaning_of_an_online_health_community.pdf

Marvin, L. E. (1995). Spoof, spam, lurk and lag: The aesthetics of text-based virtual realities. *Journal of Computer-Mediated Communication,* 1(2). Retrieved December 30, 2008, from http://jcmc.indiana.edu/vol1/issue2/marvin.html

McKenna, K.Y.A., & Seidman, G. (2005). You, me, and we: Interpersonal processes in online groups. In Y. A. Hamburger (Ed.), *The social net: The social psychology of the Internet* (pp. 191-217). New York: Oxford University Press.

McKenna, K.Y.A., Green, A. S., & Gleason, M. E. J. (2002). Relationship formation on the Internet: What's the big attraction? *Journal of Social Issues, 58,* 9-31. doi:10.1111/1540-4560.00246

Meier, A. (2004). *Technology-mediated groups.* In C. D. Garvin, L. M. Gutie'rrez, & M. J. Galinsky (Eds.), *Handbook of social work with groups* (pp. 479-503). New York: Guilford.

Moody, E. (2001). Internet use and its relationship to loneliness. *Cyberpsychology and Behavior,* 4, 393-401. doi:10.1089/109493101300210303

Murguía, E., Tackett-Gibson, M., & Lessem, A. (2007). *Real drugs in a virtual world: Drug discourse and community online.* Lanham, MD: Lexington Books.

Murphy, L., MacFadden, R., & Mitchell, D. (2008). Cybercounseling online: The development of a university-based training program for e-mail counseling. *Journal of Technology in Human Services, 26* (2,3,4), 447-469. doi:10.1080/15228830802102081

Murray, C. D., & Fox, J. (2006). Do Internet self-harm discussion groups alleviate or exacerbate self-harming behaviour? *Australian e-Journal for the Advancement of Mental Health,* 5(3) 1-9. Retrieved December 30, 2008, from http://www.auseinet.com/journal/vol5iss3/murray.pdf

Nelson, J. A. (1995). The Internet, the virtual community and those with disabilities. *Disability Quarterly, 15* (2), 15-20.

O'Boyle, E. J. (2002). An ethical decision-making process for computing professionals. *Ethics and Information Technology,* 4(4), 267-277. doi:10.1023/A:1021320617495

Prior, T. I. (2004). Suicide methods from the Internet. *American Journal of Psychiatry, 161,* 1500-1501. doi:10.1176/appi.ajp.161.8.1500-a

Radin, P. (2006). "To me, it's my life": Medical communication, trust, and activism in cyberspace. *Social Science and Medicine, 62,* 591-601.

Rajagopal, S. (2004). Suicide pacts and the Internet. British Medical Journal, 329(7478), 1298-1299. revisited. *Journal of Social Issues, 58,* 49-74. doi:10.1136/bmj.329.7478.1298

Ralston J. D, Carrell D, Reid R, Anderson M, Moran M, & Hereford J. (2007). Patient web services integrated with a shared medical record: Patient use and satisfaction. *Journal of the American Medical Informatics Association, 14*(6). doi:10.1197/jamia.M2302

Riegelsberger, J., Sasse, M. A., & McCarthy, J. D. (2003). The researcher's dilemma: Evaluating trust in computer-mediated communication. *International Journal of Human Computer Studies, 58,* 759-782. doi:10.1016/S1071-5819(03)00042-9

Segal, S. P., Silverman, C., & Temkin, T. (1993). Empowerment and self-help agency practice for people with mental disabilities. *Social Work, 38*(6), 705-712. Retrieved December 30, 2008, from http://eric.ed.gov/ERICWebPortal/recordDetail?accno=EJ482963

Stoppard, M. (2008, December 9). How safe are Internet health forums? – *Dear Miriam – Mirror.co.uk*. Retrieved December 23, 2008, from http://blogs.mirror.co.uk/dearmiriam/2008/12/how-safe-are-internet-health-f.html.

Spears, R., Postmes, T., Lea, M., & Wolbert, A. (2002). When are net effects gross products? The power of influence and the influence of power in computer-mediated communication. *Journal of Social Issues, 58*, 91–107. doi:10.1111/1540-4560.00250

Southworth, C., Finn, J., Dawson, S., Fraser, C., & Tucker, S. (2007). Intimate partner violence, technology, and stalking. *Violence Against Women, 13*(8), 842–856. doi:10.1177/1077801207302045

Suler, J. R. (2004). The online disinhibition effect. *CyberPsychology and Behavior, 7*, 321–326. doi:10.1089/1094931041291295

Sullivan, C. F. (2003). Gendered cybersupport: A thematic analysis of two online cancer support groups. *Journal of Health Psychology, 8*, 83–103.

Sum, S., Mathews, M. R., Pourghasem, M., & Hughes, I. (2008). Internet technology and social capital: How the internet affects seniors' social capital and wellbeing. *Journal of Computer Mediated Communication* [Electric Edition],*14*(1), 202–220. doi:10.1111/j.1083-6101.2008.01437.x

Tavani, H. T., & Grodzinsky, F. S. (2002). Cyberstalking, personal privacy, and moral responsibility. *Ethics and Information Technology, 4*(2), 123–132. doi:10.1023/A:1019927824326

Tichon, J. G., & Shapiro, M. (2003). The process of sharing social support in cyberspace. *CyberPsychology and Behavior, 6*, 161–170.

Tierney, S. (2006). The dangers and draw of online communication: Pro-Anorexia websites and their implications for users, practitioners, and researchers. *Eating Disorders: The Journal of Treatment & Prevention, 14*(3), 181–190. doi:10.1080/10640260600638865

Vallee, J. (1982). *The network revolution: Confessions of a computer scientist*. Berkeley, CA: And/Or Press.

van Dam, H. A., van der Horst, F. G., Knoops, L., Ryckman, R. M., Crebolder Harry, F. J. M., & van den Borne Bart, H. W. (2005). Social support in diabetes: A systematic review of controlled intervention studies. *Patient Education and Counseling, 59*, 1–12.

Vasisht, D. (2003, April 11). E-medicine is just what the doctor didn't order. Delhi Times-Cities-The Times of India. T*he Times of India*. Retrieved December 23, 2008, from http://timesofindia.indiatimes.com/articleshow/43007827.cms.

Waldron, V., Lavitt, M., & Kelley, D. (2000). The nature and prevention of harm in technology mediated self-help settings: Three exemplars. *Journal of Technology in Human Services, 17*(1, 2, 3), 267–294. doi:10.1300/J017v17n02_09

Walther, J. (1997). Group and interpersonal effects in international computer-mediated communication. *Human Communication Research, 23*, 342–369. doi:10.1111/j.14682958.1997.tb00400.x

Weis, R., Stamm, K., Smith, C., Nilan, M., Clark, F., Weis, J., & Kennedy, K. (2003).Communities of care and caring: The case of MSWatch com. *Journal of Health Psychology, 8*, 135–148.

Woolley, D.R. (1994). DR. PLATO: The emergence of online community. Retrieved November 5, 2008 from http://thinkofit.com/plato/dwplato.htm.

Worotynec, Z. S. (2000). The good, the bad and the ugly: Listserv as support. *CyberPsychology and Behavior, 3*, 797–810.

Wright, K. B., & Bell, S. B. (2003). Health-related support groups on the Internet: Linking empirical findings to social support and computer-mediated communication theory. *Journal of Health Psychology, 8*, 39–54. doi:10.1177/1359105303008001429

Yalom, I (1985). *Theory and practice of group psychotherapy*. New York: Basic Books.

Young, K. S. (1998). *Caught in the Net*. New York: Wiley.

Zhou, L., Burgoon, J. K., Zhang, D., & Nunamaker, J. F. (2004). Language dominance in interpersonal deception in computer-mediated communication. *Computers in Human Behavior, 20*(3), 381–402. doi:10.1016/S0747-5632(03)00051-7

Chapter 6
An Overview of Mutual Support Groups for Family Caregivers of People with Mental Health Problems: Evidence on Process and Outcomes

Wai-Tong Chien

Abstract This chapter summarizes the literature from a systematic search and assesses the evidence on the effectiveness and therapeutic ingredients of mutual support groups for helping family caregivers of people with severe mental health problems. This review used a combined free-text and thesaurus approach to search relevant research articles within major electronic databases and System for Info on gray literature for the period 1988–2008 and reference lists of all retrieved literature. Twelve research studies were selected for inclusion in the analysis on the basis that they were family-led support group programs for caregivers of people with severe mental health problems. Many studies reported different benefits of group participation such as increasing knowledge about the illness and enhancing coping ability and social support. However, there is little evidence supporting the significant long-term positive effects of mutual support groups on families' and consumers' psychosocial health conditions except illness relapse. Qualitative studies identified four potential therapeutic mechanisms of family mutual support groups. The authors also discuss lessons learned from development of and evaluation on family-led support groups including the major principles in establishing and strengthening a support group, barriers to its development and families who are likely to attend and benefit from group participation.

6.1 Introduction

With the current emphasis on community care for people with mental health problems, family intervention, particularly in a group format using a diverse range of modalities, is thought to help satisfy the families' health needs (Cuijpers, 1999) and enhance their coping abilities to take care of their relative with severe mental

W.-T. Chien (✉)
The School of Nursing, Faculty of Health & Social Sciences, The Hong Kong Polytechnic University, Hong Kong SAR, China
e-mail: chinwaton@yahoo.com.hk; hschien@inet.polyu.edu.hk

health problems (Chien & Wong, 2007), and hence reduce mental health consumers' illness relapses (Pharoah, Mari, & Streiner, 2001). Demands for family interventions in the community have also substantially increased as a result of changes in the organization of mental health services in both western and Asian countries (Budd & Hughes, 1997; Pearson & Ning, 1997). All family intervention programs offer psycho-education and psychosocial support to family members, and some include the consumer, although the theoretical orientation of these interventions varies considerably.

Recent systematic reviews of family interventions in schizophrenia (Barbato & D'Avanzo, 2000; Pharoah et al., 2001) suggest that psychological models such as psycho-educational family groups (Hogarty et al., 1991) and behavioral family management (Falloon et al., 1982) can be effective in reducing illness relapse but unable to improve a family's health condition and burden of care. Surprisingly, few clinical trials of family intervention have assessed family-related outcomes (Barbato & D'Avanzo, 2000), and those that had reported inconsistent findings with regard to any significant improvement in family functioning. It is not clear which particular treatment model or technique is the most beneficial for family members or their relatives with schizophrenia on psychosocial well-being. In addition, most family intervention studies have focused on Caucasian populations; few have included Hispanics or Asians (McFarlane et al., 1995; Teller et al., 1995).

The use of mutual support groups as an approach to family intervention for consumers with severe mental health problems was relatively uncommon in Western countries until the late 1980s. Mutual support groups for family caregivers provide information about mental illness, treatment, and community resources; opportunities to openly share feelings and experiences with group members; and emotional support and empathy. National Alliance for Mental Illness (NAMI) groups are well-established in the United States. Participation in a support group is a social action process by which individuals can gain a greater sense of personal control over issues of concern, adopt a more proactive approach to life, and develop an in-depth understanding of their social environment (Zimmerman, 1995).

Peer-led mutual support groups for families of people with schizophrenia have recently been subjected to a few cross-sectional descriptive and cohort studies, which evidenced their apparent benefits of maintaining the psychological and social well-being of families (Heller et al., 1997; Pearson & Ning, 1997). It is unknown whether there is evidence to support enthusiastic claims for their benefits in improving family functioning and satisfying families' psychosocial needs. In Western and Asian communities, a few studies have used mutual support and sharing as a major component of their family psycho-education programs (Asen, 2002; Li & Arthur, 2005). There is a need to review the use of mutual support groups for family caregivers of people with mental health problems, to improve understanding of the health outcomes and therapeutic components for both consumers and their family caregivers. It is also important to better understand the important issues in development of and evaluation on family-led mutual support groups such as the main principles of establishing and strengthening a support group and the obstacles to group development.

6.2 The Conceptual Basis of Mutual Support Groups

The use of mutual support to families of people with severe mental illness is grounded in the stress-vulnerability and coping model (Lazarus & Folkman, 1984). The model states that family's ability to cope with the immediate stress of hospitalization is determined by the extent to which the illness and hospitalization is perceived as a threat to their well-being. In addition, family adaptation of the ongoing stress in caring for people with mental illness is associated with the perceived difficulty of the care-giving task. The moderating effect of social support to family caregivers is emphasized in the model on: facing the stressful experiences of social stigma (Bernheim & Lehman, 1985), reducing social isolation due to constraints from care-giving and guilty feelings due to having a relative with severe mental health problem (Turnbull et al., 1994), and enhancing emotional support and practical assistance in care-giving (Wituk et al., 2000).

Theoretical concepts of social relationships and empowerment, social comparison theory, and principles of social learning can provide partial but insightful explanations of how the supportive groups work. Social relationships have been found to be most helpful to people who have a small or loosely related social network and, thus, they are unable to obtain the help they need from people in their network. Important social relationships are the means by which the individual acquires a social identity and receives social, emotional, and material support (Penney, 1997). As the natural networks may not be able to protect families caring for a relative with mental illness from stigmatization and social isolation, new social relationships may be useful to uphold a different set of values and norms while simultaneously accepting persons with the similar problems (Borkman, 1999). The mutual support group can be an important asset to develop such new relationships in an accepting social environment and especially important if the families have been isolated by their problems related to care-giving to people with severe mental health problems. These groups provide an informal but consistent parallel system of peer support to complement professional help and social support from relatives and friends (Wituk et al., 2000).

In viewing the mutual help processes within a support group for family caregivers, psychological empowerment is purported to build on the supportive social context and by making connections with people outside the group. This is a social action process by which the family carers as group participants learn to gain mastery over issues of concern to them (i.e., perceptions of personal control), while learning a proactive approach to life and a critical understanding of their intrapersonal, social, and societal environment (Maton & Salem, 1995). The aspects of empowerment applied to a mutual support group can be: the provision of a peer-based support system, the availability of an opportunity role structure (i.e., allows individuals to take on meaningful roles within the group), and the inculcation of a belief system that inspires members to strive for better mental health (Perkins & Zimmerman, 1995).

Social comparison theory provides another theoretical basis of studying mutual support groups. This theory postulates that social behavior in a group can be predicted largely on the basis of the assumption that individuals seek to maintain a sense of normalcy and accuracy about their world (Festinger, 1954; Kessler, Mickelson & Zhao, 1997). In times of uncertainty and high level of anxiety, affiliative behaviors will increase as people seek others' opinions about how they should be thinking. Basing on the findings of a study on illness experiences in four metropolitan areas and online forums in the United States (Davidson, Pennebaker & Dickerson, 2000), support seeking is highest for illnesses viewed as socially stigmatizing and embarrassing such as AIDS, schizophrenia, and other severe mental illnesses, or disfiguring such as eating disorder and breast cancer, leading people to seek the support of others in similar situations. In addition, this support seeking applies to the family members caring for these mental health consumers. On the other hand, help-seeking behavior is lowest for less embarrassing and equally devastating disorders such as heart and neurological diseases. Therefore, people with a diagnosis of mental illness, long-term psychiatric treatment, and various kinds of life disruptions prompt their willingness and motivation to talk with others undergoing a similar challenge; and this motivated socialization can also apply to their family members.

Similar to some other group interventions or therapies, mutual support group members can learn new adaptive behavior from other peer members with three major elements of social learning: clear instructions, adequate reinforcement, and the effect of good model behavior (Bandura, 1977). A support group typically employs mutual sharing and learning from each other's lived experiences during the group sessions. The group uses carefully considered suggestions, action plans, or mutually agreed instructions to help the individual eliminate or live more comfortably with their life problems. This is similar to the major component of social learning – giving instructions of new behavior (Zimmerman & Schunk, 2003), which can motivate and give direction to participant's actions to achieve his/her goal(s). The effort of behavior change is usually reinforcing as the group and the social environment positively appraises and approves the development of new skills and extinction of undesirable habits.

Group reinforcement nurtures a positive social environment for individual family caregivers to appreciate their accomplishment for overcoming unwanted behaviors or responses to the mental health consumers, and on the other hand, to admit their faults and problems in care-giving (Mankowski, Humphreys & Moos, 2001). Helgeson and Gottlieb (2000) suggested that the contributing factors of vicarious learning among support group members were: (a) the problems of the role models are similar to those of the relatively inexperienced group members; (b) the veteran members can describe the specific means used to bring about changes, thus facilitating the success of problem-solving behavior; (c) those veterans can demonstrate desirable behavior and effective communication skills in real situations; and (d) the veterans invite more interactions with other members because they admit freely that their well-being depends upon being able to mutually share their experience of care-giving with others.

In viewing these theoretical perspectives, mutual support groups are complex entities that differ in important ways from professionally delivered help. As suggested by Penney (1997), familiarity with mutual support groups is a crucial skill for professionals that need to provide the most flexible and low-cost service for their clients. Therefore, with no similar literature review identified, this literature review will be important and useful in understanding evidence on the efficacy of peer-led mutual support groups for family caregivers of people with severe mental health problems in the past two decades.

6.3 Literature on Mutual Support Groups for Families of People with Severe Mental Illness

Literature reviews examining the effects of family interventions in people with severe mental illness have focused primarily on a few approaches of intervention frequently used and empirically tested in mental health research such as psychoeducation and behavioral management programs (Barbato & D'Avanzo, 2000; Dixon, Adams & Luckstead, 2000; Pharoah et al., 2001). There is a notable omission of other alternative approaches of family intervention such as mutual support groups, given the increasing emphasis of self-help programs and family-based interventions in mental health services in the United States, the United Kingdom, and other western countries. The aim of this literature review was to establish what is known about the effectiveness of peer-led mutual support groups for family caregivers of people suffering from severe mental illness and thus to answer two important questions of family care: "Are the mutual support groups effective in promoting health and other benefits for families of people with psychotic disorders?" and "What are the therapeutic components of mutual support groups for these families?"

6.3.1 Literature Search Strategy

This review of the research literature was based on the procedures suggested by the National Health Service Centre for Reviews and Dissemination (2001). Databases searched were Medline, Embase, CINAHL, OVID full text, PsycINFO, Cochrane Library, NHS National Research register, and System for Info on gray literature. *The British Journal of Psychiatry*, *Schizophrenia Bulletin*, *Schizophrenia Research*, *American Journal of Psychiatry*, and other psychiatry and psychology journals available at the university libraries (i.e., both English and Chinese languages) were hand-searched and reference lists of all retrieved literature were also searched to identify studies that may have been missed. Leading researchers of current studies, as identified on the National Research Register, were contacted to ascertain if a research report or paper relating to this intervention was due for publication during this review.

For electronic databases searching, a combined free-text and thesaurus approach was adopted. "Population" search terms included: serious mental disorder, severe mental illness, mood or affective disorder, dementia, psychos*, and schizophreni*. "Intervention" search terms included: mutual support or aid, social or peer support, self help, group therap*, family therap*, family work, and family intervention. The search strategy was restricted to English-language, research articles published in the past-20 years (from 1989 to 2008).

With an expectation of a small number of research articles being identified, three inclusion criteria were used to guide the search strategy: (1) the intervention used should be a family-led support group program for families of a relative with severe mental illness; (2) prospective or retrospective evaluation studies on a mutual support group program, and (3) qualitative studies on group participants' perceived benefits and limitations of a support group program were selected. In addition, systematic reviews and meta-analyses of this topic would also be included but none were identified. A total of 728 articles were retrieved from the electronic databases, of which one-fifth ($n = 151$) was found relevant and appropriate for further review. Hand searching, tracing unpublished or in press research reports, and screening reference lists increased of the total number of articles retrieved for critical review to 172. After critical appraisal of these retrieved articles, 160 were excluded mainly because they were psycho-education family groups ($n = 97$) with much didactic education, cross-sectional descriptive and single-group cohort studies ($n = 29$), professional-driven support group programs ($n = 25$), or mainly one component of client intervention ($n = 9$) in which the programs focused on consumer outcomes only. Finally, 12 studies are reviewed in this paper, consisting of: five studies using experimental or randomized controlled trial design; three using quasi-experimental design (non-equivalent comparison groups); and four using qualitative design (on perceived benefits and limitations of group participation).

6.3.2 Methodological Quality of the Studies Reviewed

The 12 studies reviewed are summarized in Table 6.1 for experimental studies, Table 6.2 for quasi-experimental studies, and Table 6.3 for qualitative studies. Overall, most of the seven quantitative (experimental or quasi-experimental) studies focus on families of people with various types of chronic and severe mental illnesses in community mental health care. The majority of the family caregivers were female (50–88%), middle age (40–58 years; 48–70%), parent or spouse (58–68%), elementary or high school education (48–54%), and Chinese (20–100%, two studies did not report). Six studies indicated that the families were from mainly the middle social class (about 53% of total number of subjects in the six studies); only two studies reported that the families had low household income and two reported that 25 and 46% of the caregivers were employed.

More than half of the mental health consumers in the quantitative studies were male (mean 66%, range 40–75%), with more than 9 years of illness (mean 9.2 years, range a few months to 20 years). Psychiatric diagnoses of the consumers were mainly schizophrenia (range 40–100%), schizoaffective disorder and bipolar

Table 6.1 Summary of experimental studies on family-led mutual support groups

Study	Country	Sample	Intervention	Method	Instrument	Major Findings	Attrition
Albramowitz, and Coursey, (1989)	US	Forty-eight families of people with schizophrenia were recruited at 4 community mental health centers in Baltimore and Washington, DC. Twenty-four families in treatment group and another 24 in control group. *Family carers*: >70% female; >60% white; mean age = 51 years; 75% parent. *Consumers*: 29 male and 19 female; 67% aged 25–35 years; illness duration = 1–30 years	*Treatment group*: consisted of six 2-h, weekly group sessions led by family caregivers, with 5–17 caregivers in each group. Group content, which was based on a needs assessment, included: introduction and discussion of current problems; information of the illness; consumers' coping with symptoms, medication, and environment; managing problem behaviors; community resources; and review of learning and future plans. *Control group*: routine community mental health care (its content was not specified)	Experimental, pre-test and post-test design, using questionnaire	State-Trait Anxiety Inventory Relatives' Stress Scale Nine-item scale for community resources use Generalized self-Efficacy Scale	Treatment group indicated significant improvements on personal distress and management of home life, a reduction of anxiety, and an increase of community resources utilization	Not specified

Table 6.1 (continued)

Study	Country	Sample	Intervention	Method	Instrument	Major Findings	Attrition
Fung, and Chien (2002)	HK	Sixty family caregivers from two dementia care centers in Kwai Chung district participated in the clinical trial. Thirty families were randomly assigned to either a mutual support or a routine care group. Families: 55% female; 100% Chinese; mean age = 50 years; 43% spouse and 25% child; >50% employed. Consumers: 60% male; mean age 68 years; average duration of illness = 1.1 years	*Mutual support group*: met regularly weekly, for a total of 12 1-h sessions, led by one peer leader and facilitated by one trained psycho-geriatric nurse. All group sessions consisted of education, sharing and discussion, psychological support, and problem-solving, similar to Toseland, Rossiter, & Labrecque (1989) group program. A protocol was designed by the researchers to guide the progress and development of the group.	Experimental, pre-test and post-test design, using questionnaire	Neuropsychiatric Inventory – Caregiver Distress scale WHO Quality of Life Measure – Brief version Mental Health Services Index Demographic data sheet	Significant differences were found for distress levels and quality of life, with the mutual support group having greater improvements than the routine care group at post-test	13%

6 An Overview of Mutual Support Groups for Family Caregivers 115

Table 6.1 (continued)

Study	Country	Sample	Intervention	Method	Instrument	Major Findings	Attrition
			Routine care group: received the usual family services provided by the dementia care centers. The services included: medical consultation by a visiting psychiatrist, advices and referrals of financial aids, and social welfare provided by a social worker, educational talk and social recreational activities organized by the nurses and other staff at the centers				

Table 6.1 (continued)

Study	Country	Sample	Intervention	Method	Instrument	Major Findings	Attrition
Chien et al. (2005)	HK	Ninety-six of 300 family carers of schizophrenic outpatients in two psychiatric outpatient clinics were recruited. Thirty-two in mutual support group, 33 in psycho-education group, and 31 in standard care. *Family carers*: 68% male; mean age = 40.6–43.2 years, range 22–60 years; 23% parent, 20% spouse, and 15% child. *Consumers*: 66% male; mean age = 29.3 years, range 20–49 years; average illness duration = 2 years	*Mutual support group*: contained 12 bi-weekly sessions, consisting of discussion, role-play and rehearsals of care-giving problems and providing peer support. The groups were facilitated by a trained mental health nurse. *Psycho-education group*: contained 12 bi-weekly sessions, consisting of psychological support and education, based on McFarlane et al. (1995). *Standard care group*: received medical consultation, consultation and financial support by social worker and psychiatric nurses at outpatient department	Randomized controlled trial, 3-group and repeated measures design (1 week prior to intervention, and 1 week and 6 months after intervention), using questionnaires	Family Assessment Device Family Support Services Index Consumers' Specific Level of Functioning Scale Length of re-hospitalization	Mutual support group indicated significantly greater improvements on family and consumers' functioning at 1 week and 6 months follow-up, than the psycho-education and control group	~8 and 13% at 1 week and 6 months after intervention, respectively

Table 6.1 (continued)

Study	Country	Sample	Intervention	Method	Instrument	Major Findings	Attrition
Chien et al. (2006a)	HK	Ninety-six families of people with schizophrenia or psychotic disorders were recruited. Thirty-two in mutual support group, 33 in psycho-education group, and 31 in standard care. Family carers: 64% male; mean age = 41.6 years, range 23–58 years; mainly parent, child, or spouse. Consumers: 67% male; mean age = 27.8 years, range 20–48 years; average illness duration = 2 years	Mutual support group: contained 12 bi-weekly, 2-h sessions (consumers excluded). It was led by on family carers and co-facilitated by one psychiatric nurse, using Wilson's (1995) principles. Psycho-education group: contained 12 bi-weekly, 2-h sessions focusing on psychological support and education, modified from Anderson, Reiss, & Hogarty (1986) program. It was led by 2 mental health nurses. Standard care: received medical consultation, individual consultation, and financial support at outpatient department	Randomized controlled trial, 3-group and repeated measures design (at recruitment and 6 and 18 months after intervention), using questionnaires	Family Burden Interview Schedule Family Support Services Index Specific Level of Functioning Scale Brief Psychiatric Rating Scale Dosage of anti-psychotic medication Number and length of psychiatric re-hospitalization	Mutual support group indicated significantly greater improvement on consumer and family functioning, and caregiver burden at both 6-month and 18-month follow-up, when compared to the other two groups. The lengths of consumer re-admissions in both Mutual Support Group and Psycho-education Group significantly reduced at 6 months but not 18 months after intervention, while re-admission in control group slightly increased	~10% at 18-month follow-up

Table 6.1 (continued)

Study	Country	Sample	Intervention	Method	Instrument	Major Findings	Attrition
Chien et al. (2008)	HK	Seventy-six families of people with schizophrenia were recruited Thirty-eight families in both mutual support group and standard care *Family carers*: 55% female; mean age = 35.9 years, range 20–62 years; mainly parent or spouse Consumers: 58% female; mean age = 25.4 years, range 19–26 years; average illness duration = 2.7 years	*Mutual support group*: contained 12 bi-weekly, 2-h sessions (consumers excluded). It was led by family carers and co-facilitated by one psychiatric nurse, using Wilson's (1995) principles *Standard care*: received medical consultation, individual consultation, and financial support at outpatient department	Randomized controlled trial, 2-group and repeated measures design (at recruitment and 1 week and 12 months after intervention), using questionnaires	Family Burden Interview Schedule Family Support Services Index Family Assessment Device 6-item Social Support Questionnaire Brief Psychiatric Rating Scale Dosage of anti-psychotic medication Number and length of psychiatric re-hospitalization	Mutual support group indicated significantly greater improvement on family functioning, social support, and burden at both 1-week and 12-month follow-up, when compared to the standard care group The lengths of consumer re-admissions in the mutual support group significantly reduced at 12 months after intervention, while re-admissions in the control group mildly increased	~10% at 18-month follow-up

Table 6.2 Summary of quasi-experimental studies on family-led mutual support groups

| Winefield, H.R. and Harvey, E.J. (1995) | Australia | Thirty-six of 56 family caregivers of people with schizophrenia were recruited in Adelaide metropolitan area. Sixteen in discussion group and 15 in waiting-list controls. *Family carers*: 89% female; mean age = 58.9 years; 86% parent. *Consumers*: average illness duration = 2.1 years; otherwise no other demographic information specified | *Discussion group*: 8 weekly family-led meetings consisting of: introduction; family communication and problem-solving; information sharing about the causes and nature of the illness, medication and community resources; awareness of early signs of an episode and management and guidance; sharing of care-giving experiences and how to maintain hope; and summary and follow-up. *Waiting-list Controls*: received community services (details not specified) | Quasi-experimental, non-equivalent groups, 1 pre-test and 2 post-tests (at recruitment and immediate and 8 weeks after intervention), using questionnaires. Open-ended questions for caregivers to comments on group participation | Multidimensional Support Scale and 10 questions on taking care of own well-being. Profile of Mood States. Family Attitudes scale. Process of group meetings: audio recordings of sessions; group attendance; and reasons for absence | Discussion group indicated significant greater improvements on availability and adequacy of family and peer support at immediate and 8-week after intervention, when compared to waiting-list controls. Over 50% of the participants expressed that they enjoyed the group participation, experienced positive changes in feelings or behavior toward consumer, and gained confidence from sharing their problems with other group members | Not clearly specified. High attendance rate once they were engaged in the group indicated |

Table 6.2 (continued)

Pickett-Schenk, S.A. and Heller, T. (1998)	US	One hundred and thirty-one families recruited from 14 support groups in Chicago and southern Illinois. Thirty-seven in four professional-led support groups and 94 in ten family-led support groups. *Family members*: 72% female; mean age = 56 years; mainly Caucasian; mainly parents (78% vs. 59%) and siblings; >3 years group participation. *Consumers*: 69% male; mean age = 35 years, average illness duration = 15 years	*Professional-led vs. family-led support groups*: both types of groups contained 4–26 members (mean = 13) in each group. They met weekly or monthly, at one participant's home or mental health care center, using an 8-step model adapted from a 12-step approach. The groups consisted of: sharing of information about mental illness, discussion about care-giving situations and problems, and providing psychological support	Quasi-experimental, non-equivalent comparison groups design (professional-led vs. family-led), using questionnaires	Group Benefits Scale (information and relationship benefits) Five-item Coping Ability Scale Participants rated extent of discussion (e.g., medication, consumer's illness and behavior, and financial concerns)	No significant differences between two groups on provision of information about the illness and treatment and improvement of relationship with consumer. Professional-led groups indicated greater improvements in rating of consumers' behavior problems and coping with emotions, whereas family-led groups showed better rating of advocacy	Not specified
Chou, K.R., Liu, S.Y., and Chu, H. (2002)	Taiwan	Eighty-four primary family caregivers of people with schizophrenia were recruited from community	*Family-led support group*: contained eight 1.5-h sessions on Saturday, using Zarit et al.'s	Quasi-experimental time series non-equivalent control group design (at baseline, immediate and one	Caregiver Burden Inventory Beck Depression Inventory Physical Self-Maintenance	Support group indicated significant greater improvements in depression and caregiver burden at	Not specified

Table 6.2 (continued)

agencies, social services, visiting home health agencies, or self-referrals Forty-two in both support group and routine care *Family carers*: 65% female; 65% parents; middle class *Consumers*: average illness duration = 10 years; average BPRS score = 9.8; otherwise, no other demographic information specified	Caregiver Support Group Procedure Manual. Its content mainly included: introduction and orientation; caregivers' emotion and feelings toward care-giving; consumers' reactions and behavior problems to illness; taking care of self and doing positive things with consumer; information of resources, financial issues, and service and medical needs; and review and future planning *Routine Care Group*: received community mental health care (its content was not specified)	month after intervention), using questionnaires	Scale Instrumental ADL Care-giving Self-Efficacy Scale Brief Psychiatric Rating Scale Participants' perceived benefits questionnaire	immediate and 1-month after intervention than routine care From the data of perceived benefits, the group participants indicated high level of satisfaction with support group experiences, especially for having someone listen to their concerns, helping with emotional feelings of the illness; and providing strategies in stress coping

Table 6.3 Summary of qualitative studies on family-led mutual support groups

Lemmens, G.M., Wauters, S., Heireman, M., Eisler, I., Lietaer, G., and Sabbe, B. (2003)	Belgium	Twelve family carers and 10 people of different mental illnesses (e.g., major depression and schizoaffective disorder) in two family discussion groups of a psychiatric day clinic *Carers*: mainly spouse and mother; otherwise, no other demographic information specified *Consumers*: 60% female; mean age = 34 years	*Family discussion group*: family-led support groups, contained 5–6 bi-weekly sessions (1.5 h each), using a systemic multiple-family therapy model. Its content focused on families' coping and problem-solving, impacts of the illness on family interactions, resources and family life-cycle issues; and 4–6 family members (consumer included) in each group. After 6 sessions, there were monthly regular meetings over 2 years	Qualitative, exploratory study, using questionnaire Questionnaires were completed by family members, therapists and observers	Open-ended questions for perceptions of therapeutic factors in group, and experiences that the participants considered helpful for individual, family, and the group	Therapeutic team and families diverged in their perceptions of which factors are important in the discussion group The team members indicated that the relational climate, involvement and support from the group were more helpful. The families placed more emphasis on the process aspects (experiencing communality and gaining insight)	N/A

Table 6.3 (continued)

McCann, G. (1993)	UK	Twenty-one relatives or friends of mental health consumers participated in a relative support group (>1 year) at Ashworth Special Hospital, Merseyside. Relatives & Consumers: no demographic information was specified	Relatives' support group: contained monthly 1.5-h sessions. Its content mainly focused on enhancing support networks. Participants took turns writing up the minutes of each meeting	Cohort study, retrospective qualitative study, using the minutes of meetings and questionnaires	Qualitative analysis of the minutes of 12 meetings. A self-designed questionnaire with 7 questions to evaluate the group	From the minutes, consumer care within hospital, preparation for discharge, and after-care were the most predominant issues identified. Perceived benefits of group participation included: information of the illness and its treatment, maintaining hope, and more involvement in consumer care	N/A

Table 6.3 (continued)

Winefield, H., Barlow, J., and Harvey, E. (1998)	Australia	Thirty-six family members of a relative with schizophrenia were recruited. Eight from extreme positions on 4 criteria: (1) length of time since consumer's diagnosis; (2) amount of carer–consumer contact; (3) level of psychological distress; and (4) level of rejecting attitudes to consumer. *Family carers*: 19% parent and 2% spouse; otherwise, no other demographic information specified. *Consumers*: no demographic information specified	*Discussion-based support groups*: contained 8 sessions in 3 series. Group content mainly included: introduction and discussion about carers' worst problems; update on psychiatric models, medication, and community resources; recognition of early warning signs of relapse; communication and problem-solving; how carers care for themselves and maintain hope; lobbying for resources; and summary and follow-up plans. Family participants led the group discussions	Exploratory, qualitative design, using tape recording of group sessions	Participants' responses to group participation, short- and long-term effects, and suggestions on how groups might be selected and structured for optimal effectiveness	Support group participants emphasized the importance of accurate information on the illness, respect from health professionals, and duration of care-giving experience. Their short-term needs addressed by the group included: understanding mental health services, knowledge of medication, and consumer's problem behavior. Their long-term needs addressed by regular participation included greater sense of control in caring and less perceived care-giving burden	N/A

Table 6.3 (continued)

Chien et al. (2006b)	HK	A convenience sample of 30 family carers and 10 people with schizophrenia participated in a 12-session mutual support group in psychiatric clinics *Carers*: 53% female; mean age = 39.1 years; 100% Chinese; 90% child, parent or spouse *Consumers*: 60% female; mean age = 24.1 years; average illness duration = 2 years	*Mutual support group*: contained 12 bi-weekly, 2-h sessions facilitated by a trained psychiatric nurse and a peer leader. A protocol was designed to guide the 5-phased group development: orientation; sharing of feelings and concerns; understanding about self and consumer needs; adopting new care-giving roles; and preparation for future	Exploratory, qualitative study design, using interviews and tape recording of group sessions	Semi-structured interview (34 first and follow-up interviews) at 2 weeks after completion of intervention, and audiotape recording of 12 sessions Appraisals of the group process and feelings toward the group, benefits, and difficulties in group participation	Three main themes from interview and group session data included: positive personal changes attributed to group participation (e.g., enhanced acceptance of care-giving role and increased knowledge of the illness); positive group characteristics (e.g., explicit group ideology and consensus and social empowerment; and inhibitors of group development	10%

Table 6.3 (continued)

(e.g., enhanced acceptance of care-giving role and increased knowledge of the illness); positive group characteristics (e.g., explicit group ideology and consensus and social empowerment; and inhibitors of group development (e.g., peer pressure and intense negative feelings) affective disorder (range 15–32%), and dementia (about 5%); however, two studies did not report the consumers' psychiatric diagnosis. Consumers mean age was about 31 years (age range 18–76 years). Five studies reported the consumers' hospitalizations, ranging from 2.5 to 7 times, or 0–40 days in the past 6 months; and only four of them reported the education level and working status of the consumers (mainly primary school education and unemployed).

For the four qualitative studies, one of them (McCann, 1993) did not report about any characteristics of the families and mental health consumers. For the other three studies (Chien, Norman, & Thompson, 2006b, Lemmems et al., 2003; Winefield, Barlow, & Harvey, 1998), only Chien et al. had more detailed description of the characteristics of the caregivers, who were mainly female (53% in Chien et al., study only) and parents or spouses (70%), with mean age of 39 years. The people with mental health problems in studies by Chien et al. and Lemmens et al. had a mean age 24 and 34 years, respectively, and a short duration of illness (1–2 years).

The 12 studies mainly used one type of data collection method – a set of questionnaire or a qualitative interview; and only three studies used two types of methods – a set of questionnaire and qualitative analysis of group process (Pickett-Schenk & Heller, 1998; Winefield & Harvey, 1995) or semi-structured interviews and audio-taped recordings of group sessions (Chien et al., 2006b). Nearly all ($n = 6$) of the quantitative studies reviewed measured a variety of families' psychosocial conditions using standardized measures such as family burden, social support, levels of stress and coping ability, community service utilization, and knowledge of mental illness. The remaining one study measured family outcomes, using self-designed or non-standardized research instruments such as perceived group benefits, information, coping, and social support (Pickett-Schenk & Heller, 1998). In addition, five studies measured specific client outcomes such as relapse, psychiatric symptoms, and functioning.

For the 12 studies reviewed, two were conducted in the United States, two in Australia, one in the United Kingdom, and one in Belgium. Six studies were conducted in Asia (five in Hong Kong and one in Taiwan).

With regard to methodological limitations, only five studies reviewed included experimental designs with randomized samples. Thus, there is limited empirical evidence on the effects of mutual support groups to families of people with mental illness and clear implications for future research and practice. Most of the eight quantitative studies used a great variety of standardized or self-designed family-related measures and very brief descriptions of the development, structure, and content of the intervention used. Only three studies (Chien, Chan, Morrissey, & Thompson, 2005; Chien, Chan, & Thompson, 2006a; Chien, Thompson, & Norman, 2008) made reference to a power calculation, and whether the other studies are sufficiently powered is open to question.

Four of the eight quantitative studies reviewed did not report the attrition rate, while reported attrition rates varied (range 10–100%). A few reasons for discontinuation from the support groups were reported (Chien et al., 2006a; Winefield & Harvey, 1995), including inconvenient or insufficient time to attend, inadequate leadership, lack of comfort with other group members, and not having another person to take care of the mental health consumer.

It is noteworthy that the structure and content of the family-driven mutual support groups reported in the studies reviewed varied substantially. For example, the period of intervention varied from four 2-h weekly sessions at a psychiatric unit to continuous, 1–2-h weekly or monthly sessions affiliated to the Alliance of the Mentally Ill in the United States. Despite a few common topics including knowledge of the illness and its treatment, principles of managing mental health consumer's problem behavior and information about community resources, major components and format of the group sessions within the support group programs were not clearly described or structured. This limits the potential for generalization and replication of the intervention in future research and practice. It is also important to recognize that in more than half of the studies reviewed, the mutual support groups only included the family members or main carers; and the consumers were excluded from attending the group meetings. There was no explanation of the rationale for the exclusion of consumers' group participation.

6.3.3 Major Findings on the Effects and Process of Mutual Support Groups

6.3.3.1 Four Experimental Studies Reviewed

Table 6.1 summarizes the five studies that used an experimental design (Albramowitz & Coursey, 1989, in the United States; Chien et al., 2005, 2006a, 2008, and Fung and Chien, 2002, in Hong Kong). One of them followed up the sample for 6 months (Chien et al., 2005), one for 12 months (Chien et al., 2008), and one for 18 months (Chien et al., 2006a). The outcome measures used in these studies varied but most of them were family-related outcome measures, particularly family burden, functioning, self-efficacy, knowledge about the illness and its treatment, stress and coping ability, and social support measures. Only Chien et al. (2005) and Chien et al.'s (2006a) study consisted of a few consumer outcome measures, including mental state, symptom severity, functional level, and medication compliance assessment.

Albramowitz and Coursey's (1989) study reported that the support group showed significant greater improvement in personal distress and management of family life, reduction of anxiety, and increase of community resources utilization, when compared to routine community care. Three controlled trials in Hong Kong (Chien et al., 2005, 2006a, 2008; Fung & Chien, 2002) reported that Chinese family carers and consumers in the mutual support groups indicated statistically significant improvements on family and consumers' psychosocial functioning and/or mental state at 1 week, 6, 12, and/or 18 months after completion of the intervention, when compared with their counterparts in the psycho-education and routine care groups. However, these studies suggested that difficulties in engaging family members to group participation and reducing their attrition in the group process imposed limitations to the findings of the mutual support group studies (Chien et al., 2006a).

6.3.3.2 Quasi-Experimental Studies Using a Non-Equivalent Comparison Group

Table 6.2 summarizes the three quasi-experimental studies (Winefield & Harvey, 1995; Pickett-Schenk & Heller, 1998; Chou et al., 2002) which were conducted in different countries (i.e., the United States, Australia, and Taiwan) and compared the effects between mutual support group and routine psychiatric care or another type of multiple-family group intervention (i.e., psycho-education and professional-led education) for family members of people with schizophrenia or other severe mental illnesses. The outcomes measured varied substantially, focusing mainly on family's psychosocial conditions such as social support, depression, and burden.

Pickett-Schenk and Heller (1998) compared the effects of a professional-led and a family-led support group for 131 families of people with mental illness in Chicago and Southern Illinois. Despite the lack significant differences on coping ability and group benefit ratings between groups, the two groups indicated that the intervention provided the participants with needed information about the mental illness and its treatment and improved their relationship with their consumer family member. The researchers recommended that a joint collaboration between mental health professionals and peer family as co-leaders that can share both experience and expertise in care-giving might work best for a family support group.

Significant positive family-related outcomes of mutual support groups were identified in three of the five studies reviewed. Outcomes included an increase in knowledge about the illness after intervention (Chou et al., 2002), family and peer support and positive attitudes toward consumer family members over 2-month follow-up (Winefield & Harvey, 1995), and a reduction of depression and burden over 1-month follow-up (Chou et al., 2002).

Two studies (Chou et al., 2002; Winefield & Harvey, 1995) collected qualitative data of families' feedback on mutual support group participation and its benefits using one open-ended question. Findings summarized from the written feedback indicated that most of the participants expressed satisfaction with the group experience and perceived several benefits from their group participation, including: increased confidence from sharing with others their concerns, emotions, and difficulties in care-giving; learning some effective strategies and skills to cope with caring situations; and receiving useful information of mental illness and its management.

6.3.3.3 Qualitative Exploratory Studies

Little is known about the various factors that are beneficial to the participants of mutual support groups for family caregivers of people with severe mental illness. The four qualitative exploratory studies reviewed attempted to increase the understanding of the factors perceived as helpful by family caregivers in support group participation. Two of the studies were conducted in European countries, one in Hong Kong, and one in Australia. Several different methods of data collection were used, including questionnaires, tape-recording of group sessions, and open-ended interviews. McCann (1993) evaluated the group progress and benefits to 21 relatives of people with severe mental health problems in a psychiatric hospital in the United Kingdom, using the minutes of 12 monthly sessions of a support group. Chien et al. (2006b) interviewed (once or twice) a convenience sample of 30 family caregivers and 10 people with schizophrenia or psychosis who had participated in a 12-session mutual support group at a psychiatric outpatient clinic in Hong Kong and tape-recorded all 12 support group sessions for content analysis. Winefield et al. (1998) tape-recorded 36 participants' responses during meetings of support groups for family caregivers of people with schizophrenia in Australia, whereas Lemmens et al. (2003) in Belgium collected data on the perceived therapeutic factors and positive experiences in a support group from 12 family caregivers of consumers with different types of severe mental illnesses, group facilitators, and group observers using a self-report, open-ended questionnaire. From these studies, several common perceived benefits of group participation were identified, including: information on the illness, its treatment, available services, and effects of medication; respect and support from group members and professionals; and better coping with care-giving situations.

McCann (1993) indicated that family caregivers emphasized their confidence in conducting and managing the group themselves; and from group participation, they gained more hope of consumer recovery and involvement in consumer care. Winefield et al. (1998) indicated that frequent and consistent support group participation increased caregivers' sense of control in care-giving and reduced their burden of care. However, length of caring experience may affect their involvement and responsiveness to group discussions and activities. The results of the study showed that the caregivers with more care-giving experience were more involved in the support group and perceived group participation to be more beneficial.

However, Lemmens et al. (2003) found that the perceptions of a support group may differ between family participants and health professionals as facilitators or observers. The caregivers indicated that the process aspects of a support group, such as experiencing communality of caring situations and gaining insight from others' sharing of experiences and coping methods of difficult situations are very important and helpful to them. Professionals emphasized the importance of group structure and climate, such as enhancing group involvement, ensuring adequate support from the group, and the provision of specific interventions to meet every member's health needs.

6.4 Discussion

Mutual support groups are informal networks of individuals who share a common experience or issue. Despite the widespread use of different self-help programs and initiatives across Canada, the United States, and the United Kingdom for a range of problems, such as grief and bereavement, chronic physical diseases, and substance abuse (Carpenter, 1997; Lorig et al., 2000; Mankowski et al., 2001), there is little research evidence in the past two decades supporting its effectiveness or identifying its therapeutic elements. What emerges from the research articles reviewed in this chapter is that they can be potentially effective in building family participants' personal skills, empowerment and social support. In addition, only 12 research studies hitherto have investigated the helping and supportive process or the short-term effects of mutual support groups for family members in caring for a relative with severe mental illness. In fact, family mutual support studies for severe mental illnesses in Western and Asian countries is replete with cross-sectional surveys, prospective cohort studies, and quasi-experimental approaches with non-equivalent groups (i.e., more than 40 studies of those excluded in this literature review), emphasizing the apparent benefits of group participation in maintaining the psychological and social well-being of family caregivers (Chien et al., 2005; Heller et al., 1997).

Nevertheless, there exists a solid foundation of support group research in both the quantitative and qualitative approaches used in the 12 studies reviewed, describing some types of problems within these families typically addressed through their group participation, such as improved access to information and community resources and perceptions of greater social support (Winefield et al., 1998). These research findings in the last two decades support further investigation of the benefits of support groups in improving both family and client functioning, and in satisfying families' long-term psychosocial health needs (Szmukler et al., 2003). This may also explain why in the recent reviews of clinical trials of family intervention for schizophrenia by the Cochrane Review Group (Barbato & D'Avanzo, 2000; Pharoah et al., 2001) do not include any studies with a mutual support group approach.

Only two of the four experimental studies or clinical trials reviewed (Chien et al., 2005, 2006a) showed that mutual support groups were more effective in producing long-term health or other benefits for family members, compared with other treatment models. Nevertheless, all of these studies demonstrated that mutual support groups could produce consistent short-term positive impacts to the family caregivers such as knowledge about the illness and family burden and functioning. Significant longer-term benefits (i.e., at least 1 year following intervention) have not been demonstrated possibly because of methodological limitations on study design and organization, facilitation, and progress monitoring of the intervention. For example, Fung and Chien (2002) pointed to the difficulties of getting families to engage in the support group with the result, that the support group participants in their study reported a low rate of group attendance (30% attended less than half of the group meetings). In addition, the length of the support groups varied substantially, ranging from 2 months to more than 9 months. The content and format of the intervention, including peer leadership, group facilitation by professionals, and mutual helping between participants within and outside group meetings were not clearly defined. As suggested by Biegel, Elizabeth, and Kennedy's (2000) review of family caretaker studies (single-family or group work), the variations and ambiguities identified in the design of the educational and supportive programs in recent studies might have affected findings on the effectiveness of a mutual support group in promoting family health.

The four qualitative studies reviewed attempted to explore the perceived benefits of family members participating in a mutual support group and their feedback on the strengths and limitations of the group. Four potential therapeutic mechanisms of the family-driven mutual support groups are identified and their key elements summarized in Fig 6.1. The four mechanisms were

> M1: Reconstructing a new positive self-image (role identity) in relation to care-giving;
> M2: Establishing and focusing on clear, realistic common goals, and tasks within group;
> M3: Psychological empowerment of caregivers through the acquisition of knowledge and skills for care-giving; and
> M4: Extending social support network both within and outside the group.

The flow diagram in Fig. 6.1 also presents the stages of group development used in a few reviewed experimental studies (Chien et al., 2005, 2006b, 2008), associated with and the potential outcomes achieved by each mechanism. The five phases or stages of group development have been used in this modality of support group intervention and are generally accepted by mental health professionals (Chien et al., 2005; Galinsky & Schopler, 1995; Wilson, 1995). The use of phases, instead of definite tasks or topics of each group session, allows flexibility in time and task achievement, and is thought to foster the development of trust, autonomy, closeness, and interdependence, and even successful termination of group (Wilson, 1995).

Some of the potential outcomes outlined in Fig. 6.1 were demonstrated by the findings of the three experimental studies conducted by the authors (Fung & Chien, 2002; Chien et al., 2005, 2006b). These included: decreased family burden, which might be enhanced through construction of a new positive self-image for care-giving (M1); increased perceived social support, which might result from the psychological empowerment of carers through the acquisition of knowledge and skills for care-giving (M3); extending social support network both within and outside the mutual support group (M4); and improved family functioning, which might be promoted by establishing and focusing on clear, realistic common goals and tasks within the group (M2). These four therapeutic mechanisms of mutual support groups suggested by the author are subject to testing and evaluation in future research.

In addition, one major hindrance to the success of the support group was also identified within one of the four mechanisms. The expression of intensive and negative emotions at an early stage of the group and the presence of dominant and forceful behavior of a few experienced caregivers might negatively affect some family caregivers' reconstruction of their positive identity (M1), and increase their difficulty in engaging in group participation. These caregivers might need individualized psychological support and encouragement by peer members and group facilitators to have better engagement in the support group.

6 An Overview of Mutual Support Groups for Family Caregivers

Mechanisms	Related factors identified in 5 stages of group development	Potential outcomes
M1: Reconstructing a new positive self-image (role identity) in relation to caregivng - Building trust, mutual respect and understanding between group members - Sharing of information and views of schizophrenia - Sharing of positive and successful experiences of caregiving	Stage 1 - Orientation and engaging in the group: - Orientation and increasing involvement in group participation - Building trust and mutual acceptance - Facing difficulties in engaging to the group	- Better engagement and involvement in group activities - Improved self-image and responsibility for caregiving - *Decreased burden of care*
Negative factors: - Expression of intense and negative emotions at early stage of the group - Dominant and forceful behavior of a few experienced carers (group members)		Increased difficulty in engaging to group participation: - need more individualized psychological support and encouragement
M2: Establishing and focusing on clear, realistic common goals and tasks within group - Discuss and agree on explicit goal and direction in the first and/or second session - Task orientation and focusing on goal achievement	Stage 1 to 2 – Orientation and engaging in the group; Being aware of own feelings and concerns regarding caregiving - Setting clear realistic common goals - Perception of better control over own life situation	- Creating altruism and commitment to achieve the purposes of participation in the support group - Enhanced learning of problem solving and caregiving skills - Improved family functioning
M3: Psychological empowerment of carers through the acquisition of knowledge and skills for caregiving - Sharing of information about the illness, its treatment and services available - Sharing of positive and successful experiences in caregiving - Learning of problem solving and practical skills for caregiving from other members	Stage 3 – Understanding about family needs and available support services - Learning and adoption of effective coping strategies - Effective communication with patient and family - Participation in decision making	- Increased knowledge, supportive resources and skills for caregiving - Enabled to have control over patient and family care - Increased social support
M4: Extending social support network both within and outside the support group - Internal supportive environment from group members considered 'family members' - External supportive environment from family members, close friends and health professionals	Stage 4 & 5 – Adoption of new roles and challenges in caregiving; preparation for separation and future life - Recognizing support and learning from the group as rewarding - Discussing about future planning and ongoing group meetings - Evaluation of learning from the group	- Received more psychological support and practical assistance from others - Continued family support after termination of the group - Increased social support and its network

(Mutual Support Group)

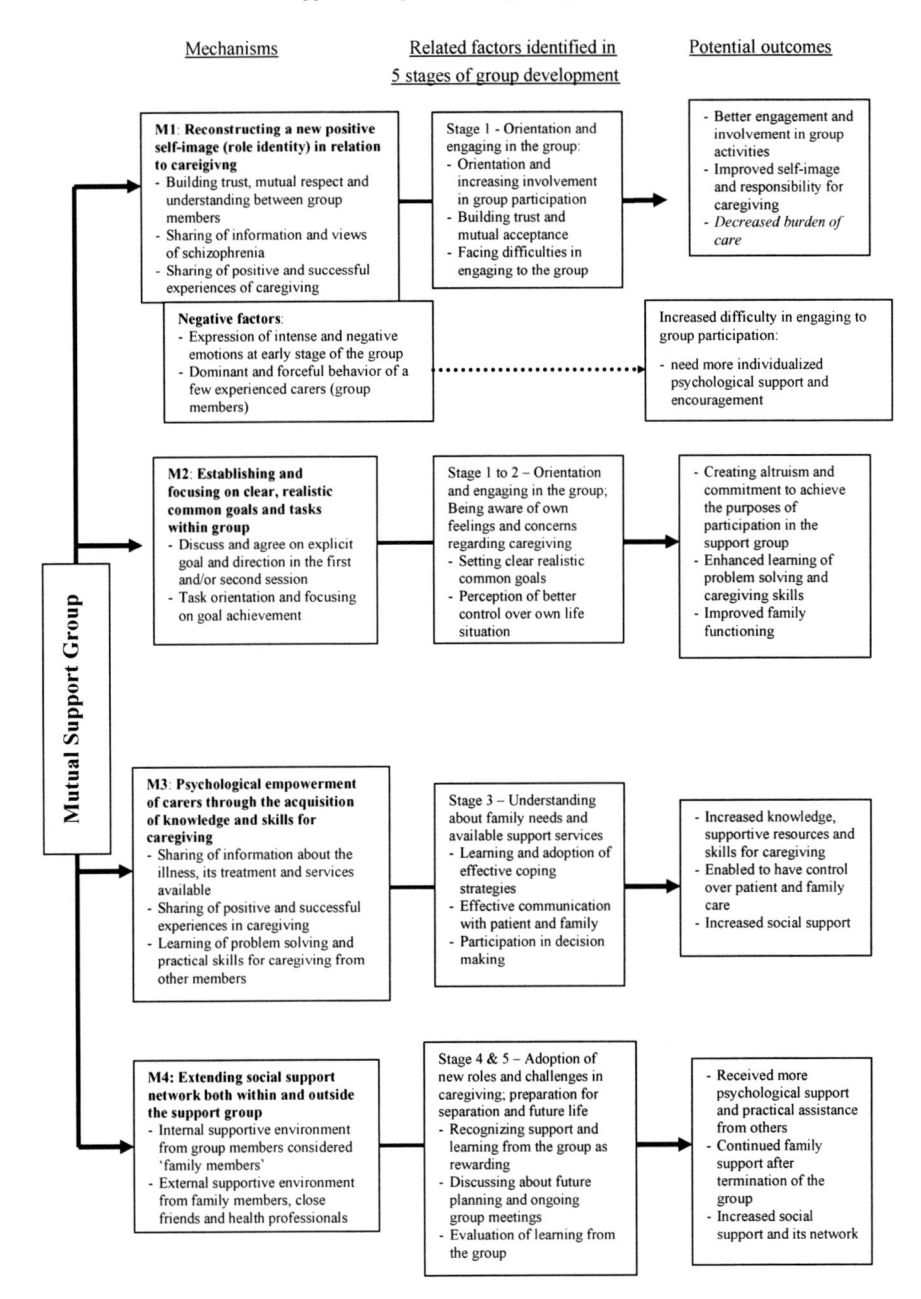

Fig. 6.1 Four therapeutic mechanisms of mutual support groups

Lemmens et al. (2003) acknowledged that there has been little research on the process of change in family group interventions for schizophrenia and other severe mental illnesses. The described curative factors and positive changes in the four studies consist of impressionistic accounts by therapists of what they believed to be the most important factors according to their clinical experience, such as generating new illness perspectives and family roles (Stein & Wemmerus, 2001) and experiencing hope and identification with other group members (Asen, 2002).

In fact, the nature of mutual support groups and other approaches of family intervention are multi-faceted and complex (Pharoah et al., 2001). Brooker (2001) suggested that the hesitation of clinicians to use family group intervention might be attributed to inadequate knowledge of the researcher on the key therapeutic components within groups. It is noteworthy that little is known about the therapeutic components of mutual support groups as well as other approaches to family intervention, which may facilitate the design of family caretaker interventions and thus produce optimal benefits for consumers and their families.

6.4.1 Cultural and Methodological Issues in Family Mutual Support Groups

Six of the 12 studies reviewed were conducted in a sample of Asian populations (Chien et al., 2005, 2006a, 2006b, 2008, and Fung and Chien, 2002 in Hong Kong; Chou et al., 2002 in Taiwan). Despite the fact that psycho-education programs are the most common approach to family intervention used in western and Asian countries, these five studies provide evidence that mutual support groups can be an effective approach to family intervention for non-Caucasian populations (Xiong et al., 1994; Chou et al., 2002). In Hong Kong and mainland China, mutual support groups have been organized as very brief programs with only three to four sessions held at health care centers and residential homes by community psychiatric nurses (Ma & Yip, 1997) and often lack well-structured guidelines and constant monitoring of the group process (Pearson & Ning, 1997). Therefore, there is a need for formal evaluation of both short- and long-term effects of the support groups, which originated from the West, on families and consumers' health conditions in Asian populations.

Most of the studies reviewed focused on mainly chronic mental illness in community care settings (an average of more than 8 years of mental illness) and the support groups were mostly facilitated by social workers, psychiatrists, or psychologists rather than psychiatric nurses. Due to the methodological limitations of most of the studies reviewed, including non-probability samples, non-equivalent groups, and a wide variety of research instruments, the effects of the support group programs on family health remains inconclusive. In addition, about two-thirds of the studies did not test the long-term effects of participation. As a result, many questions about the effects of mutual support groups for family caregivers of people with severe mental illness on either the families' health condition or consumers' recovery remain unanswered.

The majority of the studies reviewed had very brief descriptions of the group intervention used; no specific protocol or clear guidelines for the group sessions, and unknown procedures or mechanisms for monitoring the group progress. Failure to provide a clear description of the content and process of mutual support groups reduces understanding of the intervention and may limit replication of the intervention and its evaluation in other samples. In addition, limited attention to the establishment of trust, belongingness, and harmony in the early stages of group development along with the provision of continuous encouragement and support to each family caregiver throughout group participation may have reduced the motivation and interest of the caregivers in attending the group, thus increasing dropout.

6.4.2 Learning from Development of and Evaluation on Family Mutual Support Groups

The authors of this chapter have conducted a few evaluation studies on family mutual support groups for Chinese people with schizophrenia in Hong Kong (e.g., Chien et al., 2005, 2006a, 2006b, 2008 reviewed). The mutual support groups designed for family caregivers of people with schizophrenia in their clinical trials consisted of 12–18 bi-weekly, 2-h sessions over 6–9 months, which is an optimal duration of the family intervention suggested in systematic reviews by Barbato and D'Avanzo (2000) and Pharoah et al. (2001). Similar to other support groups, those groups aimed to provide reciprocal support and assistance among the family caregivers participating in the group, which might not be provided by health professionals. A few important issues are raised below for consideration in developing mutual support groups for family caregivers of people with severe mental health problems.

First, the mutual support group programs designed by the authors were clearly structured and organized. The support groups were developed mainly in terms of five phases. In discussing theories of small-sized group intervention, the concept of developmental phases generally arises when exploring the pattern of group development (Yalom, 1998). Throughout the five phases of group development (i.e., engaging, recognition of caregivers' own psychological needs, dealing with psychosocial needs of self and family, adopting new roles and challenges, and ending), group members perform a variety of roles, mainly group building, group maintenance, task performance, and individual caring and counseling. Therefore, they themselves share the power of self-determination, information and skills exchange, group dynamic, and participative management (Yalom, 1998; Sampson & Murtha, 1997). Indeed, groups have a natural history of development; these five phases of group development used in the mutual support group intervention were the generally accepted ones for group therapy in the literature of health, social, and behavioral sciences (Cragan & Wright, 1999). The use of this phased development in the mutual support group was preferred to the identification of definite tasks or topics for each group session; on the other hand, this allowed flexibility in time, task achievement, development of trust, autonomy, closeness, interdependence, and termination of the group (Akinson & Coia, 1995; Wilson, 1995). Furthermore, the group members could have more control in the group development, although the peer leader(s) needed to assist in the smooth and efficient progression of group functions and achievement.

Throughout each group phase, the peer leader of the group made great efforts to maintain telephone contacts with individual group members weekly and encouraged each member to attend the next meeting. When any members of the group found difficulty in attending a group session, the peer leader was responsible for raising these issues in the group meeting and ensuring the group members negotiated a mutually agreed time and venue of the meeting.

Similar to other phase theories in support groups, Wheelan (1994) and Kimberly (1997) delineated the group development in terms of at least five stages, which were incorporated into the 12- or 18-session mutual support group programs used in their studies. The five phases used are: engagement (2–3 sessions), recognition of psychological needs of the whole family (3–4 sessions), dealing with psychosocial needs of self, consumer and other family members (3–5 sessions), adopting new roles and challenges (3–4 sessions), and ending or preparation for group continuation (1–2 sessions). The number of sessions cited in the parentheses was tentative and subject to change in accordance with the group progress and the mutual agreement among the group members. The details of these five phases are described in Table 6.4.

Second, the content and themes of group sessions were reviewed and modified after each group meeting as necessary, based on a few important aspects identified in previous research: careful consideration of the participants' involvement and personal development in the group; the inhibitory factors influencing group and individual benefits; the establishment of group ideology and consensus; and the use of professional and additional support outside the group (Chien et al., 2006b; Schiff & Bargal, 2000).

Third, the timing of meetings for the support groups was decided through common agreement of the group members during the group sessions. Content of the group sessions also varied depending on group decisions. It consisted of group discussion, the provision of information about schizophrenia and treatment by one group member, watching a video and giving feedback, sharing experiences of care-giving and methods of consumer management, role play, and behavioral rehearsal of learned skills from group members or the facilitator. All group sessions involved supportive interventions such as ventilation of feelings, sharing stressful experiences, validation of care-giving experiences, encouragement and praise for providing care, affirmation of the family's coping ability, and support for struggles with difficult situations and disturbing behaviors of consumers. The support group also focused on enhancing participants' self-efficacy in coping by: (a) reviewing similar experiences from every member, whether they have dealt with them successfully or not; (b) making the care-giving situations more manageable using problem-solving strategies and social learning from models or veterans within the group; and (c) altering the cognitive and emotional reactions to these situations by

Table 6.4 Mutual support group program for family caregivers of a relative with schizophrenia

Phase/stage	Theme	Content	Format of sessions	Length of intervention[a]
1. Engagement (introduction)	Who we are; We need to share our experiences and feelings *Goal*: Establish trusting relationships and common goals	• Orientation of the group program (format, duration, content, flexibility, and so forth) by the organizer (researcher) • Introduction of the overall purposes of the group intervention and expectations of each participant • Beginning of sharing common concerns and establishing trust and acceptance; ensuring confidentiality • Negotiation of goals/objectives, rules and norms, and roles and responsibilities • Recognizing and clarifying the role of a peer leader in the group • Initial discussion of the consumers' mental illness, symptoms, behaviors, and their effects on family	• Briefing by facilitator • Discussion among group participants • Video about schizophrenia followed with discussion	2–3 sessions *1st session* *2nd and 3rd session (optional to include consumer)*
2. Recognition of psychological needs	Being aware of and accepting our feelings and reactions *Goal*: Open sharing and more understanding about individual concerns and cultural issues	• Resolution around power, control, and decision-making within group; any need of a peer leader; • Discussion about Chinese culture of their family (e.g., family structure, relationships, and communication patterns) and attitude toward mental illness • Clarifying information and misconceptions about schizophrenia and its related illness behavior	• Discussion • Explanation with leaflet • Discussion with scenarios presented by participants	3–4 sessions *4th session* *5th session*

Table 6.4 (continued)

Phase/stage	Theme	Content	Format of sessions	Length of intervention[a]
		• Exploring and verbalizing the intense emotions and feelings about the difficulties in consumer care provision and family interactions; sharing stories of success and difficulties in living and interacting with consumer family members • Discuss ways to deal with negative feelings and emotions to consumer family members • Encouraging members to face powerlessness and limitations, accepting the "self-as-is" • Focusing and paying specific attention to: (a) helping members to view themselves as "average" or "similar to others" among the group members, not exceptional; and (b) reduction of participants' exaggerated or dysfunctional sense of shame, by sharing and recognizing unrealistic self-expectations, expectations of consumer family members, and externally imposed evaluations	• Discussion and sharing and role modeling by one or two more experienced family carers • Discussion about their expectations and reaction toward social stigma and pressure	*6th session* *7th session*
3. Dealing with psychosocial needs of self and family	Understanding our relative's needs and available community resources	• Discussion about each participant's physical and psychosocial health needs (how they relate to family culture)	• Self-reporting and discussion	3–5 sessions *8th and 9th session*

Table 6.4 (continued)

Phase/stage	Theme	Content	Format of sessions	Length of intervention[a]
	Goal: Adequate understanding about important needs for self, consumer, and family	• Information about medications, management of the illness, and available mental health services for consumer and family • Learning and practice of effective communication skills with consumer; seeking social support from others, e.g., family members and friends • Exploration of appropriate home management strategies, e.g., finance and budgets, social support network, living environment and hygiene	• Explanation and information leaflet • Demonstration, role play, and giving principles • Discussion and sharing experience	(optional to include consumer) *10th –11th session* *12th session*
4. Adopting new roles and challenges	Recognizing and adapting to new roles and challenges in care-giving Goal: Learning from other participants the effective coping skills and management of people with schizophrenia	• Sharing coping skills for the demands of care, family dysfunction and conflict, and positive experiences with consumer family member • Identifying supportive persons who can reduce the burden of care in their social environment • Enhancing problem-solving skills in care-giving and minimizing family conflicts and burden, by working on some individual consumer management situations • Conducting behavioral rehearsals of interactions with consumer and other family members within group	• Discussion • Explanation, case study, and discussion • Role play • Home assignment and evaluation	3–4 sessions *13th and 14th session*

Table 6.4 (continued)

Phase/stage	Theme	Content	Format of sessions	Length of intervention[a]
		• Practicing coping skills learned during the sessions to real family life (in-between group sessions) and evaluate the results • Re-evaluating their family role and responsibility and shared responsibility of care-giving among family members	• Discussion	*15th session* *16th session*
5. Ending	Conclusions – Where will I go from here? *Goal:* Preparing for group termination or continuation	• Preparation and discussion on termination issues, e.g., separation anxiety, independent living, and use of coping skills learned • Evaluation of learning experiences and goals achievement • Discussion about the continuity of care after this group program and the utilization of community supporting resources • Explanation of post-intervention assessment and follow-up taken in the following months	• Discussion	1–2 sessions *17th and 18th session*

Note: [a] A total of 24- or 36-week group intervention was carried out, on a bi-weekly basis. Achievement of the content and themes was reviewed following each group session by the facilitator and researcher.

The mutual support group program was reviewed by an expert panel (including psychiatrists, psychiatric nurses, clinical psychologists, and social workers) and 10 group participants in the pilot testing: One extra session would be conducted for those who were interested in group continuation to discuss for detail arrangement.

clearing up any misconceptions and unrealistic expectations, and getting the members to see themselves as "average" or "similar" when dealing with the difficulties in care-giving faced commonly by all families. The caregivers in the support groups were permitted, and were sometimes encouraged, to meet with each other outside the formal group meetings.

Fourth, nine principles to strengthen mutual support were emphasized within the group and served as the basis of interactions between the group members during meetings.

These principles included: "all-in-the-same boat," "mutual aid and support," "reciprocal demands of giving help and being helped," "self-determination," "sharing information and personal assets," "dialectical process," "discussing a taboo area," "individual problem solving," and "behavioral rehearsal," and are described in Table 6.5.

Fifth, there should be clear definition of the roles of the peer participant as a group leader. Recent studies of mutual support groups have reported that success in any program correlates with more intense mutual help involvement (Kessler et al., 1997). Therefore, it was very important for the peer leader(s) to encourage the group participants to be as actively involved in the group as possible. A training workshop such as the one used by the author that were largely derived from the practical experience and guidelines reported by Akinson and Coia (1995) and Gazda, Ginter, and

Table 6.5 Nine principles to strengthen mutual support groups

Nine principles used in mutual support groups strengthened mutual help and support and served as a guide and ground rules to the facilitator and peer leaders in running the group, as recommended by researchers (Wilson, 1995; Schiff & Bargal, 2000). These principles reflected the demands on families of caring for people with schizophrenia in a non-pathological way. Caring of consumers by the family caregivers in the support group refers to specific actions and interactions that make the consumer feel valued as a person; and the caregivers themselves and their consumers were not blamed to be responsible for the mental illness and its problematic behavior. They consisted of:

1. All-in-the-same boat
There might be differences among the family caregivers who faced a common difficult situation within the group, but above all, they shared this unity of situation, which was the source of their common pain. Therefore, the participants of this mutual support group, similar to family members caring for another consumer population, possessed social homogeneity. They did gain strength as individuals and as a group by coming together and struggling against a common plight and a new way of looking at themselves and how they regarded those outside the group

2. Mutual aid and support
The commonality of situation encouraged empathic feelings flowing among the group members. They needed to care for each other in order to experience release from the stress of the situation, and benefit from the therapeutic effect and understanding of being helped by, and helping others. Having others in the group with the same problem was one of the key strengths of the support group. The peer leader needed to ensure the members to not only consider their own pain, but also reach out to others in empathic ways (Wilson, 1995)

Table 6.5 (continued)

3. Reciprocal demands of giving help and being helped
A productive group culture should be developed, in which there are mutual expectations that the members risk their real thoughts and ideas, listen to each other, and put their own concerns aside at times to help one another. Taken together, mutual support and mutual demand were powerful forces in helping group members in a dialectical fashion, both giving and caring on the one hand, and expecting oneself and others to work on the other (Powell, 1994). Helping others gave the helpers a sense of control: "I can't be helpless if I can help someone else"

4. Self-determination
Group members largely determined social and interpersonal activities within the mutual support group internally. This mechanism allowed a new dimension of participatory democracy to emerge. Self-governance of the group was enhanced by individual contribution and involvement in the process of helping others in the group (Winefield et al., 1998)

5. Sharing information and personal assets
Imparting information (factual, psychological, or personal) and disclosing personal capacities and success in caring can be a meaningful way to build mutual trust and caring. Group building started with the process of locating the assets, skills, and strengths of group members. These strengths and knowledge could then be put to work on individual problems

6. Dialectical process
Participants have opportunities to consider the different ideas and different ways of accomplishing responsibilities with the group, discussing their pros and cons. Where affirmations and doubts about a topic or problem could be challenged, both individuals and the group stood to gain from each other in a dialectical relationship

7. Discussing a taboo area
The shared secret (taboo area) was the basis for the formation of the support group, and the small community of mutual helpers was the source of strength for surmounting an internalized stigma. There could be catharsis, examination of feelings of guilt and shame, expressions of hate and hostility toward consumer family members, grieving over the absence of a needed social relationship, and appraisal of a non-stigmatized helping environment (Galinsky & Schopler, 1995). All of these issues could be ventilated within the group of similar people who did understand and could help one another regain self-respect and self-esteem

8. Individual problem-solving
The mutual support group could serve as a healing agent to help an individual member to deal with his/her own unique troubles. The group leader and members became consultants, assuming the roles of supporter (showing empathy), clarifiers (helping to think through a problem), challengers (help to think and do things in new ways), and listeners (show that they care). As a result of what the members learned from the group, they might be able to initiate or work out self-care and problem-solving strategies for their own use

9. Behavioral rehearsal
Rehearsal of what had been taught frequently took the form of role-playing. The support group was a safe place to risk some "run-throughs" of anxiety-provoking social situations, particularly managing the consumer's problematic and disturbing behaviors. The group could provide support, guide, and offer criticism of the individual's role-playing responses, which were new and unfamiliar

6 An Overview of Mutual Support Groups for Family Caregivers

Horne (2001) should be provided to the peer leader(s). As suggested in the literature, a trained group leader was considered an appropriate person to serve as a facilitator of the group process, particularly giving more guidance and assistance in the early stage of group development (Steinberg, 2004). As suggested by Kurtz (1997) and Stein and Wemmerus (2001), although using different labels for the therapeutic endeavors in the literature, the role of the peer leader in this mutual support group included:

a. Encouraging and modeling information giving and sharing, while relating this process to goals of building trust and a caring context;
b. Eliciting, and if necessary, mediating differing opinions, while pointing out the group's ability to build individuality within group solidarity;
c. Giving guidance and facilitation to discuss taboo areas, while strengthening the group's commitment to confidentiality and safety;
d. Insisting firmly that the need for lifestyle change includes finding an appropriate support system;
e. Calling attention to members' shared situations, thus emphasizing the common bond;
f. Reinforcing and demonstrating empathic responses, with the intention of building mutual support and not blaming or indicting families or consumers for their problems;
g. Supporting individual's demands, while reviewing the expectations for all members about the functions and goals of participation in the group;
h. Allowing individual problem-solving to take place, while helping group members assume consultant roles in dealing with stress, emotional distress, and burden;

The peer leader also takes on these functions, in order to enhance the mutual helping and support atmosphere within the group. Instead of being dependent on the peer leader, the participants should be assisted to find peers who could help them achieve a life of continuing growth through the group intervention (Kyrouz, Humphrey, & Loomis, 2002). Nevertheless, the group leader sought to remain available to the group members if something emotionally and psychologically negative or harmful happened. It was important to recognize and resolve any harm experienced by individual members, which was often related to destructive group dynamics, if a family caregiver was rejected by other group members or felt they had nothing to offer or gain from the group.

Although the leading or facilitating work of the peer leader might not be acknowledged and formalized as a "leader" position, their informal role of coordination and facilitation of the group intervention was considered very important. As suggested by Sampson & Murtha (1997) and Nichols and Jenkinson (2006), these informal group leaders during the group meeting were also able to:

a. Assist and encourage the group to be more transparent and more apt to engage in self-disclosure;

b. Accentuate socially approved behavior through positive reinforcement and encouragement (i.e., focusing on supportive rather than interpretative issues of members);
c. Encourage increased control and the helping function among group members;
d. Reinforce interdependence by pointing out the similarities and differences between members, in the services of increased group cohesion;
e. Act as a role model to nourish an attitude of trust and confidence in participants.

6.4.3 Families Who are Likely to Attend and Benefit from Group Participation

As identified in this review, the majority of the family caregivers benefited from participation in the mutual support groups were female (50–88%) and middle age between 40 and 58 years (48–70%). More than half of them were the parent or spouse (58–68%) of the mental health consumers and had completed elementary or high school education (48–54%). As five of the 12 studies were conducted in Hong Kong or Taiwan, about 30% of the total samples were Chinese (20–100%). Half of the families were from the middle social class (53%); and only one study reported that the families had low household income. These socio-demographic characteristics of family caregivers in the mutual support groups are quite similar to those in other family- and professional-driven support groups in the United States and other western countries. However, there are only 12 studies identified in this review. The samples in these studies were demographically non-representative. In particular, western populations were under-represented. Previous research has also suggested that the experience of having a family member with severe mental health problems may differ among ethnic groups (Solomon et al., 1997; Telles et al., 1995). Therefore, our acceptance of these specific families as the main groups of caregivers who would be likely to attend and benefit from the group participation should be cautious.

In half of the studies reviewed with significant positive results in the mutual support groups (four experimental studies by Fung & Chien, 2002; Chien et al., 2005, 2006a, 2008, in Hong Kong; one quasi-experimental study by Winefield & Harvey, 1995, in Australia; and two qualitative studies by Winefield et al., 1998; Chien et al., 2006b), the patients' illness had been of a relatively short duration (i.e., 77% of them had been ill for less than 3 years). These families might have been more optimistic and motivated about the potential for change (Schiff & Bargal, 2000) than families of patients who had a more chronic illness. This also emphasizes the need for family support services to offer accessible and early intervention after discharge from hospital (Craig et al., 2004). The peer leader of the support group contributed much time and effort in encouraging and assisting group members to attend the meetings; for example, in Chien et al.'s studies, the peer leaders used telephone calls and face-to-face contacts with the participants, and the provision of transport and practical help to facilitate attending group meetings. As a result, there were very low dropouts from the groups (5–10%) over the initial 6–9 months period. The follow-up and constant encouragement by the peer leaders (and other group members) served to reinforce and maintain the effects of the intervention over the follow-up period (Dixon et al. 2000).

In addition, those family caregivers in the mutual support groups (Chien et al., 2005, 2006a, 2006b, 2008) who emphasized the importance of individual problem-solving and the provision of practical aids to one another, both within and outside the group, perceived group participation to be more beneficial. The degree of contact and support received outside the formal group sessions identified from Chien et al.'s study groups were greater than in other types of support group researched previously. The perceived benefits of social contact and practical assistance between the group members outside the group meetings in dealing with immediate and important care-giving difficulties and problems was emphasized and positively appraised by the family caregivers during their individual interviews. There was evidence for this also from the tape-recorded data of the group sessions. These unique features might explain the fact that, even though the mutual support group sometimes only included the primary caregivers and excluded the patients, the benefits of their participation in the support group were able to extend to the consumer and the entire family. These mechanisms are also consistent with Chinese culture and family practices, in that Chinese people have a strong sense of kinship and cohesiveness with their extended families (Lee & Liu, 2001); and they prefer and benefit more from collective, inter-dependent, and practical assistance and support than from frequent discussions and sharing of problem-solving techniques and successful care-giving experiences during the group sessions.

6.4.4 Barriers to Development of Mutual Support Groups

There were a wide variety of obstacles to the group development and contingency plans identified in relevant literature and research. The group facilitator and the group members set out to build mutual support and should be cognizant of the potential obstacles for mutual aid such as conflicts and dominance, which might exist in the support group. Additionally, the group facilitator and researcher should be aware of over-identifying with the family caregivers' resistance to attending the group meetings. They should help and encourage them to find an adequate and effective social support system, and thus better cope with their care-giving role (Steinberg, 2004; Buchkremer et al., 1995). The findings of the mutual support group research conducted by the authors highlighted a few potential obstacles to group development, which are similar to other support group studies and experiences (Borkman, 1999; Nichols & Jenkinson, 2006; Pickett-Schenk & Heller, 1998), are discussed as follows.

6.4.4.1 An Irregular or Low Attendance by Group Members

It has been commonly but inappropriately accepted that attendance of a social or therapeutic group may be poor. There are various reasons for poor attendance, and people with low attendance can be more difficult to integrate into the mutual-aid social world. Problems such as difficulties with transportation, inconvenient meeting location, and other barriers to attendance need to be carefully considered and resolved. Family caregivers with low group attendance in the evaluation studies discussed several difficulties due to low attendance, such as: "building a more trusting relationship and an intimate and open social climate," "achievement of common goals and contracts," and "positive behavioral changes and effective coping skills for care-giving" (Chien et al., 2006b, pp. 7–12). Therefore, more attention needs to be paid to encouraging regular and continued attendance of group members, in particular by ensuring flexibility in the time of group meetings, and by regularly contacting group members and encouraging participation. Contacts should come not only from the facilitator, but also from the more enthusiastic group members (Luke, Roberts, & Rappaport, 1993; Steinberg, 2004).

6.4.4.2 Difficulty of Inexperienced or Young Caregivers in Establishing Social Relationships

When starting a group, there might be a few young or inexperienced caregivers who find it difficult to express their own concerns and needs in care-giving or identify with the troubles and suffering of other group members (i.e., inability to form caring relationships). More help and support should be directed to these members in the first and second meetings with the more experienced caregivers discussing their caring experiences, both successful and failed. The inexperienced caregivers may then be more confident and willing to share their views and experiences following the sharing of the experienced caregivers.

6.4.4.3 A General Failure Concerning Group Development

Certain unspoken rules and roles within the group may prevent sustained cooperative efforts. For example, unspoken rules about what may or may not be talked about within the support group oppose the value of openness among group members. Therefore, groups need to be flexible in allowing personal interests and issues to be discussed during the group meetings. Tasks and activities should be done collaboratively among group members, instead of being a single member's work.

6.4.4.4 Difficulty in Establishing the Norm of Open and Honest Communication

Open and honest communication is an important group norm. However, some of the group members might find it embarrassing and uncomfortable to expose some personal, unpleasant events, or the harmful or painful consequences for which they were responsible. Participants needed time and encouragement to open themselves up to others. It is also important to have active group members' mutual sharing and concern, which is critical to diminishing embarrassment and suspicion.

6.5 Implications for Research and Practice

This literature review highlights the need for more empirical evidence on the effectiveness of mutual support groups for family caregivers of people with severe mental illnesses, especially with regard to its effects over time (e.g., at least 2 years follow-up) on families and consumers' health statuses. The review also indicates a need for investigations on the benefits and therapeutic mechanisms of the support group as perceived by the group participants and to describe the stages of group development. Insight into these processes is currently limited by the availability of only a few qualitative studies. Future research can address several important issues indicated in this review that most other studies neglected, as follows:

a. Research should pay attention to treatment integrity, which is known to enhance the effect of an intervention and increase the power of the study and the validity of results. More randomized controlled trials can be used, with a treatment protocol to guide the group development and process, to evaluate the effectiveness of the mutual support group compared to routine psychiatric care and/or other intervention approaches.
b. Studies need to conduct a long-term follow-up of psychosocial health data from both family caregivers and their mental health consumers in order to understand the substantive effect of mutual support groups. Future research can examine a variety of psychosocial outcomes, using standardized and valid measures such as family burden and functioning, perceived social support, and mental health care services utilization by these families; and consumers' psychosocial functioning, medication compliance, and symptom improvement.
c. Regarding feasibility in practice, it is also important to test whether a health professional (e.g., a community psychiatric nurse) who only received a brief training in support group facilitation can manage the group well and thus produce significant positive outcomes; compared with other approaches of family intervention such as cognitive behavioral therapy (e.g., Haddock et al., 1999) and psycho-education groups (McFarlane, 2002), in which group facilitators received substantially more training.
d. Further practice and research on support groups should carefully consider socio-cultural conditions, which may influence the structure and process of the group. Successful family group work requires adaptation of the intervention in response to relevant cultural factors. For example, as suggested by Bae and Kung (2000), in working with Chinese families, it is important to recognize the family functions and processes (e.g., emphasis on mutual respect and positive practical help and actions for family members rather than talking), and take advantage of these cultural factors in group work.
e. The evaluation research experiences of the authors on mutual support groups for Chinese families of people with schizophrenia indicate a few important issues in the design and implementation of a mutual support group. The principles, stages of development, training of facilitators, roles of facilitator and peer leader, and the potential inhibitors of mutual support groups can be considered or adopted by

health professionals interested in supporting these groups and family caregivers who lead the groups.

f. Finally, it is useful to conduct a concurrent and retrospective process evaluation of the group intervention process, using rigorous qualitative methods such as grounded theory or ethnographic approaches, to identify the perceived benefits, group integrity and development, and therapeutic components and mechanisms of a support group from the participants' perspective, and any changes in the experience of individual members and the group overall, in the course of the intervention.

6.6 Conclusion

An increasing recognition and acceptance of mutual support groups as a means of helping people with chronic and severe mental illness and their families is part of a broader self-help movement that has progressed worldwide, particularly in the United States, attracting people who encounter common problems to group together for mutual help and emotional support. Theoretical models discussed in the background for this literature review such as stress-vulnerability and coping, social comparison, and social learning theories highlighted the important concepts applied to and the potential effects of the support group. These included providing an appropriate social environment in which they can affiliate with other family caregivers to explore a new adaptive role in care-giving; and explaining why it helps to develop a new belief system that corrects each member's understanding of the mental health problems and difficulties in care-giving. In viewing these theoretical perspectives, mutual support groups are complex entities that differ in important ways from professionally delivered help and highlight the importance and benefits of social support to the caregivers as group participants.

From the review of studies from January 1989 to December 2008 described in this report on mutual support groups for family caregivers of people with severe mental disorders, there is little empirical evidence supporting the significant long-term effects of mutual support groups on families' psychosocial well-being and their consumers' health conditions. Even though increasing numbers of non-experimental and qualitative studies on mutual support groups conducted in Western countries demonstrated a variety of benefits of group participation reported by the participants such as increasing knowledge about the illness and coping ability and reducing care-giving burden, these studies lacked rigorous control, did not use standardized instruments as outcome measures, and did not schedule longer-term (e.g., 1 year or more) follow-up investigations of the effects of support groups to these families. In addition, only a few studies were conducted in non-western populations, even though the findings of the studies reviewed indicated positive effects of mutual support groups to Chinese families of people with schizophrenia and other psychotic disorders. This review also highlights the need for further research to examine the benefits and therapeutic mechanisms of support groups as perceived by the group participants, which have been highlighted as the major limitations of research in the past decades. This understanding of the relevant literature on mutual support groups adds to existing knowledge of family interventions for severely mentally ill people and may be drawn upon in the selection and design of appropriate interventions for families providing care to a relative with severe mental health problems, and also in future evaluation research.

References

Abramowitz, I. A., & Coursey, R. D. (1989). Impact of an educational support group on family participants who take care of their schizophrenic relatives. *Journal of Consulting & Clinical Psychology, 57*(2), 232–236.

Akinson, J. M., & Coia, D. A. (1995). Families coping with schizophrenia: A practitioner's guide to family groups. New York: Wiley.

Anderson, C., Reiss, D., & Hogarty, G. (1986). *Schizophrenia and the family: A Practitioner's guide to psychoeducation and management*. New York: Guilford Press.

Asen, E. (2002). Multiple family therapy: An overview. *Journal of Family Therapy, 24*, 3–16.

Bae, S. W., & Kung, W. W. M. (2000). Family intervention for Asian Americans with a schizophrenic patient in the family. *American Journal of Orthopsychiatry, 70*(4), 532–541.

Bandura, A. (1977). *Social learning theory*. Englewood Cliffs, NJ: Prentice Hall.

Barbato, A., & D'Avanzo, B. (2000). Family interventions in schizophrenia and related disorders: A critical review of clinical trials. *Acta Psychiatrica Scandinavica, 102*(2), 81–97.

Bernheim, K. F., & Lehman, A. F. (1985). *Working with families of the mentally ill*. New York: Norton.

Biegel, D. E., Robinson, E. A., & Kennedy, M. J. (2000). A review of empirical studies of interventions for families of persons with mental illness. *Research in Community and Mental Health, 11*, 97–130.

Borkman, T. J. (1999). *Understanding self-help/mutual aid: experiential learning in the commons*. New Brunswick, NJ: Rutgers University Press.

Brooker, C. (2001). Decade of evidence-based training for work with people with serious mental health problems: Progress in the development of psychosocial interventions. *Journal of Mental Healthm, 10*, 17–31.

Buchkremer, G., Schulze, M. H., Monking, H., Holle, R., & Hornung, W. P. (1995). The impact of therapeutic relatives' group on the course of illness of schizophrenic patients. *European Psychiatry, 10* (1), 17–27.

Budd, R. J., & Hughes, I. C. T. (1997). What do relatives of people with schizophrenia find helpful about family intervention? *Schizophrenia Bulletin, 23*(2), 341–347.

Carpenter, J. S. (1997). Self-esteem and well-being among women with breast cancer and women in an age-matched comparison group. *Journal of Psychosocial Oncology, 15*(3/4), 59–80.

Chien, W. T., Chan, S., Morrissey, J., & Thompson, D. (2005). Effectiveness of a mutual support group for families of patients with schizophrenia. *Journal of Advanced Nursing 51*(6), 595–608.

Chien, W. T., Chan, W. C. S., & Thompson, D. R. (2006a). Effects of a mutual support group for families of Chinese people with schizophrenia: 18-month follow-up. *British Journal of Psychiatry 189*, 41–49.

Chien, W. T., Norman, I., & Thompson, D. R. (2006b). Perceived benefits and difficulties experienced in a mutual support group for family carers of people with schizophrenia. *Qualitative Health Research, 16*(7), 962–981.

Chien, W. T., Thompson, D. R., & Norman, I. (2008). Evaluation of a peer-led mutual support group for Chinese families of people with schizophrenia. *American Journal of Community Psychology, 42*, 122–134.

Chien, W. T., Wong, K. F. (2007). The family psycho-education group program for Chinese people with schizophrenia in Hong Kong. *Psychiatric Services, 58*(7), 1003–1006.

Chou, K. R., Liu, S. Y., & Chu, H. (2002). The effects of support groups on caregivers of patients with schizophrenia. *International Journal of Nursing Studies, 39*(7), 713–722.

Craig, T. K. J., Garety, P., Power, P., Rahaman, N., Colbert, S., Fornells-Ambrojo, M., & Dunn, G. (2004). The Lambeth Early Onset (LEO) Team: Randomized controlled trial of the effectiveness of specialized care for early psychosis. *British Medical Journal, 329*(7474), 1067–1071.

Cragan, J. F., & Wright, D. W. (1999). *Communicating in small groups: Theory, process and skills* (5th ed.). Belmont, CA: Wadsworth Publications.

Cuijpers, P. (1999). The effects of family interventions on relatives' burden: A meta-analysis. *Journal of Mental Health, 8*(3), 275–285.

Davidson, K. P., Pennebaker, J. W., & Dickerson, S. S. (2000). Who talks? The social psychology of illness support groups. *American Psychologist, 55*(2), 205–217.

Dixon, L., Adams, C., & Luckstead, A. (2000). Update on family psycho-education for schizophrenia. *Schizophrenia Bulletin, 26* (1), 5–20.

Falloon, I. R. H., Boyd, J. L., McGill, C. W., Razani, J., Moss, H. B., & Gilderman, A. M. (1982). Family management in the prevention of exacerbations of schizophrenia: A controlled study. *New England Journal of Medicine, 306*(4), 1437–1440.

Festinger, L. A. (1954). A theory of social comparison processes. *Human Relations, 7*(2), 117–140.

Fung, W. Y., & Chien, W. T. (2002). The effectiveness of a mutual support group for family caregivers of a relative with dementia. *Archives of Psychiatric Nursing, 14*, 134–144.

Galinsky, M. J., & Schopler, J. H. (Eds.) (1995). *Support groups: Current perspectives on theory and practice*. New York: Harworth Press.

Gazda, G. M., Ginter, E. J., & Horne, A. M. (2001). Group counselling and group psychotherapy: Theory and application (pp. 33–94). Boston, MA: Allyn and Bacon.

Haddock, G., Tarrier, N., Morrison, A. P., Hopkins, R., Dake, R., & Lewis, S. (1999). A pilot study evaluating the effectiveness of individual in-patient cognitive behavioral therapy in early psychosis. *Social Psychiatry and Psychiatric Epidemiology, 34*(5), 254–258.

Helgeson, V. S., & Gottlieb, B. H. (2000). Support groups. In: S. Cohen, L. G. & Underwood (Eds.), *Social support measurement and intervention: A guide for health and social scientists* (pp. 221–245). London: Oxford University Press.

Heller, T., Roccoforte, J. A., Hsieh, K., Cook, J. A., & Pickett-Schenk, S. A. (1997). Benefits of support groups for families of adults with severe mental illness. *American Journal of Orthopsychiatry, 67*(2), 187–198.

Hogarty, G. E., Anderson, C. M., Reiss, D. J., Kornblith, S. J., Greenwald, D. P., Ulrich, R. F., & Carter, M. (1991). Family psycho-education, social skills training, and maintenance chemotherapy in the aftercare treatment of schizophrenia, II: Two-year effects of a controlled study on relapse and adjustment. *Archives of General Psychiatry, 48*(5), 340–347.

Kessler, R. C., Mickelson, K. D., & Zhao, S. (1997). Patterns and correlates of self-help group membership in the United States. *Social Policy, 27*(3), 27–46.

Kimberly, K. C. (1997). *Group processes and structures: A theoretical integration*. Lanham, MD: University Press of America.

Kurtz, L. F. (1997). *Self-help and support groups: A handbook for practitioners*. Thousand Oaks, CA: Sage.

Kyrouz, E. M., Humphreys, K., & Loomis, C. (2002). A review of research on the effectiveness of self-help mutual aid groups. In: B. J. White, & E. J. Madara (Eds.), *The American self-help clearinghouse self-help group sourcebook* (7th ed.). Cedar Knolls, NJ: American Self-help Clearinghouse.

Lazarus, R. S., & Folkman, S. (1984). *Stress and coping*. New York: Springer.

Lee, R. M., & Liu, T. H. T. (2001). Coping with intergenerational family conflict: Comparison of Asian American, Hispanic, and European American college students. *Journal of Counseling Psychology, 48* (4), 410–419.

Lemmens, G. M., Wauters, S., Heireman, M., Eisler, I., Lietaer, G., & Sabbe, B. (2003). Beneficial factors in family discussion groups of a psychiatric day clinic: perceptions by the therapeutic team and the families of the therapeutic process. *Journal of Family Therapy, 25*, 41–63.

Li, Z., & Arthur, D. (2005). A study of three measures of expressed emotion in a sample of Chinese families of a person with schizophrenia. *Journal of Psychiatric & Mental Health Nursing, 12*(4), 431–438.

Lorig, K., Holman, H., Sobel, D., & Laurent, D. (2000). *Living a healthy life with chronic conditions: Self-management of heart disease, arthritis, stroke, diabetes, asthma, bronchitis, emphysema and others* (2nd ed.). Boulder: Bull Publishing.

Luke, D. A., Roberts, L., & Rappaport, J. (1993). Individual, group context, and individual-group fit predictors of self-help group attendance. *Journal of Applied Behavioral Science, 29*(2), 216–238.

Ma, K. Y., & Yip, K. S. (1997). The importance of an effective psychiatric community care service for chronic mental patients in Hong Kong. *Hong Kong Journal of Mental Health, 26*(1), 28–35.

Mankowski, E. S., Humphreys, K., & Moos, R. H. (2001). Individual and contextual predictors of involvement in Twelve-step self-help groups after substance abuse treatment. *American Journal of Community Psychology, 29*(4), 537–563.

Maton, K. E., & Salem, D. A. (1995). Organizational characteristics of empowering community settings: A multiple case study approach. *American Journal of Community Psychology, 23*(5), 631–656.

McCann, G. (1993). Relatives' support groups in a special hospital: An evaluation study. *Journal of Advanced Nursing, 18*(12), 1883–1888.

McFarlane, W. R. (2002). *Multifamily Groups in the Treatment of Severe Psychiatric Disorders.* New York: Guilford Press.

McFarlane, W. R., Lukens, E., Link, B., Dushay, R., Deakins, S. A., Newmark, M., et al. (1995). Multiple-family groups and psycho-education in the treatment of schizophrenia. *Archives of General Psychiatry, 52*(8), 679–687.

National Health Service Centre for Reviews and Dissemination. (2001). *Undertaking systematic reviews of research on effectiveness: CRD's guidance for those carrying out or commissioning reviews* (CRD Report No. 4, 2nd Ed.). York, UK: University of York.

Nichols, K., & Jenkinson, J. (2006). *Leading a support group: A practical guide.* Maidenhead: Open University Press.

Pearson, V., & Ning, S. P. (1997). Family care in schizophrenia: An undervalued resource. In: C. L. W.Chan, & N. Rhind (Eds.), Social Work Intervention in Health Care. The Hong Kong Scene (pp. 317–336). Hong Kong SAR, China: Hong Kong University Press.

Penney, D. (1997). Friend or foe: The impact of managed care on self-help. *Social Policy, 27*(4), 48–53.

Perkins, D. D., & Zimmerman, M.A. (1995). Empowerment theory, research, and application. *American Journal of Psychology, 23*(5), 569–579.

Pharoah, F. M., Mari, J. J., & Streiner, D. (2001). Family intervention for schizophrenia. *The Cochrane Library Reviews, Issue 3, 2001.* Oxford: Cochrane Library Update Software [Electronic database].

Pickett-Schenk, S. A., & Heller, T. (1998). Profession-led versus family-led support groups: Exploring the differences. *Journal of Behavioral Health Services and Research, 25*(4), 437–443.

Powell, T. J. (Ed.) (1994). *Understanding the self-help organization: Framework and findings.* Thousand Oaks, CA: Sage Publications.

Sampson, P., & Murtha, R. (1997). *Group process for the health professional* (3rd ed.). Albany, NY: Delmar Publishers.

Schiff, M., & Bargal, D. (2000). Helping characteristics of self-help and support groups: Their contribution to participants' subjective well-being. *Small Group Research, 31*(3), 275–304.

Solomon, P., Draine, J., Mannion, E., & Meisel, M. (1997). Effectiveness of two models of brief family education: Retention of gains by family members of adults with serious mental illness. *American Journal of Orthopsychiatry, 67*(2), 177–186.

Stein, C. H., & Wemmerus, V. A. (2001). Searching for a normal life: Personal accounts of adults with schizophrenia, their parents and well-siblings. *American Journal of Community Psychology, 29*(5), 725–746.

Steinberg, D. M. (2004). *The Mutual-aid Approach to Working with Groups: Helping People Help One Another* (2nd ed.). New York: Haworth Press.

Szmukler, G., Kuipers, E., Joyce, J., Harris, T., Leese, M., Maphosa, W., et al. (2003). An exploratory randomized controlled trial of a support programme for carers of patients with psychosis. *Social Psychiatry & Psychiatric Epidemiology, 38*, 411–418.

Telles, C., Karno, M., Mintz, J., Paz, G., Arias, M., Tucker, D., et al. (1995). Immigrant families coping with schizophrenia: Behavioural family intervention vs. case management with a low-income Spanish-speaking population. *British Journal of Psychiatry, 167*(4), 473–479.

Toseland, R. W., Rossiter, C. M., & Labrecque, M. S. (1989). The effectiveness of peer-led and professionally led groups to support family caregivers. *Gerontologist, 29*(4), 465–471.

Turnbull, J. E., Galinsky, M. J., Wilner, M. E., & Meglin, D. E. (1994). Designing research to meet service needs: An evaluation of single-session groups for families of psychiatric inpatients. *Research on Social Work Practice, 4*(2), 192–207.

Wheelan, S. A. (1994). *Group processes: A developmental perspective*. Boston, MA: Allyn and Bacon.

Wilson, J. (1995). *How to Work with Self-Help Groups: Guidelines for Health Professionals*. Aldershot, UK: Arena.

Winefield, H., Barlow, J., & Harvey, E. (1998). Responses to support groups for family caregivers in schizophrenia: Who benefits from what? *Australian and New Zealand Journal of Mental Health Nursing, 7*(30), 103–110.

Winefield, H. R., & Harvey, E. J. (1995). Tertiary prevention in mental health care: effects of group meetings for family caregivers. *Australian and New Zealand Journal of Psychiatry, 29*, 139–145.

Wituk, S., Shepherd, M. D., Slavich, S., Warren, M. L., & Meissen, G. (2000). A topography of self-help groups: An empirical analysis. *Social Work, 45*(2), 157–165.

Xiong, W., Philips, M. R., Hu, X., Wang, R., Dai, Q., Kleinman, J., & Kleinman, A. (1994). Family-based intervention for schizophrenic patients in China. A randomized controlled trial. *British Journal of Psychiatry, 165*(3), 239–247.

Yalom, I. D. (1998). *The Yalom reader: Selections from The work of a master therapist and storyteller.* New York: Basic Books.

Zimmerman, M.A. (1995). Psychological empowerment: Issues and illustrations. *American Journal of Community Psychology, 23*(5), 581–599.

Zimmerman, B. J., & Schunk, D. H. (Eds.) (2003). *Educational psychology: A century of contributions*. Mahwah, NJ: Erlbaum.

Part III
Consumer-Delivered Services

Chapter 7
Consumer-Run Drop-In Centers: Current State and Future Directions

Louis D. Brown, Scott Wituk, and Greg Meissen

Abstract Consumer-run drop-in centers are a popular form of mental health self-help that typically requires external funding. The drop-in center can serve as a foundation for many other organizational pursuits. In addition to organizing recreational activities, drop-in centers can host self-help groups, bring in speakers from the community, offer classes to members, organize public awareness campaigns about mental illness, volunteer in the community, and work with policy makers to improve the public mental health system. This chapter will review research on several different facets of these organizations including their activities, organizational structure, evidence base, funding support, and community relations. Strategies to enhance the organizational effectiveness and peer support of consumer run drop-in centers are outlined with attention to enhancing empowerment and recovery. The chapter concludes by considering future directions for research and practice.

7.1 Consumer-Run Drop-In Centers: Current State and Future Directions

Consumer-run drop-in (CRDI) centers provide participants with many opportunities for peer support and leadership while also addressing issues of social isolation and stigma. Drop-in centers are a place where mental health consumers can socialize, organize recreational activities, exchange mutual support, and organize community initiatives. These centers are similar to self-help groups in that participants can benefit from giving and receiving social support in an informal setting. Operation of a CRDI center also provides mental health consumers with numerous opportunities to fill leadership positions within the organization. Approximately 1400 CRDI centers operate in the United States, according to data from a national survey of consumer

---

L.D. Brown (✉)
Prevention Research Center, The Pennsylvania State University, 135 E, Nittany Ave, Suite 402, State College, PA 16801, USA
e-mail: ldb12@psu.edu

and family driven initiatives (Goldstrom et al., 2006). The goal of this chapter is to provide an overview of CRDI centers and a review of research on the topic. Issues addressed in the following sections include: (a) organizational activities; (b) organizational capacity needs; (c) organizational structure; (d) evidence base; (e) organizational strategies for success; (f) the challenge of maintaining appropriate funding support; (g) community relations; and (h) future directions for research and practice.

7.1.1 Organizational Activities and Characteristics

CRDI centers are a popular form of mental health self-help that typically maintains more structure than a self-help group. CRDI centers are frequently incorporated nonprofits that maintain a board of directors, have paid staff, and depend on grant funding. Their emphasis on mutual support is similar to that of a self-help group, however, they also provide numerous leadership opportunities for members (Brown, Collins, Shepherd, Wituk, & Meissen, 2004). In addition to operating a drop-in center with recreational activities, CRDI centers often organize educational activities, host support groups, advocate for consumers, initiate public education efforts about mental illness, and conduct volunteer projects in the community (Trainor, Shepherd, Boydell, Leff, & Crawford, 1997).

7.1.2 Organizational Capacity Needs

Although the needs of CRDI centers have not been extensively studied, a retrospective analysis of 13 consumer-operated programs found that their organizational capacity needs were similar to that of other small nonprofits. The study suggested that these organizations needed capacity assistance "focused on all areas of nonprofit organization management, including board development, fiscal management, staff supervision, conflict resolution, strategic planning, fundraising, managed care, and cultural diversity/competency" (Van Tosh & del Vecchio, 2000, p. 82).

Using an organizational framework based on the work of Connolly and York (2002), a more recent study by Wituk, Vu, Brown, Shepherd, & Meissen (2008) also highlighted the organizational capacity needs of CRDI centers. The framework categorizes several specific organizational capacities essential to operating a nonprofit into four core areas: (1) technical (e.g., grant writing, quarterly reporting), (2) management (e.g., business management, staffing issues, conflict resolution), (3) adaptive (e.g., activity planning, strategic planning), and (4) leadership capacity (e.g., board development). Overall, the most frequent organizational capacity needs of CRDI centers were related to management ($N = 687$), followed by technical needs ($N = 686$), adaptive needs ($N = 276$), and leadership needs ($N = 222$). The most often cited specific organizational capacity needs were: (1) grant writing ($N = 287$), (2) quarterly reporting ($N = 223$), (3) board development

($N = 222$), and (4) business management ($N = 198$). Increases in organizational capacity needs from 2004 to 2006 occurred in the following areas: (1) grant writing, (2) quarterly reporting, (3) board development, (4) business management, (5) staffing issues, (6) conflict resolution, (7) policy development, (8) activity planning, (9) financial mismanagement, and (10) strategic planning. Gradual decreases in organizational capacity needs from 2004 to 2006 occurred in the following areas: (1) attracting new members and (2) attaining nonprofit status. This study further documents that the organizational capacity needs of CRDI's are similar to many other small nonprofits.

7.1.3 CRDI Organizational Structure

The organizational structure of CRDI centers typically fall in the middle of a continuum between unstructured grassroots associations operated by volunteers on one end (e.g., self-help groups) and formal nonprofit agencies operated by paid staff (e.g., Red Cross) on the other. These two types of organizational structures have different strengths and weaknesses (Smith, 2000). Grassroots associations benefit from flexibility in purpose along with the passion and warmth that accompany volunteerism. Nonprofits with paid staff may not only be more efficient and productive, but also more rigid. CRDI centers frequently manifest some characteristics of both structures because they started as a small group of passionate but often inexperienced volunteers that exemplify unstructured grassroots associations and developed into more structured nonprofit organizations operated using a mixture of paid and volunteer support. If CRDI centers begin to receive grant funding or reimbursement for services, they often struggle to maintain the advantages of an unstructured association while managing the unintended consequences of becoming a nonprofit with a budget and paid staff. CRDI centers need adequate structure to be accountable without compromising the grassroots camaraderie and passion that inspires the organization.

Previous research on the goals of CRDI centers in Kansas provides insight into where these organizations fall on the continuum between formal nonprofit organizations and informal grassroots associations (Brown, Shepherd, Wituk, & Meissen, 2007). With respect to funding, CRDI centers resemble structured nonprofits in their reliance on grant funding to continue operations, whereas grassroots associations remain financially independent (Smith, 2000). Furthermore, CRDI centers are similar to structured nonprofits in their focus on maintaining or increasing their days and hours of operation. Grassroots associations typically have more intermittent rather than continuous activity (Smith, 2000). Several goals of CRDI centers do reflect their grassroots heritage. Their reliance of voluntarism remains substantial and most implement organizational strategies to increase the number of members contributing voluntary leadership. The internal focus of CRDI centers on reducing social isolation among members and celebrating member accomplishments is further reflective of their grassroots nature (Brown et al., 2007; Fischer, 1982).

7.1.4 Research on the Effectiveness of CRDI Centers

Overall, evidence supporting the effectiveness of CRDI centers is encouraging. The strongest evidence comes from the SAMHSA/CMHS Consumer-Operated Service Program (COSP) multisite randomized control trial. Intent-to-treat analyses indicate that assignment to the CRDI center condition significantly improved well-being, with a moderate effect size of .39 (Teague, Johnsen, Rogers, & Schell, 2005). Other evaluations of CRDI centers were also positive, but the findings are more difficult to interpret because analyses mix participation in CRDI centers with other types of grant-funded consumer initiatives. For example, research by Trainor et al. (1997) documented a 91% decline in the use of inpatient services after participation in grant-funded consumer/survivor initiatives began. In addition, the Trainor study found that, on average, people with psychiatric disabilities considered their organization the single most helpful component of the mental health system. Furthermore, Yanos, Primavera, & Knight (2001) found that participants involved in consumer-run services had better social functioning and used more coping strategies than those involved only in traditional mental health services. Finally, in a longitudinal observational study of four consumer/survivor initiatives, two of which operated a drop-in center, Nelson et al. (2006) found that after 18 months, active participants experienced increased social support, improved quality of life, and decreased psychiatric hospitalization, whereas non-active participants did not change on these outcomes.

Mowbray and Tan (1993) found that when compared to community mental health services, 77% of consumers perceived CRDI centers more favorably. Frequently cited differences included having more freedom, more support and caring, and less structure. Consumers also reported having organizational control (87%), feeling accepted (99%), and coming to their CRDI center out of their own free will (98%). According to members, CRDI involvement led to increases in volunteer work, paid employment, and school involvement while decreasing institutionalization, substance abuse, and the use of professional mental health services (Mowbray & Tan, 1993).

People with mental health problems appear to be eager to get involved in CRDI centers once funding becomes available. From 2000 to 2003, as the availability of funding for CRDI centers in Kansas increased, the number of organizations increased 75% from 12 to 21 and the number of members involved increased 114% from 582 to 1,244 members (Center for Community Support & Research, 2003).

Research also suggests that CRDIs are cost efficient because of their small budgets and reliance on voluntary leadership, operating on approximately $8 daily per person in Michigan (Holter & Mowbray, 2005) and $11.51 daily per person in Kansas (Brown et al., 2007). In addition to being relatively inexpensive compared to traditional mental health services, previous research indicates that CRDI centers achieved 69% of goals they set (Brown et al., 2007). This rate of organizational goal achievement suggests general organizational competence. Member perceptions of CRDI environments are consistent with the self-help ideology of providing a supportive environment, opportunities for active involvement in the organization, and the encouragement of individual autonomy (Segal, Silverman, & Temkin, 1997).

Considering the low cost of these organizations, their ability to operate effectively, the benefits of participation, and their popularity among people with mental illness, CRDI centers have the potential to become a major component of the mental health system.

7.1.5 Developing More Effective CRDI Centers

CRDI centers can enhance organizational decision-making with the use of accurate logic models that explain how people benefit from participation. Numerous theories explain how people can benefit from CRDI centers and other types of self-help. Prominent perspectives are described in Chapter 2, including the helper therapy principle (Riessman, 1965), empowerment theory (Maton & Salem, 1995; Segal, Silverman, & Temkin, 1993), social networks (Biegel, Tracy, & Corvo, 1994; Goldberg, Rollins, & Lehman, 2003), social support (Cohen, Gottlieb, & Underwood, 2000), experiential expertise (Borkman, 1999), and the role framework (Brown, 2009a, 2009b).

The role framework suggests that consumers who get involved in helper roles at a CRDI can benefit by acquiring more resources, obtaining positive appraisals, developing new skills, and embracing a healthier identity. Two types of helper roles available at a CRDI center are socially supportive friendship roles and empowering leadership roles. Previous research suggests that both of these roles promote recovery (Brown, Shepherd, Merkle, Wituk, & Meissen, 2008). The role framework also indicates that the development of these roles depends upon person–environment interaction. CRDI environments need to encourage the development of both socially supportive friendship roles and empowering leadership roles in order to promote the recovery of their members. In order to promote empowering and supportive CRDI environments, the Center for Community Support and Research (CCSR) at Wichita State University has been providing CRDI centers with training and technical assistance for more than a decade. CCSR's experience working with CRDI centers to improve organizational functioning has led to the identification of several strategies that CRDI centers use to encourage the development of socially supportive friendships and empowering leadership roles. Drawing from this experiential knowledge base, the following two subsections outline strategies CRDI centers can use to build empowering and socially supportive environments.

7.1.6 Promoting an Empowering Environment

Promoting member involvement in organizational operations is challenging but critical to organizational success, as the task of sustaining a CRDI center can easily overwhelm a small leadership base. Adding to the challenge is the fact that, in the short term, it often takes longer to train an individual to complete a task than it does to complete the task without support. Once new volunteers gain training and experience, however, they can begin to make valuable contributions to the organization independently. Investing in the skill development of volunteers not only promotes organizational functioning, but also an empowering sense of ownership and commitment to the CRDI center. The learning opportunities may also help members with problem solving in other situations. To avoid replicating a disempowering professional environment where paid staff members take care of consumers, the following subsections discuss several strategies that can help get members contributing to organizational operations early and often.

7.1.6.1 Volunteer Opportunities

Regularly recruiting members to complete small but recurring organizational duties provides all members with immediate opportunities to contribute to the daily operations of the organization. Through tasks such as meal preparation, transportation assistance, and cleaning/building maintenance, everyone can make substantial contributions to their CRDI center. The use of sign-up sheets can help to promote accountability and commitment. Publicly recognizing and rewarding members for their contributions can help to encourage continued volunteerism, enhance camaraderie, and promote the self-esteem of recognized members. Establishing shared social norms with respect to organizational contribution and instilling those attitudes early when members join a CRDI center can help to get everyone involved.

7.1.6.2 Organizational Decision-Making

Keeping meetings open, encouraging everyone to attend, and seeking the perspectives of all attendees during discussions can both improve organizational decision-making and help to get all members invested in shaping the policies and practices of their organization. Maintaining non-confrontational discussions, where all perspectives are valued, can help keep meetings welcoming and productive. Furthermore, when tackling major organizational decisions such as voting for board of directors positions, it is especially important to advertise and schedule the meeting at a convenient time. Involving the majority of the members in such decisions is critical to keeping the CRDI center operating in a manner consistent with the interests and priorities of the general membership.

7.1.6.3 Planning and Organizing Activities

Providing members with opportunities to plan, organize, and facilitate activities that interest them can be one of the most rewarding voluntary leadership roles offered by CRDI centers. The activities undertaken are only limited by the imagination of members (and the availability of an activity budget), but include game tournaments, group outings, crafts, parties, meals, and learning opportunities (e.g., gardening, cooking, or computer classes). Organizing group activities can be both enjoyable and an excellent opportunity to develop leadership skills. Forming several small collaborative groups who organize activities on a rotating or ad hoc basis can help to prevent burnout and provide the CRDI center with a larger pool of members ready to make organizational contributions.

7.1.6.4 Formal Leadership Positions

CRDI participants can also occupy formal leadership roles such as board member, shift manager, or director. These positions typically entail more responsibility and some may require substantial training on topics such as grant writing and completing quarterly reports. Organizations may benefit from spreading a full time paid staff position across several interested CRDI members who can each contribute using their own unique talents. This can help prevent burnout and over reliance on a single member. If one paid staff member becomes sick, other experienced staff can temporarily fill in. Another strategy CRDI centers can use to promote shared leadership is to rotate positions on the board of directors every year. This can encourage the development of new leaders and prevent entrenched hierarchies from forming.

7.1.6.5 Promoting a Socially Supportive Environment

The social support available at CRDI centers provides both a powerful incentive for participation and promotes recovery (Brown et al., 2008; Mowbray & Tan, 1993). In the CRDI context, social support may be particularly valuable because members can share experiential knowledge in managing mental illness. This shared background promotes mutual understanding and empathy (Borkman, 1999). Although CRDI centers have natural advantages in promoting socially supportive relationships, such relationships will not develop without substantial effort from the organizational leadership. The follow subsections review several organizational strategies that can promote a more socially supportive environment.

7.1.6.6 Recognize Member Accomplishments

Recognizing members for their personal accomplishments and contributions can help members develop a sense of self-worth as a capable and valued member of the organization. Furthermore, the act of recognizing member accomplishments can promote mutual affection between the recipient and the recognizer. Accomplishments can be honored through both private interactions (e.g., letters, compliments, tokens of appreciation) and publicly (e.g., banquets, birthday parties). Habitual recognition of member accomplishments by organizational leaders can be particularly effective because CRDI leaders have a powerful influence on the atmosphere of the organization. When leaders model supportive interactions, others will often follow their example, enhancing a socially supportive environment.

7.1.6.7 Organize a Variety of Interesting Activities

By organizing fun and interesting activities, CRDI centers provide a medium for the development of close friendships. Providing members with engaging activities enables comfortable social interaction with reduced pressure to maintain conversation. Although each CRDI center will want to tailor their activities to the interests of members, some commonly successful activities include hosting holiday parties, providing craft making opportunities, organizing friendly competitions such as pool tournaments, having group meals such as potlucks, and taking field trips. CRDI centers that offer multiple activity options at a given point in time may be the most successful, as members can gravitate toward the activities best suited for their interests while avoiding activities they find boring. Scheduling activities on a weekly basis and mailing a monthly activity calendar to participants can also help regularly attract members who are particularly fond of one activity but otherwise disinclined to participate. Maintaining a dynamic and engaging environment is especially important for attracting and retaining new CRDI members because they have not established close relationships with fellow members that can make any activity enjoyable.

7.1.6.8 Prevent and Resolve Conflict with a Code of Conduct

As with any open social setting, conflicts between members occur at times. If left unchecked, such conflict can negatively impact the well-being of members, deter attendance, erode the socially supportive nature of the CRDI environment, and eventually threaten the existence of the organization (Mohr, 2004). To avoid these consequences, CRDI centers must prioritize conflict prevention and resolution. Developing a code of conduct that provides members with a shared set of behavior expectations during CRDI participation can help to prevent and resolve conflicts. For codes of conduct to be effective, all members must be familiar with and accept their content. Effective codes of conduct can develop through group discussions that use of consensus-driven decision-making to determine acceptable and unacceptable behaviors at the CRDI center, along with the consequences for violating rules. Revisiting and updating the code of conduct on a regular basis can help maintain member buy-in and ensure new members also have the opportunity to influence its content. Within a code of conduct, it can be useful to outline a process for conflict resolution that focuses on addressing the behavior in question rather than criticizing the individual offender. At times, problems may arise that the code of conduct does not address. As such, it may be useful to describe a process for resolving unanticipated problems within the code of conduct.

7.1.6.9 Develop Self-Help Groups and/or Peer Counselors

Regardless of the self-help group's focal issue, participation encourages mutual self-disclosure and the formation of intimate, trusting relationships between members. The relationship dynamics developed in a self-help group carry over to other CRDI activities. The explicit emphasis on sharing personal struggles and mutual encouragement in a self-help group can promote socially supportive exchanges that may not occur in relationships developed through purely social activities. The use of peer counselors is another strategy CRDI centers can use to promote empathic listening and discussions focused on problem solving. Additionally, the fact that peer counselors have faced similar mental health challenges provides them with a natural strength that non-consumer counselors do not have. The lived experience of coping with mental illness can help peer counselors provide practical and appropriate support.

Although the preceding sections have presented numerous strategies for promoting socially supportive and empowering environments, many more yet unmentioned approaches exist. Some suggested strategies will inevitably work well in some settings and not in others, thus it is important for CRDI centers to consider their own unique situation when selecting strategies. Furthermore, CRDI centers may need to develop entirely new strategies if the proposed strategies prove insufficient. With limited time and resources to devote to any particular challenge or activity, it is important for CRDI centers to find overlap and synergy between efforts to promote empowerment and social support. Balancing both appears to be an important component of effective CRDI operation based in the philosophy of recovery.

7.1.6.10 Funding Support

Nonprofits that depend on external funding continually face the challenge of maintaining consistent funding without losing sight of the organization's original mission. To meet this challenge, nonprofits must find appropriate funding agencies who are interested in supporting their mission. With good fit, a healthy collaborative relationship can be sustained if the needs of both the nonprofit and the funding agency can be met.

One central need for funding agencies is to ensure the accountability of funding recipients, which allows funding agencies to make informed decisions about how to effectively distribute their resources. Funding agencies typically establish accountability using grant requirements that mandate nonprofits to report on their execution of grant-related activities. Cumbersome or rigid requirements can conflict with the organizational mission and operational philosophy of the funded nonprofits. When nonprofits face this conflicting situation, they may have to make an uncomfortable choice in favor of either obtaining money or maintaining mission integrity. Rejecting grant requirements may lead to organizational dissolution whereas accepting grant requirements may compromise the organizational mission and philosophy.

The imposition of grant requirements by a funding agency can erode the autonomy of a nonprofit and operate as a form of cooptation or coercive cooperation, especially if the nonprofit is heavily dependent on a single funding agency. The introduction of new grant requirements restricting the independent decision-making of the organization can occur both gradually over funding cycles and suddenly in a major overhaul of grant requirements. If grant contracts prohibit established organizational activities or funding becomes contingent upon the completion of specific activities that compromise the nonprofit's philosophy, needs, goals, or methods, then cooptation begins.

CRDI centers and other consumer initiatives must be particularly vigilant against cooptation because it has historically been a problem (Kasinsky, 1987). Avoiding cooptation is particularly important for CRDI centers because consumer control is a central tenet of their operation, which helps to promote empowerment and recovery (Holter, Mowbray, Bellamy, MacFarlane, & Dukarski, 2004; Brown et al., 2008). Although coercive grant requirements are clearly problematic, funding agencies typically have no desire to control a nonprofit. Instead, funding agencies create grant requirements in an effort to ensure accountability and the effective allocation of resources. Thus, developing strategies to establish accountability without compromising the independence of consumer initiatives is an important policy issue for mental health systems to address.

One strategy that demonstrates promise in establishing accountability while maintaining consumer control is the use of goal tracking. The use of goal tracking allows organizations to provide individually defined, context appropriate markers of success while still enabling the objective tracking and reporting of organizational goal achievement. Developing concrete, objectively determinable goals that serve as milestones of progress toward the fulfillment of the organizational mission can also facilitate planning and create a shared understanding of the logic behind tasks (Bryson, 1995). Periodically conducting an audit of goal achievement can serve to establish organizational accountability while also providing the organization with corrective feedback on their progress (Kiresuk & Lund, 1978). Finally, the process of setting goals and tracking organizational progress can also enhance organizational focus and achievement motivation (Rodgers & Hunter, 1991). The use of goal tracking among CRDI centers has been successful in Kansas (Brown et al., 2007) and may generally be an effective strategy for demonstrating the accountability of grant-funded consumer initiatives, especially when technical assistance is available to support the development of appropriate goals.

7.1.7 Organizational Networks and Community Relations

Through inter-organizational collaboration, CRDI centers and other nonprofits can gain resources, knowledge, and influence (Hardy, Phillips, & Lawrence, 2003). Research suggests CRDI centers with more organizational connections have more financial resources, more members, and organize more activities (Center for Community Support & Research, 2004). However, this study found no relation between organizational network size and progress toward recovery attributable to CRDI participation. Thus, the benefits of inter-organizational collaboration may be more important for CRDI centers with an external focus on social change rather than inward focus on personal change.

Social change oriented system-level activities that influence the human service system, the broader community, and social policy are also more likely to require strong community relations and inter-organizational collaborations. Popular system-level activities among CRDI centers include public education about mental illness, political advocacy, and community planning focused on improving supports and services available to mental health consumers (Janzen, Nelson, Trainor, & Ochocka, 2006). Research suggests CRDI involvement in these system-level activities can be both effective in achieving system-level change and in enhancing the credibility, awareness, and respect for consumer voices in the community (Janzen et al., 2006).

7.1.8 Implications for Research and Practice

Consumer leaders who are seeking funding support for a CRDI center can use the evidence based outlined in this chapter to support funding applications. Although rigorous research suggests participation in a CRDI center is beneficial, we know relatively little about the conditions necessary for CRDI centers to succeed. Future research needs to examine which individuals are most likely to engage in and benefit from CRDI participation. Research also needs to identify setting characteristics that enhance engagement and the benefits derived from participation. Furthermore, evidence-based outreach practices and implementation support systems need to be developed.

Consumers who operate CRDI centers need to be intimately involved in research studies that address these issues. Only through close collaboration will research efforts succeed in developing and testing practical hypotheses about the conditions necessary for CRDI success. One important component of CRDI success lies in its provision of an empowering and socially supportive environment (Brown et al., 2008). This chapter outlines several promising strategies CRDI centers can use to promote empowering and socially supportive CRDI environments. Although CRDI centers can draw on this experiential knowledge base for guidance, further research is necessary to test the effectiveness of the identified strategies.

7.1.9 Conclusion

CRDI centers are a low-cost strategy for promoting the well-being of mental health consumers (Holter & Mowbray, 2005; Teague et al., 2005). Participation in the friendship and leadership roles available in these settings may promote recovery (Brown et al., 2008). Common organizational needs include help with grant writing, quarterly report writing, board development, business management, and staffing issues (Wituk et al., 2008). Strategies for success include offering numerous volunteer opportunities, holding open business meetings, organizing a variety of interesting activities, using a code of conduct, recognizing member accomplishments, and hosting support groups. We know relatively little about how CRDI centers can best collaborate with other organizations in the community. However, when interacting with funding agencies, the use of goal tracking appears to be a promising method for establishing accountability without compromising independence. CRDI centers using this strategy achieved 69% of their organizational goals, suggesting general organizational competence (Brown et al., 2007). Although CRDI centers appear to be a viable and effective type of mental health self-help, their penetration across communities is limited. Future work needs to develop effective dissemination models that can ensure the implementation of high-quality CRDI centers.

Acknowledgements Support for this research comes from Kansas Social and Rehabilitation Services, Division of Mental Health.

References

Biegel, D. E., Tracy, E. M., & Corvo, K. N. (1994). Strengthening social networks: Intervention strategies for mental health case managers. *Health and Social Work, 19*, 206–216.

Borkman, T. J. (1999). *Understanding self-help/mutual aid: Experiential learning in the commons.* New Brunswick, NJ: Rutgers University Press.

Brown, L. D. (2009a). How people can benefit from mental health consumer-run organizations. *American Journal of Community Psychology, 43*, 177–188.

Brown, L. D. (2009b). Making it sane: Using life history narratives to explore theory in a mental health consumer-run organization. *Qualitative Health Research, 19*, 243–257.

Brown, L. D., Collins, V. L., Shepherd, M. D., Wituk, S. A., & Meissen, G. (2004). Photovoice and consumer-run mutual support organizations. *International Journal of Self-Help and Self-Care, 2*, 339–344.

Brown, L. D., Shepherd, M. D., Merkle, E. C., Wituk, S. A., & Meissen, G. (2008). Understanding how participation in a consumer-run organization relates to recovery. *American Journal of Community Psychology, 42*, 167–178.

Brown, L. D., Shepherd, M. D., Wituk, S. A., & Meissen, G. (2007). Goal achievement and the accountability of consumer-run organizations. *Journal of Behavioral Health Services and Research, 34*, 73–82.

Bryson, J. M. (1995). *Strategic planning for profit and nonprofit organizations: A guide to strengthening and sustaining organizational achievement.* San Francisco: Jossey-Bass.

Center for Community Support & Research. (2003). An analysis of consumer-run organization quarterly reports [Electronic Version], 2009 from http://www.kansascro.com/includes/downloads/article_feedback.pdf.

Center for Community Support & Research. (2004). *Network analysis of consumer-run organizations.* Wichita, KS: Wichita State University Center for Community Support & Research.

Cohen, S., Gottlieb, B. H., & Underwood, L. G. (2000). Social relationships and health. In S. Cohen, L. G. Underwood, & B. H. Gottlieb (Eds.), *Social support measurement and intervention: A guide for health and social scientists* (pp. 3–28). Oxford, UK: Oxford University Press.

Connolly, P. M., & York, P. J. (2002). Evaluating capacity-building efforts for nonprofit organizations. *OD Practitioner, 34*, 33–39.

Fischer, C. S. (1982). *To dwell among friends: Personal networks in town and city.* Chicago: University of Chicago Press.

Goldberg, R. W., Rollins, A. L., & Lehman, A. F. (2003). Social network correlates among people with psychiatric disabilities. *Psychiatric Rehabilitation Journal, 26*, 393–402.

Goldstrom, I. D., Campbell, J., Rogers, J. A., Lambert, D. B., Blacklow, B., Henderson, M. J., et al. (2006). National estimates for mental health mutual support groups, self-help organizations, and consumer-operated services. *Administration and Policy in Mental Health and Mental Health Services Research, 33*, 92–103.

Hardy, C., Phillips, N., & Lawrence, T. (2003). Resources, knowledge and influence: The organizational effects of interorganizational collaboration. *Journal of Management Studies, 40*, 289–315.

Holter, M. C., & Mowbray, C. T. (2005). Consumer-run drop-in centers: Program operations and costs. *Psychiatric Rehabilitation Journal, 28*, 323–331.

Holter, M. C., Mowbray, C. T., Bellamy, C. D., MacFarlane, P., & Dukarski, J. (2004). Critical ingredients of consumer run services: Results of a national survey. *Community Mental Health Journal, 40*(1), 47–63.

Janzen, R., Nelson, G., Trainor, J., & Ochocka, J. (2006). A longitudinal study of mental health consumer/survivor initiatives: Part 4–Benefits beyond the self? A quantitative and qualitative study of system-level activities and impacts. *Journal of Community Psychology, 34*, 285–303.

Kasinsky, J. (1987). Cooptation. In S. Zinman, H. T. Harp & S. Budd (Eds.), *Reaching across: Mental health clients helping each other* (pp. 177–181). Sacramento, CA: California Network of Mental Health Clients.

Kiresuk, T. J., & Lund, S. H. (1978). Goal attainment scaling. In C. C. Attkisson, W. A. Hargreaves, M. J. Horowitz & J. E. Sorensen (Eds.), *Evaluation of human service programs*. New York: Academic.

Maton, K. I., & Salem, D. A. (1995). Organizational characteristics of empowering community settings: A multiple case study approach. *American Journal of Community Psychology, 23*, 631–656.

Mohr, W. K. (2004). Surfacing the life phases of a mental health support group. *Qualitative Health Research, 14*, 61–77.

Mowbray, C. T., & Tan, C. (1993). Consumer-operated drop-in centers: Evaluation of operations and impact. *Journal of Mental Health Administration, 20*, 8–19.

Nelson, G., Ochocka, J., Janzen, R., & Trainor, J. (2006). A longitudinal study of mental health consumer/survivor initiatives: Part 2–A quantitative study of impacts of participation on new members. *Journal of Community Psychology, 34*, 261–272.

Riessman, F. (1965). The "helper" therapy principle. *Social Work, 10*, 27–32.

Rodgers, R., & Hunter, J. E. (1991). Impact of management by objectives on organizational productivity. *Journal of Applied Psychology, 76*, 322–336.

Segal, S. P., Silverman, C., & Temkin, T. (1993). Empowerment and self-help agency practice for people with mental disabilities. *Social Work, 38*, 705–712.

Segal, S. P., Silverman, C., & Temkin, T. (1997). Program environments of self-help agencies for persons with mental disabilities. *The Journal of Mental Health Administration, 24*, 456–464.

Smith, D. H. (2000). *Grassroots associations*. Thousand Oaks, CA: Sage.

Teague, G. B., Johnsen, M., Rogers, J. A., & Schell, B. (2005). Research on consumer-operated service programs: Effectiveness findings and policy implications of a large multi-site study. Retrieved March 10, 2009, from http://www.power2u.org/cosp.html

Trainor, J., Shepherd, M., Boydell, K. M., Leff, A., & Crawford, E. (1997). Beyond the service paradigm: The impact and implications of consumer/survivor initiatives. *Psychiatric Rehabilitation Journal, 21*, 132–140.

Van Tosh, L., & del Vecchio, P. (2000). *Consumer-operated self-help programs: A technical report*. Rockville, MD: U.S. Center for Menal Health Services.

Wituk, S. A., Vu, C., Brown, L. D., & Meissen, G. (2008). Organizational capacity needs of consumer-run organizations. *Administration and Policy in Mental Health and Mental Health Services Research, 35*, 212–219.

Yanos, P. T., Primavera, L. H., & Knight, E. L. (2001). Consumer-run service participation, recovery of social functioning, and the mediating role of psychological factors. *Psychiatric Services, 52*, 493–500.

Chapter 8
Certified Peer Specialists in the United States Behavioral Health System: An Emerging Workforce

Mark S. Salzer

Abstract A unique discipline of persons who provide peer support and mutual-aid has grown exponentially over the past decade. Individuals with personal experience with mental illnesses from across the country are receiving specialized training and certification as Peer Specialists and an increasing number of states have approved the supports they provide for Medicaid reimbursement. This chapter will provide an historical overview and discuss this movement as a significant evolutionary step in the involvement of peers-as-staff in the traditional service system, programs, and workforce. A review of current knowledge about certified peer specialist (CPS) training programs will be offered along with research findings on the benefits associated with participating in such training on well-being, knowledge, and employment. Finally, national findings pertaining to CPS wages, hours worked per week, and number of persons they support, as well as job titles and work activities will be presented. Evidence of continuing implementation barriers are also discussed, suggesting that knowledge among non-peers about recovery and the value of peer support have not yet had as big of an effect as one might like. Emerging policy, program, and practice issues will be discussed, as well as future research topics of greatest priority.

Peer[1] support involves an intentional relationship between individuals with mutually perceived similarities based on personal characteristics and experiences and the open acknowledgement and sharing of these experiences. Consumer-delivered programs and services involving peer support in behavioral health services have been touted as a best practice based on a solid theory, policy, and growing research support (Salzer & MHASP Best Practices Team, 2002).

Peers are present among traditional behavioral health disciplines (e.g., psychiatry, psychology, nursing, social work) and have always worked within the mental

---

M.S. Salzer (✉)
Department of Psychiatry, University of Pennsylvania, Philadelphia, PA, USA
e-mail: mark.salzer@uphs.upenn.edu

[1] The term "peer" will be used to describe an individual who has personal experience with a mental illness.

health system, but generally not openly, thereby negating the possibility of offering peer support. Fear of discrimination, such as a mental health diagnosis being used as evidence of being an "impaired provider," or being shunned by non-peer colleagues are likely reasons. In fact, among traditional mental health disciplines the notion of using one's own personal experiences, including experiences with mental health issues, as a therapeutic tool through disclosure is viewed as highly controversial (Kottsieper, 2009).

As a result of these and other factors it is not surprising that peer support services often occur outside traditional mental health agencies and programs. The most obvious examples are self-help/mutual-aid groups and stand alone consumer-operated services that are planned, managed, and delivered by persons in recovery. However, there have also been smatterings of initiatives in which peers have openly been employed in traditional programs, such as vocational, case management, or partial hospital programs (see Solomon & Draine, 2001 for a categorization of peer-delivered services).

Peer support within traditional mental health agencies and programs is viewed as potentially valuable in developing positive therapeutic relationships between program staff, in this case a peer, and a program participant, as a result of the staffperson's willingness to share their personal experiences with mental health issues. Peers may also express greater empathy, or at least empathy that the program participant views as more authentic. The peer staffperson may also be more effective in normalizing the experience of the program participant (i.e., "We are not alone"), inspiring hope, and modeling alternative ways of thinking and behaving while living successfully and productively in the community with a mental illness.

Funding for all peer support services has conventionally been modest and unstable. This is possibly due to perceptions that peer support and other forms of self-help/mutual-aid are less helpful and valuable compared to professionally led services (Salzer et al., 1994, 2001). However, the status and funding stability of peer support services took a revolutionary turn in 2001 when Georgia became the first state to specifically identify peer support as a Medicaid-fundable service (Sabin & Daniels, 2003). Peers were provided with opportunities to participate in a 2-week training program to become a "Certified Peer Specialist" and could then be hired to provide Medicaid billable, direct services to their peers. The primary responsibility of the certified peer specialist as specified in the authorization is to "... assist consumers in regaining control over their own lives and control over their recovery processes ... model competence and the possibility of recovery ..." and "... .assist consumers in developing the perspective and skills that facilitate recovery" (Georgia Division of Mental Health as cited in Sabin & Daniels, 2003). Such a funding approach offers long-term financial stability for the provision of peer support, recognition of peer support as a legitimate form of help on equal footing with services provided by more traditional behavioral health disciplines (i.e., psychiatrists, psychologists, social workers), and augments the voice and opportunities for self-determination of persons in recovery within mental health policy, agencies, and programs. It also dramatically expands opportunities for peers as valued and essential members of the behavioral health workforce.

The goal of this chapter is to review current knowledge related to peers as paid employees in the behavioral health system. The literature in this area lacks uniformity in the definition of this emerging workforce and specificity about what they do. For example, as will be described later, even the basic job titles for these individuals vary dramatically. For the purposes of this chapter we will use the generic term "peer specialist" to describe a peer who is explicitly hired because of their personal experience with mental health issues and willingness to share these experiences for the benefit of others. The intention of this chapter is to primarily focus on those peer specialists who have completed specialized training leading to some form of certification, often referred to as certified peer specialists (CPSs), and describe such training and their outcomes. This focus does not necessarily reflect a belief that non-CPSs are less qualified. Instead, it recognizes the significance of Medicaid reimbursement for peer support and the training requirement for such reimbursement. Moreover, it is believed that CPS training also further legitimizes peers as an important and valuable new behavioral health workforce. Current knowledge on the following topics will be addressed in this chapter:

(1) Current status of peer support funding in state-approved Medicaid programs
(2) Certified peer specialist training initiatives and training content
(3) Certified peer specialist training outcomes
(4) Certified peer specialist and peer specialist employment, hours, and pay
(5) Certified peer specialist job titles, work activities, and job satisfaction
(6) Implementation issues pertaining to certified peer specialists and peer specialists

Finally, we will end with a discussion of emerging policy, program, practice, and research issues in this area. In addressing these questions it is important to recognize that some current research includes results from peer specialists who have not received specialized training (i.e., certification as a peer specialist), peer specialists who work as volunteers instead of paid employees, and those who are compensated through funding other than Medicaid. Nonetheless, we believe the results that are presented are relevant to the future of this vital new workforce.

8.1 Current Status of Peer Support Funding in State-Approved Medicaid Programs

As noted earlier, the state of Georgia, quickly followed by Arizona, was the first to approve peer support as a Medicaid billable service in 2001. Since that time a number of other states have moved to include peer support under their Medicaid programs using the following authorities: Section 1905(a)(13), 1915(b) Waiver Authority, 1915(c) Waiver Authority. The Center for Medicare and Medicaid Services (CMS) has developed further guidance to states on what is required under these authorities (CMS Operations, 2007). CMS specifically comments on the need for supervision of peer support providers by a "competent mental health professional," that peer support services should be coordinated with other services in order to achieve person-centered, individualized goals, and that "Peer support providers must complete training and certification as defined by the State," and, like other certified providers, obtain continuing education.

Gene Johnson, President and CEO of one of the pioneering certified peer specialist training programs in the country, Recovery Innovations, wrote a comprehensive report about the current status of Medicaid funding for peer support services across the nation as of 2008 (Johnson, 2008). Johnson identified three types of peer support service initiatives across the various states. The first he described as peer support delivered as a "discrete service," where the focus is on the credentials of the individual providing peer support (i.e., a CPS) without consideration of the agency or program in which the services are embedded. Arizona, Pennsylvania, Georgia, and Washington are given as examples of states allowing for Medicaid funding for these services. The second was peer support delivered as part of another Medicaid reimbursed service, like Assertive Community Treatment or "Community Support Teams," in states such as Hawaii, North Carolina, Maine, Illinois, Wisconsin, Michigan, Oregon, and Minnesota. Finally, New Hampshire, Georgia, Arizona, and Minnesota allow for Medicaid reimbursement of peer support services provided through a licensed and credentialed "peer support organization" that exclusively provides peer support services. The specific authorization language for each state was consolidated in Johnson's (2008) outstanding report.

8.2 CPS Training Initiatives and Training Content

Some form of training for peers who provide support to other peers has existed to some extent in the past. This has been particularly evident in the self-help/mutual-aid group movement where groups like the GROW and the Depression and Bipolar Support Alliance offer training for group leaders, as well as the National Mental Health Consumers Self-Help Clearinghouse, a federally funded center that also offers training materials for self-help/mutual-aid group leaders. One of the earliest known training programs for peers who were to work as case manager aides occurred in the late 1980s (Sherman & Porter, 1991). Medicaid reimbursement for peer support services, including the requirement that peers receive specialized training in order to ensure standards of competency and quality assurance, has drawn increased attention to such training, and dramatic increases in the number of training programs available across the country.

Certified peer specialist (CPS) training programs first emerged in Georgia and Arizona, not surprisingly given that these were the first states to authorize Medicaid funding. Many more CPS training programs have since been developed. In the Summer of 2006 a compendium of known training programs was pulled together from among those who responded to requests for information (Katz & Salzer, 2007). The goal of this initiative was to develop a greater understanding of the similarities and differences in training hours and content and to provide descriptions and contact information for other states interested in developing similar initiatives. A total of 13 CPS training programs were listed.

Training programs differ in many ways, including the number of hours and days that are required, format, including use of experiential exercises and role plays, and evaluation criteria for earning a certificate. The length of CPS training, often 80 h or less, falls well below the hours required for other common behavioral health disciplines, such as that for social workers, nurses, psychologists, and psychiatrists. However, the training is seemingly on par with what is commonly received by the majority of persons employed in the mental health system. These individuals, commonly referred to as "mental health professionals," often have high school or college degrees with no specific additional academic mental health training, and commonly work in hospital settings, partial programs, case management, and residential programs.

No national standards are currently available for what competencies CPS themselves should have or what should be covered in CPS training programs. One initiative to develop national competencies has been undertaken by the Veterans Administration (VA), which has become one of the biggest employers of peer specialists nationwide. A national committee of experts, including CPS, CPS supervisors, and others, including this author, were brought together to identify competencies that peers should have in order to work as peer specialists in VA facilities and that should be covered by CPS training programs who prepare peers for employment in the VA. These criteria are not currently publicly available. The content of CPS training programs differ somewhat, but do include some overlapping areas. The Center for Mental Health Services at SAMHSA published a guide on "Establishing Medicaid-Funded Peer Support Services and a Trained Peer Workforce" (2005) in which they list CPS competencies used in the Georgia Peer Specialist Training Program. These competencies are reproduced in Table 8.1.

8.3 Certified Peer Specialist Training Outcomes

Persons who are skeptical about peers in the workforce may be equally wary about the value of CPS training programs in preparing peers for such work. Concerns have been raised about the stress of intensive training on peers, that such training programs would have little benefit, and that they are inadequate to prepare peers for roles in the behavioral health workforce. A few studies of relevance to these issues have been conducted and are reported here.

A series of studies have shown that a high percentage of peers who enroll and attend training programs successfully complete them. Ratzlaff et al. (2006) report that 100 out of 137 (73%) of the peers who were accepted and attended an intensive 15-week course plus internship program graduated. Hutchinson et al. (2006) report that all 141 individuals (100%) who enrolled in the Meta Services Peer Provider

Table 8.1 CPS training competencies (from CMHS/SAMHSA, 2005)

Competency domain	Competency standard
1. An understanding of their job and the skills to do that job	• Understand the basic structure of the State mental health system and how it works • Understand the CPS job description and Code of Ethics within the State mental health system • Understand the meaning and role of peer support • Understand the difference in treatment goals and recovery goals • Be able to create and facilitate a variety of group activities that support and strengthen recovery • Be able to do the necessary documentation required by the State • Be able to help a consumer combat negative self-talk, overcome fears, and solve problems • Be able to help a consumer articulate, set, and accomplish his/her goals • Be able to teach other consumers to create their own wellness recovery action plans • Be able to teach other consumers to advocate for the services that they want • Be able to help a consumer create a person-centered plan
2. An understanding of the recovery process and how to use their own recovery story to help others	• Understand the five stages in the recovery process and what is helpful and not helpful at each stage • Understand the role of peer support at each stage of the recovery process • Understand the power of beliefs/values and how they support or work against recovery • Understand the basic philosophy and principles of psychosocial rehabilitation • Understand the basic definition and dynamics of recovery • Be able to articulate what has been helpful and what not helpful in his/her own recovery • Be able to identify beliefs and values a consumer holds that work against his/her recovery • Be able to discern when and how much of their recovery story to share with whom
3. An understanding of and the ability to establish healing relationships	• Understand the dynamics of power, conflict, and integrity in the workplace • Understand the concept of "seeking out common ground" • Understand the meaning and importance of cultural competency • Be able to ask open-ended questions that relate a person to his/her inner wisdom • Be able to personally deal with conflict and difficult interpersonal relations in the workplace • Be able to demonstrate an ability to participate in "healing communication" • Be able to interact sensitively and effectively with people of other cultures
4. An understanding of the importance of and having the ability to take care of oneself	• Understand the dynamics of stress and burnout • Understand the role and parts of the Wellness Recovery Action Plan (WRAP) • Be able to discuss one's own tools for taking care of oneself

training program successfully completed it. Stoneking and McGuffin (2007) found that 69 out of the 73 (95%) individuals accepted in the Recovery Support Specialist Institute graduated. And Salzer et al. (2009) report that 72 out of 74 (97%) individuals enrolled in training provided by the Institute on Recovery and Community Integration successfully completed the program.

Studies have also shown that participation in these training programs is associated with positive psychological outcomes and personal growth. Hutchinson et al. (2006) conducted a pre-posttest study and found that training graduates reported higher levels of empowerment and stronger recovery attitudes and perceptions of themselves after the training compared to before. Ratzlaff et al. (2006) also gathered survey data using a pre-posttest design, but controlled for possible response shifts, in other words, changes in how the respondent interprets the questions, by including a retrospective pretest survey. Overall, they found that participants in the training program they studied reported greater levels of hope, self-esteem, and advancement in their recovery over time.

Finally, a third area of inquiry has been on the impact of training on knowledge acquisition. This is particularly relevant given Johnson's (2008) finding that a number of states require tests, including written and oral components, in order to certify someone as a peer specialist. Examples of such states are Washington, Georgia, Illinois, and Hawaii. There is currently no national certification process or test.

The findings so far in this area look promising. One study (Stoneking & McGuffin, 2007) asked respondents to rate their own knowledge, skills, and attitudes before and after the training in competency areas identified by the program and viewed as relevant to their future work as peer specialists. They found substantial increases in pre-posttest self-ratings in all areas. Their supervisors also rated them highly in these areas after being hired.

Some CPS training programs have taken it upon themselves to develop tests as part of their certification process. For example, Recovery Innovations (formerly Meta Services) developed a test and reports finding an increase in scores over time in a pre-posttest evaluation involving 15 trainees (Boston University Center for Psychiatric Rehabilitation, 2007 as reported in Johnson, 2008). Another pre-posttest evaluation found a 12% increase in correct answers on a knowledge test administered to 40 participants in the Peer Support Certification course offered by the Depression and Bipolar Support Alliance (Cook & Burke-Miller, 2004). Finally, a statistically significant increase in knowledge has also been reported for trainees of the CPS program developed by the Institute on Recovery and Community Integration (Salzer et al., 2009). In this latter study, a 60-item test assessing all areas of the curriculum, such as recovery concepts, peer support, Wellness Recovery Action Plan (WRAP), communication skills, diversity and cultural competency, motivational enhancement skills, boundary issues and ethics, workplace issues and practices, is used with identified correct and incorrect responses as part of the certification process. On the pretest items taken by respondents it was found that peers had an overall mean of 63% correct responses. This indicates fairly good knowledge in these areas, possibly as a result of the fact that many were already working in the field as peer specialists upon entering the program. The mean correct on the posttest was 85%, indicating a 22% increase in knowledge. While no benchmark is used in the Institute's certification process, it is instructive to note that only 39% scored above a 70% correct threshold on the pretest while 98% scored above that threshold on the posttest.

8.4 CPS/PS Employment, Hours, and Pay

One interesting perspective on the training of peers for positions in the behavioral health system is to view it as an employment initiative for a population of individuals that has historically had high unemployment rates. A substantial amount of knowledge is being generated in this area. Employment outcomes for individuals who have participated in CPS training programs are impressive. All trainees in the Meta Services program obtained employment, and 89% were employed 12 months later (Hutchinson et al., 2006). Similar outcomes were found for the Pennsylvania CPS study where 82% of all graduates were employed 1-year post-training (Salzer et al., 2009). Somewhat less positive employment findings were reported for the Arizona RSS training where approximately 55–60% were employed at any given time post-training (Stoneking & McGuffin, 2007). Longitudinal follow-up of the Kansas Consumers as Providers (CAP) graduates found that 60% were competitively employed at 6 months post-training, 59% at 1-year post-training, and 58% at 2 years post-training (Rapp et al., 2008).

A number of important factors are worth considering when examining CPS training as an employment initiative. For example, Salzer et al. (2009) studied employment outcomes in three regions of Pennsylvania. They found that while overall employment outcomes were good, there was variability across the regions – 100% of trainees were employed in one region, 79% in another, and 69% in a third region. The variability was partly attributed to regional differences in the prior employment status of the trainees. For example, nearly all the peers in the region that achieved 100% employment post-training were already employed prior to training, many in the same positions. Over all the regions, approximately 74% were employed prior to training. The net increase in employment among all trainees was only 8%. Rapp et al. (2008) report that 28% of the CAP graduates were competitively employed prior to the training, resulting in a 30% net increase in the number of people employed after the training.

While some obtain full-time employment as peer specialists, the current data suggest that most do not. One study (Stoneking & McGuffin, 2007) reported that several trainees began their employment working full-time with benefits, but that part-time work, around 20 h per week was most common. Another study (Hutchinson et al., 2006) reported that 29% of the jobs obtained by trainees were full-time positions, 52% were part-time, and 19% worked flexible hours. Average starting wage was $9.33/h and full-time salaries ranged between $23,566 and $40,000 with benefits. Employed CPS worked an average of 27 h per week with an average hourly wage of $10.85 in another study (Salzer et al., 2009). A study of peers employed in the Veterans Administration (Hebert et al., 2008) found hourly wages ranging from minimum wage to $20/h, and salaried positions ranging from $16,600 to $34,920 per year with benefits. The National Association of Peer Specialists (2007) conducted a national survey in which they received responses from 173 peer specialists. They found that the average respondent worked 29.5 h per week with an hourly wage of $12.13. Finally, Salzer, Schwenk, & Brusilovskiy (2010) conducted a national survey of 291 certified peer specialists from June 2008 to March 2009 and found that they worked an average of 29.6 h per week.

Results from the National Association of Peer Specialists (2007) also indicate that 37% of respondents report the loss of benefits, presumably social security entitlements and public healthcare coverage, as a major barrier to their working full-time. Seventeen percent reported their own "mental health" as a barrier and 12% report that their "physical health" is a barrier. Low wages, administrator/manager issues, and lack of demand for their services were other factors.

8.5 CPS Job Titles, and Work Activities, Job Satisfaction

Johnson's (2008) review of state Medicaid authorizations indicates great variability in where peers specialists can work and what they can do. The Georgia job description, for example, lists 17 specific activities ranging from helping consumers create a Wellness Recovery Action Plan to "support[ing] the vocational choices consumers make and assist[ing] them in overcoming job-related anxiety" and "inform[ing] consumers about community and natural supports and how to utilize these in the recovery process" (Georgia Division of Mental Health, Developmental Disabilities and Addictive Diseases as cited in Sabin & Daniels, 2003).

8.5.1 Job Titles

As reported earlier, Salzer and colleagues (Schwenk et al., 2009; Salzer, Schwenk, & Brusilovskiy, 2010), conducted a national survey in which 291 employed CPS from 28 states completed an online survey in which they were asked to report on their job titles, type of program in which they work, amount of time spent engaged in various activities, and provide a brief description of what they do. Respondents offered 105 different job titles. The most common title was "Certified peer specialist" reported by 60 individuals. Another 28 individuals reported a close variation – "Certified peer support specialist." The second most common title was "Peer support specialist" reported by 42 individuals. Thirty-five other individuals reported a job title that also started with "Peer ...," but had endings such as "advocate," "counselor," "specialist," and "mentor." A similar range of job titles was found by Hebert et al. (2008).

8.5.2 Work Settings

Survey results have documented that peer specialists work in many different types of agencies, a variety of programs within these agencies, and are engaged in different activities within these programs. The National Association of Peer Specialists (2007) survey found that most peers were working in non-profit organizations (66%), with the remaining respondents working in government agencies (20%), for-profit organizations (11%), or as independent contractors (3%). Stoneking and McGuffin (2007) report that RSS trainees were employed in multiple settings, including residential treatment programs, case management clinics, integrated dual diagnosis treatment programs, outpatient substance use programs for mothers with children, consumer-run and operated agencies, and advocacy rights programs. Respondents to the national survey of CPS (Salzer, Schwenk, & Brusilovskiy, 2010) worked in an assortment of programs: independent peer support ($N = 70$), case management ($N = 57$), partial hospital/day program, inpatient or crisis ($N = 31$), vocational rehabilitation and clubhouse programs ($N = 23$), drop-in centers ($N = 21$), education/advocacy ($N = 15$), residential ($N = 12$), and finally, therapeutic recreation/socialization or psychiatric rehabilitation ($N = 10$). The remaining respondents ($N = 52$) were categorized as working in "other" types of programs.

8.5.3 Work Activities

Peer specialists are also engaged in varied activities. Hebert et al. (2008) gathered information about what peer specialists do in 25 VA facilities. Ten facilities (40%) reported that peer specialists only led groups; nine (36%) indicated that peer specialists provided 1:1 peer mentoring, outreach, or counseling services; and six (24%) said they offered a combination of supports including one-to-one individual and group support, a warmline, and a peer drop-in center. Chinman et al. (2008) conducted focus groups at a national VA conference that involved 59 peer specialists and 34 supervisors. They found that peer roles varied across facilities, but generally involved direct service with veterans, including the following: assisting with or conducting new patient orientation; leading many types of groups (support, illness management, 12-step, and social or quality of life); completing intakes, screenings, and treatment planning; helping people find housing; accompanying people to community activities; providing advocacy for needed services; providing transportation; helping people with basic daily needs; and serving as a program "clerk."

Salzer, Schwenk, & Brusilovskiy (2010) have thus far provided the most in-depth national look at CPS activities. The results indicate that CPSs provide most of their services on-site rather than in the community. The one exception to this was CPS who worked in case management programs. CPSs also spend almost 50% of their time supporting peers individually and approximately 25% of their time in groups. However, these percentages do differ somewhat by program. CPS in case management and residential programs provide more individualized supports while those in other programs tend to spend more time providing support in groups.

CPSs were also asked to rate the frequency of which they provide various supports. Table 8.2 lists the mean frequency of supports provided (1 = "never"; 5 = "always"). Peer support was by far the most prevalent activity, followed by encouragement of self-determination and personal responsibility. Other prevalent supports, with mean frequencies ranging between 3.5 and 3.9, included dealing with health and wellness, handling hopelessness, communication with providers, illness management, addressing stigma in the community, and working on developing friendships. The considerably less focal supports (with means below 3 "Sometimes") included family relationships, citizenship, spirituality/religion, developing psychiatric advanced directives, parenting, employment, and dating.

A further analysis of these results provides an interesting picture about how CPS activities group together and the intensity of these activities across program settings. The responses about the extent to which CPSs provide various supports were entered into an exploratory factor analysis with varimax rotation using SAS Proc Factor. The principal axis method was used for factor extraction, and the scree test and factor interpretability determined the number of factors to retain. Items were considered to be part of a particular factor if the factor loading was greater than 0.40, and the loadings on all other factors were 0.40 or less. Factor stability was confirmed through additional factor analyses using randomly split samples. Factor scores were calculated by calculating the average of all variables that load on the factor. Statistical comparisons of factor scores across programs were not conducted due to small sample sizes for some programs.

The factor analysis yielded a replicable and interpretable five-factor solution (Table 8.2). The activities loading on the "Core Supports" factor correspond to the top seven supports with the highest mean frequency of occurrence. The second factor was labeled "Intimacy Supports" and included parenting, family relationships, dating, and spirituality/religion supports. The third factor, "Leisure and Social Supports," included leisure/recreation, transportation, citizenship, and developing friendships. The fourth factor, "Advocacy and Career Supports," included education and employment, and the fifth factor, "Recovery Tools," specifically included the development of WRAP plans and PADS. Supporting citizenship loaded on both the third and fourth factors in our random, split-half analyses, but otherwise the factor loadings were relatively stable.

Table 8.3 presents the overall and by-program factor scores. Not surprisingly, the first factor (Core Supports) consistently has the highest activity score overall and across all programs ($M = 3.9$). The intimacy factor had the lowest activity scores overall ($M = 2.4$) and across all programs except residential, where the Recovery Tools factor had the lowest score. Leisure/social supports were a frequent set of CPS activities in case management, residential, drop-in centers, and independent peer support programs; career supports were more heavily provided in Vocational Rehabilitation/clubhouse, education/advocacy, and independent peer support programs; and Recovery Tools were only a central activity in the PHINC programs category.

Our results, while not definitive given small samples in certain programs that prevented statistical analysis, nonetheless appear to support the influence of

Table 8.2 Rotated factor loadings

Please tell us how often you support your peers in …	N	Mean ± Std. Dev	Factor 1 Core supports	Factor 2 Intimacy supports	Factor 3 Leisure/social supports	Factor 4 Advocacy and career supports	Factor 5 Recovery tools	Final communalities
Peer support	254	4.48 ± 0.77	54*	1	28	0	18	0.41
Encouraging self-determination and personal responsibility	257	4.26 ± 0.88	79*	14	9	19	17	0.72
Health and wellness	251	3.87 ± 0.93	58*	30	19	21	24	0.56
Hopelessness	255	3.84 ± 1.08	64*	15	18	11	11	0.49
Communication with providers	256	3.68 ± 0.99	46*	38	15	20	−5	0.42
Illness management	250	3.62 ± 1.13	60*	21	9	15	26	0.50
Stigma in the community	254	3.56 ± 1.13	53*	36	8	35	12	0.55
Family relationships (e.g., with parents, siblings, cousins, etc.)	255	2.95 ± 1.11	23	72*	13	8	14	0.62
Spirituality/religion	253	2.74 ± 1.12	30	50*	9	7	25	0.42
Parenting	248	2.14 ± 1.15	12	68*	24	21	11	0.59
Dating	250	1.74 ± 0.98	10	42*	40	31	14	0.46
Developing friendships	255	3.51 ± 1.05	27	24	57*	4	34	0.57
Leisure/recreation (e.g., exercise, hobby groups, movies)	256	3.25 ± 1.14	17	14	69*	3	11	0.54
Transportation	250	3.06 ± 1.28	11	9	59*	10	−6	0.38
Citizenship (e.g., voting, volunteering, advocacy)	252	2.83 ± 1.15	15	40	43*	33	7	0.48
Education	255	3.16 ± 1.12	24	20	1	67*	29	0.62
Employment	252	2.94 ± 1.06	18	14	21	62*	15	0.50
Developing WRAP plans	256	3.04 ± 1.31	28	16	8	24	59*	0.51
Developing psychiatric advanced directives	252	2.27 ± 1.18	26	18	9	24	54*	0.46

Note: Printed loadings are multiplied by 100 and rounded to the nearest integer. Values greater than 0.4 are flagged by an asterisk (*). Observations from 205 respondents were employed in factor analysis due to missing data

Table 8.3 Factor "subscale" scores

	Statistic	Factor Core supports (1)	Intimacy suppots (2)	Leisure/social supports (3)	Advocacy and career supports (4)	Recovery tools (5)
All programs (*OVERALL*)	Mean ± St. Dev. *N*	3.9 ± 0.72 259	2.4 ± 0.87 258	3.16 ± 0.86 258	3.05 ± 0.97 258	2.66 ± 1.12 257
Case management (*CM*)	Mean ± St. Dev. *N*	3.97 ± 0.78 48	2.24 ± 0.79 48	3.32 ± 0.71 48	2.78 ± 0.8 48	2.44 ± 1.12 48
Partial hospital/day program, inpatient, or CRISIS (*PHINC*)	Mean ± St. Dev. *N*	3.83 ± 0.69 29	2.5 ± 0.81 29	2.89 ± 0.83 29	3.02 ± 0.97 29	3.03 ± 1.02 29
VR or clubhouse	Mean ± St. Dev. *N*	3.42 ± 0.82 22	2.35 ± 0.91 22	2.77 ± 0.98 21	3.21 ± 1.25 21	2.57 ± 1.1 21
Therapeutic recreation or psych. rehabilitation (*TRPR*)	Mean ± St. Dev. *N*	3.77 ± 0.5 7	2.18 ± 0.93 7	2.82 ± 0.51 7	2.57 ± 1.06 7	2.57 ± 0.79 7
Residential (*RES*)	Mean ± St. Dev. *N*	3.59 ± 0.64 10	2.03 ± 0.61 10	3.24 ± 0.78 10	2.7 ± 0.63 10	1.85 ± 0.67 10
Drop-in center (*DC*)	Mean ± St. Dev. *N*	3.87 ± 0.57 20	2.46 ± 0.68 20	3.48 ± 0.77 20	2.9 ± 1.07 20	2.43 ± 1.17 20
Education/advocacy (*ED*)	Mean ± St. Dev. *N*	3.94 ± 0.56 15	2.05 ± 0.89 14	2.82 ± 0.91 15	3.63 ± 0.69 15	2.96 ± 0.97 14
Independent peer support program (*IPSP*)	Mean ± St. Dev. *N*	3.94 ± 0.65 63	2.37 ± 0.9 63	3.26 ± 0.92 63	3.14 ± 0.87 63	2.87 ± 1.1 63

settings on CPS activities. The set of activities we described as "Core Supports" were found to be universally important in the CPS role, regardless of the program in which they work. Leisure/social supports and advocacy and career supports were a major focus in four of the eight programs. It is not surprising that CPS focused on Recovery Tools in partial hospitals/inpatient/crisis programs, as both tools support the enhancement of crisis coping skills. However, WRAP was not used as much as anticipated given how well-known it is in recovery circles. Finally, there was an almost universal lack of attention to intimacy supports among CPS across all programs.

8.5.4 Job Satisfaction

There is limited data on how satisfied peer specialists are with their positions and how well they get along with their non-peer co-workers. One study conducted in Pennsylvania found that peer specialists were highly satisfied with their positions, with an average satisfaction rating of 4.69 on a (1) "Not at all satisfied" to (5) "extremely satisfied" scale (Salzer et al., 2009). These respondents also rated their supervisors highly in terms of listening to their ideas and suggestions and providing them with a great deal of support. They also felt accepted and respected by their non-peer co-workers. The NAOPS national survey (2007) reports similar job satisfaction results, with 32% of the respondents indicating that they are "always" satisfied with their work and another 61% reporting being "mostly" satisfied. While most CPS indicated feeling respected by their co-workers, 65% – "Frequently" and another 31% – "Sometimes," almost 5% report frequent conflicts with co-workers and 37% conflict "sometimes." This is an area worthy of further study that is directly related to the implementation issues discussed in the next section.

8.6 Implementation Issues Pertaining to CPS/PS

There is ample literature on implementation issues associated with peers as employees in traditional mental health programs going back many years (e.g., Besio & Mahler, 1993; Carlson et al., 2001; Dixon Krauss, & Lehman, 1994; Felton et al., 1995; Manning & Suire, 1996; Mowbray et al., 1997; Salzer & Mental Health Association of Southeastern Pennsylvania Best Practices Team, 2002). Common implementation issues identified in this work include negative beliefs, attitudes, and behaviors toward peer staff by non-peer staff, role conflict and confusion, lack of clarity around self-disclosure and concerns about peer staff disclosing confidential information, poorly defined jobs, and lack of opportunity for networking and support. The increased hiring of peers following the current CPS revolution has led to a flurry of new work in this area. The findings from these newer studies, reviewed below, replicate past findings cited above. Many of the key barriers to successful inclusion of peers in the workforce still exist and the recommendations made by many in the past are still relevant today.

Gates and Akabas (2007) conducted a study of agency responses to hiring peers in which they interviewed staff from 27 mental health agencies in New York City and 15 peers who attended a focus group. They found that many providers maintain negative attitudes toward peers. This included viewing their presence as contributing little, or possibly watering down the effectiveness of other staff and the treatment environment, and as "cheap" labor. However, some did express appreciation for what peers can provide in promoting recovery, especially if their agency was viewed as more advanced in terms of including recovery as part of their mission. Ample evidence of role conflict was found, especially on the part of non-peer co-workers who viewed peer staff behavior through the lens of their having a mental illness and treating them as patients rather than colleagues. Expressions of any stress, including typical work stress, was met with questions about medication compliance and health rather than more normalized validation that the work being done is difficult or that stress is part of all of our lives. Non-peers also viewed the interpersonal methods used by peers as "unprofessional" rather than appreciating that the unique experiences and approaches offered by peers would have unique value in terms of making connections. Challenges were also raised by hiring peers who were also participants in agency programs.

A review of job descriptions indicated that peers were being asked to engage in many different activities, some of which overlapped with non-peer staff activities leading to concerns that "cheaper" peers would take the jobs of non-peers. Finally, they found that non-peers were not adequately trained for the inclusion of peers in the workforce and did not understand the uniqueness and benefits from their roles. Peers were also not specifically trained in workforce demands that the non-peers were expected to have upon being hired.

Much of the recent writing on implementation issues facing peers in the workforce has come from research examining efforts to incorporate peer staff in the Veterans Affairs (VA) health care system. The VA has undertaken a series of initiatives, including hiring substantial numbers of peer specialists across the country, to achieve the goals outlined in the President's New Freedom Commission Report on Mental Health (2003). Hebert et al. (2008) gathered survey data from informants at 25 VA facilities across the country in which they asked questions about a number of peer specialist implementation issues. These included how the facility dealt with self-disclosure, role boundaries, acquiring staff buy-in, addressing criticism of non-peer staff by peer specialists, and legal/liability issues associated with peer specialists. Chinman and colleagues (2006, 2008) also examined implementation issues in the VA.

Chinman et al. (2006) examined traditional PS staff perceptions about the feasibility and acceptability of peer-delivered services and staff within three VA clinics in Southern California. They conducted focus groups with non-peer and peer staff and interviewed administrators from these facilities. They also gathered survey data from the participants. Overall, stakeholders had similar, generally positive beliefs about peer staff. However, while not statistically significant given the test used by the authors, it does appear that peer staff believe more strongly than providers that they could work well with difficult patients. It also appears that non-peer providers may tend to be more skeptical about the ability of peers to fit in with co-workers and keep information confidential. In terms of appropriate roles for PS there was consensus about the following activities: support, role modeling and hope for recovery, assistance with community integration, and a bridge between patients and the mental health system. The latter activity was an area that all groups were most enthusiastic about as they observed that many consumers need guidance to negotiate the system, an advocate within the system, and encouragement to fully participate in the service delivery process.

These authors also found that many providers were uncomfortable with the notion that peer staff would have direct 1:1 contact with their peers away from their traditional provider colleagues. They were most comfortable with peer specialists running groups that could be easily observed. Peer specialists and administrators were much more open to 1:1 contact and believed it to be of great potential benefit. Providers also expressed concerns about the amount and quality of training obtained by peer staff and whether they would rely on their own experiences solely as the only "path to recovery" rather than fully utilizing their training in their work. Concerns were also raised about potential harms to peers from peer staff acting inappropriately, including direct, conflictual interactions, possibly as a result of their symptoms. Non-peer staff providers were also concerned about added burden to their own work resulting from having to address problems created by PS, added supervision burden, and needing to deal with complications associated with hiring someone who also might receive services at the same facility.

Chinman et al. (2008) obtained a broader, national picture of peer specialist implementation issues in the VA through focus groups conducted with 59 VA peer staff and 34 VA supervisors. The hiring of peer staff in the VA was found to result in a number of positive and negative outcomes. The addition of peers impacts the entire treatment team and veteran consumers in terms of helping them become more person-centered and recovery-oriented, and veterans receiving services were reportedly better able to connect to the peers, thereby enhancing trust and engagement. Peer staff also influenced the development of new services, encouraged the use of new coping strategies, and facilitated self-advocacy. The material requirements of peer staff, such as access to designated workspace, a phone, and a computer, apparently caught some programs off-guard. Additionally, the presence of peer staff required changes in team operations and the need for non-peer staff to learn how to overcome fears about peer specialist abilities and determine the best way to include them as a new team member.

Peer staff reported experiencing some challenges as they, and the other staff, figured out their roles. Job descriptions were sometimes reported to be vague and offered little direction. Peer staff also needed to work on their own discomfort from feeling isolated, as they were often the only peer on their team. Additional stress came from dealing with the transition from "patient" to "staff" roles. These stressors were occurring while PS were also attempting to overcome the overt and covert concerns about their presence from non-peer staff.

In addition to challenges in becoming a member of the team, respondents also stated that: human resources did not fully understand the position and its requirements; upper-level administrators were unfamiliar with recovery concepts and therefore, less supportive of overcoming barriers; and peer staff were poorly compensated for their work.

Gates and Akabas (2007, p. 303) provide a number of specific suggestions for addressing implementation issues. These are similar to those offered by others in the past and from non-US initiatives to include peers (a.k.a. users) in mental health service delivery (e.g., Hansen, 2001). These suggestions are listed below. To enhance staff attitudes toward recovery they recommend a clear recovery position in mission statement, leadership commitment to recovery that is well-communicated, leadership support of recovery, and communication that the peer position is viewed as essential rather than an add-on. Role conflict and confusion could be addressed through well-defined recruitment strategies, consistent application of workplace policies to peer and non-peer staff, written job descriptions for all staff including peers, supervision to ensure that actual job expectations are the same as written job expectations, training to staff and clients to provide understanding of roles, and training of new employees about the importance of peer staff. Protecting peers from unnecessary disclosure of their mental health status could be achieved by having neutral job titles that do not disclose peer status and implementing a formal disclosure process for peers. The confidentiality of their medical records could be addressed by enhanced training on policies and practices related to confidentiality, keeping previous treatment records of internally recruited peers in confidential files, and not allowing peers to receive services in the units where they are employed. Human resources-related issues could be addressed by clearly accepting experience in lieu of formal credentials as HR policy, making peer positions permanent with a clear path for promotion, applying the same performance standards to peer and non-peer staff, equal compensation, provide benefits counseling to help peers make fully informed decisions about the number of hours they want to work and the possible impact on their entitlements, and offer ADA accommodations as requested. Finally, in order to address peers feeling isolated and lacking support, agencies can provide full opportunities for peers to engage in agency life (i.e., team meetings), involvement in treatment planning and writing case notes, provide training to learn the language of the workplace, and timely and appropriate levels of supervision.

Chinman et al. (2008) offer a few additional recommendations. They suggest a readiness assessment of current staff and programs to ensure they are fully prepared to include peer staff. Such an approach may lessen this external stressor on peers early on. They also suggest identifying effective training strategies for peer staff and implementing continuous quality improvement efforts in order to assess the impact of peer staff on their peers. Further, research need to identify factors associated with PS effectiveness.

8.7 Emerging Issues Pertaining to CPS

A number of issues are emerging as a result of the increasing inclusion of peers in the workforce. State behavioral health leaders continue to struggle with the language they should use in their Medicaid authorizations to describe peer support goals and activities while ensuring that quality supports are provided. These challenges, combined with executive and legislator fears about ballooning Medicaid budgets, may stymie the continued growth of peer specialist initiatives. In a related vein, there are no current, commonly accepted certification standards for what is to be covered in CPS training. This requires every state to develop their own unique standards and approaches. In addition to further slowing down the authorization process, it also limits the portability of certification obtained in, for example, one state that accepts the training offered by 1–2 specific training programs, to another state that might not currently recognize and accept certification from that particular program. The end result is limited employment opportunities for the CPS. A national set of competencies, training standards, and certification and continuing education procedures would be useful in addressing this issue.

It is readily apparent that current efforts to educate non-peer staff about recovery and peer support have not been sufficient to ease the implementation challenges faced by peer specialists. More strategies are needed to promote the acceptance of CPS as a new behavioral health workforce member. This also means developing career ladders that offer opportunities to the same extent as other trained disciplines, and ensuring equal pay and benefits for comparable work. One exciting development is the stupendous growth in membership at the National Association of Peer Specialists. This organization can provide CPS a greater voice in national, state, and local policies, as well as influence agency practices to the same extent as other national organizations, such as the American Psychiatric, Psychological, and Nurses Associations, and the National Association of Social Workers.

Human resource issues are also an important topic. Supervisors and human resource administrators have expressed concerns that peer staff experience more work-related and personal challenges than non-peer staff that diminish productivity and require additional attention compared to non-peer staff. Work-related challenges may include decreased efficiency and problems completing paperwork, as well as difficulties with co-workers and supervisors. Personal challenges include perceived higher rates of absenteeism and the use of more sick leave. It is not clear to what extent these issues reflect negative stereotypes and prejudice, or are due to the presence of a psychiatric disability, or a combination of both. What is known is that other similarly skilled direct care professionals in the behavioral health system also experience significant challenges (Baron, 2007). It remains an open question worthy of additional study whether or not peer staff requires more attention than other staff. Regardless, persons with disabilities have a legal right to accommodations in the workplace as long as it does not interfere with their ability to do their job.

From a practice standpoint, it is clear that CPSs are engaged in a wide-range of programs and that their activities are quite varied. Acknowledging the specialization that is occurring in CPS practice requires further development of specialized training and continuing education initiatives that are tailored to the specific settings and or activities that the CPS is engaged in. For example, Bluebird (2008) has produced a document that is explicitly focused on peers who are working in inpatient settings. Other specialized training programs include those for peer specialists who are working with individuals who have come into contact with the criminal justice system, and training for people working with older adults, transition-age youth, or children.

There are a number of research questions that would be useful to address about CPS, many of which could also be asked of other mental health disciplines. The most commonly asked question pertains to the effectiveness of CPS/Peer specialist services. However, CPSs should not be expected to achieve a single common goal because they work in different settings and have different job expectations. For example, reasonable outcomes for peer staff who work in inpatient or crisis programs may be reduced use of seclusion and restraint and other coercive methods whereas a CPS on a case management team may achieve greater success in supporting someone in moving toward their career goals.

Expecting common psychosocial outcomes, such as enhanced empowerment, recovery, quality of life, social support, or even hope from a workforce with 105 different job titles is not practical. Instead, it is more reasonable to examine the contributions of CPS within specific program and activity parameters. Quasi-experimental and experimental designs have been used to examine the effectiveness of peer-as-employee initiatives *within* specific types of programs and engaged in specific activities with precise outcome goals. This includes research-examining peers as part of case management services (e.g., Chinman et al., 2000; Felton et al., 1995; Solomon & Draine, 1995), crisis and respite services (e.g., Brown, 1997; Lyons, Cook, Ruth, & Karver, 1996), vocational services (e.g., Mowbray, Rusilowski-Clover, Arnold, & Allen, 1994), or independent peer support programs (e.g., Klein, Cnaan, & Whitecraft, 1998; Min et al., 2007). It must also be kept in mind that individual-level outcomes are affected by many factors, including the use of effective practices, regardless of which discipline engages in the practice (e.g., CPS or a social worker), and the influence of other providers who are part of a team or who otherwise come into contact with an individual. Specificity in drawing causal inferences about individual-level outcomes to a single provider such as a CPS is difficult to accomplish.

It is also important to further examine the impact of peer staff on agency culture and practices. Some of the previously mentioned qualitative studies have reported anecdotal positive effects. Additional quantitative research would also be useful. Studies could examine non-peer staff changes in attitudes toward recovery over time following the inclusion of a peer specialist in a program and identify specific changes in their practice that might be directly related to the influence of the peer staffperson. Peer specialists are also serving on committees within agencies and systems and may influence non-peer staff beliefs, attitudes, and practices at those levels as well. However, the effects of these efforts would be expected to take a long-time to detect.

Some important process questions also need to be addressed. There has been much speculation about the ability of CPS to develop better working alliances and connections with their peers compared to non-peer staff. While numerous anecdotes about such connections have been offered, it is not clear if this is the norm or only occurs sporadically. The extent of this phenomenon has yet to be sufficiently confirmed in rigorous research. In such research, it would also be important to consider that CPS may be able to develop better working relationships than non-peer staff with some individuals, but not necessarily all, and the identification of the circumstances where better connections occur would be useful in targeting where CPS may have their greatest impact.

Furthermore, to-date there have been no comparative work performance or outcome studies of certified peer specialists versus non-certified peer specialists. However, while such evidence might be interesting, even if CPSs were not found to be more effective in their jobs it cannot be used as an indication that such training is not effective. Fairly convincing evidence already exists showing the positive psychological and knowledge benefits of such training (Boston University Center for Psychiatric Rehabilitation, 2007 as reported in Johnson, 2008; Cook & Burke-Miller, 2004; Hutchinson et al., 2006; Ratzlaff et al., 2006; Salzer et al., 2009; Stoneking & McGuffin, 2007). It should also be pointed out that studies comparing licensed/certified versus unlicensed/certified practitioners in other areas also do not exist.

8.8 Summary

Medicaid reimbursement for peer support services has clearly spurred the development of a new behavioral healthcare workforce – the Certified Peer Specialist. As this review attests, we currently know a lot about this workforce in terms of the type of training they are receiving, the psychological and knowledge benefits of such training, and employment outcomes. We are also gaining a better sense of the diversity of roles they are playing in the behavioral health system, as well as the continued implementation barriers that systems, as well as peer and non-peer staff alike, still face. The increased hiring of CPS heightens the potential of actually achieving true and long-lasting system transformation goals of promoting recovery and community integration. The infusion of CPS may lead to the creation of innovative programs and practices. Additionally, their unique experiential knowledge, skills, and support shows promise for enhancing program and system effectiveness in achieving these goals. Moreover, the mental health system struggles with recruiting a committed and motivated direct care workforce that is open to the possibility of recovery and the importance of community integration. Peers represent a large potential workforce of people who can fill present employment gaps as individuals motivated to support their peers while living the goals we wish to create opportunities for everyone to achieve.

Acknowledgement The author would like to acknowledge Eugene Brusilovskiy and Edward Schwenk for their assistance in this analysis.

References

Baron, R. C. (2007). A review of current information about the careers of the direct support professional workforce in the mental health, developmental disabilities, and substance abuse delivery systems. A report from the Southeastern Pennsylvania Behavioral Health Industry. Available at http://www.upennrrtc.org/var/tool/file/143-FINAL1199C%20Report[1].pdf.

Besio, S. W., & Mahler, J. (1993). Benefits and challenges of using consumer staff in supported housing services. *Hospital and Community Psychiatry, 44*(5), 490–491.

Bluebird, G. (2008). *Paving new ground: Peers working in in-patient settings*. Alexandria, VA: National Technical Assistance Center, National Association of State Mental Health Program Directors.

Brown, L. (1997). The benefits and stresses for consumers providing respite to their peers. In C. T. Mowbray, D. P. Moxley, C. A. Jasper, & L. L. Howell (Eds.), *Consumers as providers in psychiatric rehabilitation* (pp. 243–246). Columbia, MD: International Association of Psychosocial Rehabilitation Services.

Boston University Center for Psychiatric Rehabilitation (2007). *Program evaluation results peer employment training*, Unpublished report, October, 2007. Boston University Center for Psychiatric Rehabilitation.

Center for Mental Health Services, Substance Abuse and Mental Health Services Administration. (2005). *Building a foundation for recovery: How states can establish medicaid-funded peer support services and a trained peer workforce*. DHHS Pub. No. (SMA) 05-8088. Rockville, MD.

Chinman, M. J., Rosenheck, R., Lam, J. A., & Davidson, L. (2000). Comparing consumer and nonconsumer provided case management services for homeless persons with serious mental illness. *Journal of Nervous & Mental Disease, 188*, 446–453.

Chinman, M., Lucksted, A., Gresen, R., Davis, M., Losonczy, M., Sussner, B., & Martone, L. (2008). Early experiences of employing consumer-providers in the VA. *Psychiatric Services, 59*,(11) 1315–1321.

Chinman, M., Young, A.S., Hassell, J., & Davidson, L. (2006). Toward the implementation of mental health consumer provider services. *The Journal of Behavioral Health Services and Research 33*, 2.

CMS Operations (2007). Letter to State Medicaid Director (SMDL #07-011). Available online at http://www.cms.hhs.gov/SMDL/downloads/SMD081507A.pdf.

Cook, J. A., & Burke-Miller, J. K. (2004). Evaluation of the peer support certification training program: Depression and Bipolar Support Alliance. Retrieved 7/07/09 from http://www.psych.uic.edu/MHSRP/dbsalliance.PPRC.final.rpt.pdf

Dixon, L., Krauss, N., & Lehman, A. (1994). Consumers as service providers: The promise and the challenge. *Community Mental Health Journal, 30*(6), 615–625.

Felton, C. J., Stastny, P., Shern, D. L., Blanch, A., Donahue, S. A., Knight, E., & Brown, C. (1995). Consumers as peer specialists on intensive case management teams: Impact on client outcomes. *Psychiatric Services, 46*(10), 1037–1044.

Gates, L. B., & Akabas, S. H. (2007). Developing strategies to integrate peer providers into the staff of mental health agencies. *Administrative Policy in Mental Health and Mental Health Services Research, 32*, 293–306.

Hansen, C. (2001). *Strengthening our foundations: The role and workforce development requirements of service-users in the mental health workforce*. Prepared for the New Zealand Mental Health Commission. Retrieved August 30, 2008 from http://www.oregon.gov/DHS/mentalhealth/publications/ser-user-work-dev.pdf

Hebert, M., Rosenheck, R., Drebing, C., Young, A. S., & Armstrong, M. (2008). Integrating Peer Support Initiatives in a Large Healthcare Organization. *Psychological Services, 5*(3), 216–227.

Hutchinson, D. S., Anthony, W. A., Ashcroft, L., et al. (2006) The personal and vocational impact of training and employing people with psychiatric disabilities as providers. *Psychiatric Rehabilitation Journal, 29*, 205–213.

Johnson, E. (2008). Minnesota Peer Support Implementation Consultant's Report. Available from Recovery Innovations, Phoenix, AZ.

Katz, J. & Salzer, M. S. (2007). Certified peer specialist training program descriptions. Philadelphia, PA: University of Pennsylvania Collaborative on Community Integration.

Klein, A. R., Cnaan, R. A., & Whitecraft, J. (1998). Significance of peer social support with dually-diagnosed clients: Findings from a pilot study. *Research on Social Work Practice, 8*, 529–551.

Kottsieper, P. (2009). Experiential knowledge of serious mental health problems: One clinician and academic's perspective. *Journal of Humanistic Psychology, 49*, 174–192.

Lyons, J. S., Cook, J. A., Ruth, A. R., Karver, M. (1996). Service delivery using consumer staff in a mobile crisis assessment program, *Community Mental Health Journal, 32*, 33–40.

Manning, S. S., & Suire, B. (1996). Consumers as employees in mental health: Bridges and roadblocks. *Psychiatric Services, 47*(9), 939–943.

Min, S-Y., Whitecraft, J., & Rothbard, A. & Salzer, M. S. (2007). Peer support for persons with co-occurring disorders and community tenure: A survival analysis. *Psychiatric Rehabilitation Journal, 30*(3), 207–213.

Mowbray, C. T., Moxley, D. P., Jasper, C. A. & Howell, L. L. (1997). *Consumers as Providers in Psychiatric Rehabilitation*. Columbia, MD: International Association of Psychosocial Rehabilitation Services.

Mowbray, C. T., Rusilowski-Clover, G., Arnold, J., Allen, C. (1994). Project WINS: Integrating vocational services on mental health case management teams. *Community Mental Health Journal, 30*, 347–362.

National Association of Peer Specialists (2007). Peer Specialist Compensation/Satisfaction 2007 Survey Report. Accessed online at http://www.naops.org/id22.html on 6/13/09.

Rapp, C. A., McDiarmid, D., Marty, D., Ratzlaff, S., Collins, A., & Fukui, S. (2008). A two-year longitudinal study of the Kansas Consumers as Providers Training Program. *Psychiatric Rehabilitation Journal, 32*(1), 40–46.

Ratzlaff S, McDiarmid D, Marty D, et al. (2006) The Kansas consumer as provider program: Measuring the effects of a supported education initiative. *Psychiatric Rehabilitation Journal, 29*, 174–182.

Sabin, J. E., & Daniels, N. (2003). Strengthening the consumer voice in Managed Care: VII. The Georgia peer specialist program. *Psychiatric Services, 54*, 497–498.

Salzer, M. S., Katz, J., Kidwell, B., Federici, M., & Ward-Colasante, C. (2009). Pennsylvania Certified Peer Specialist Initiative: Training, Employment, and Work Satisfaction Outcomes. *Psychiatric Rehabilitation Journal, 32*, 293–297.

Salzer & Mental Health Association of Southeastern Pennsylvania Best Practices Team (2002). Consumer-delivered services as a best practice in mental health care delivery and the development of best practice guidelines. *Psychiatric Rehabilitation Skills, 6*, 355–382.

Salzer, M. S., Rappaport, J., & Segre, L. (2001). Professional support of self-help groups. *Journal of Community and Applied Social Psychology, 11*, 1–10.

Salzer, M. S., McFadden, L., & Rappaport, J. (1994). Professional views of self–help groups. *Administration and Policy in Mental Health, 22*, 85–95.

Salzer, M. S., Schwenk, E., & Brusilovskiy, E. (2010). Certified peer specialist roles and activities: Results from a national survey. *Psychiatric Services, 61*, 520–523.

Schwenk, E. B., Brusilovskiy, E., & Salzer, M. S. (2009). *Results from a national survey of certified peer specialist job titles and job descriptions: Evidence of a Versatile behavioral health workforce*. Philadelphia, PA: The University of Pennsylvania Collaborative on Community Integration.

Sherman, P. S., & Porter, R. (1991). Mental health consumers as case management aides. *Hospital and Community Psychiatry, 42*, 494–498.

Solomon, P., Draine, J. (1995). The efficacy of a consumer case management team: Two year outcomes of a randomized trial. *Journal of Mental Health Administration, 22*, 126–134.

Solomon, P., & Draine, J. (2001). The state of knowledge of the effectiveness of consumer provided services. *Psychiatric Rehabilitation Journal, 25*, 20–27.

Stoneking, B. C., & McGuffin, B. A. (2007). A review of the constructs, curriculum and training data from a workforce development program for recovery support specialists. *Psychiatric Rehabilitation Journal, 31* (#2, Fall), 97–106.

Chapter 9
The Development and Implementation of a Statewide Certified Peer Specialist Program

Emily A. Grant, Nathan Swink, Crystal Reinhart, and Scott Wituk

Abstract Over the past several decades, peer support services have received increasing attention and support. Recently mental health peer support has become more formalized through the development and implementation of certified peer specialist (CPS) programs. While CPS programs vary from state to state, the basic premise of a CPS program is to train mental health service consumers so that they can provide support to other mental health service consumers who want to follow a path toward recovery. Late in 2007, a certified peer specialist (CPS) program emerged in Kansas following the model set forth in Georgia. This chapter traces the roots of the CPS program from Georgia to Kansas with particular focus on the benefits and crucial facets of the programs thought to be linked to program success. This chapter reports on findings from surveys conducted with over 100 Kansas CPSs. Reported findings include a description of job activities and services, workplace integration, satisfaction, and organizational support. Findings indicate that Kansas CPSs are well-received by many mental health centers, report high job satisfaction, and perceive positive organizational support. Limitations of current research and suggestions for future research are also discussed.

9.1 History of Certified Peer Specialists

Where peer counselors in the substance abuse field have grown increasingly specialized and sophisticated over the past few decades (White, 2000), peer counselors in the mental health field have not been developed as fully. According to Davidson et al. (1999), an early proponent of the valuable role peer support could play in a mental health context was Harry Stack Sullivan. In the 1920s, Sullivan recruited men who had recovered from their psychiatric disorders to be aides at a psychiatric

---

S. Wituk (✉)
Center for Community Support and Research, Wichita State University, Wichita, KS 67260-0201, USA
e-mail: scott.wituk@wichita.edu

hospital. Sullivan felt that the experiences of the recovered men qualified them to assist their peers in working through similar situations.

While inpatient settings started to encourage peer support and mentoring beginning in the 1950s (Davidson, et al., 1999), peer support expanded more rapidly outside the traditional mental health system. Peer support in mental health often took the form of self-help groups, consumer operated services, programs, and organizations, and related structures where mental health consumers supported one another. In the past 20 years, the Mental Health Consumer Movement has revitalized the concept of peer support within the mental health system. It is not uncommon for consumers to hold a number of positions in the mental health system, including as case manager, attendant care worker, mental health technician, janitor and driver (Fricks, 2005; Reinhart & Grant, 2008). Yet, in most of these positions peer support is not central to the position and disclosing personal stories of recovery are not part of the job descriptions.

One of the most recent incarnations of peer support within the mental health system are certified peer specialists (CPS). New York was a forerunner in the CPS movement as the first state where peer support specialists were trained, certified, and hired (Mental Health Association of Southeastern Pennsylvania, 2006). Georgia then emerged as a model state CPS program when it became the first state to make CPS services reimbursable by Medicaid (Mental Health Association of Southeastern Pennsylvania, 2006) leading other states, including Kansas, to continue following suit. Currently, many CPS programs in the United States are modeled after the Georgia Peer Specialist Certification Project, in part because they were the first state with CPS services reimbursed by Medicaid (Mental Health Association of Southeastern Pennsylvania, 2006). The Georgia Peer Specialist Certification Project "identifies, trains, certifies, and provides ongoing support and education to consumers of mental health services to provide peer supports as part of the Georgia Mental Health Service System, and to promote self-determination, personal responsibility, and empowerment inherent in self directed recovery." (US Department of Health and Human Services, 2003, p. 30).

9.2 CPS Purpose and Rationale

CPSs promote skills for coping with and managing psychiatric symptoms while facilitating the utilization of natural resources and the enhancement of community living skills. The role of a CPS is distinct from the roles of existing mental health services such as case management, attendant care, or crisis intervention. The CPS role differs from these and other mental health positions in that experiential knowledge or lived experience is honored as an education that, once honed through skill development, qualifies one to help peers with recovery-oriented goals. CPSs are recovery-oriented, using human-experience language, rather than being maintenance-orientated and utilizing clinical terminology and nomenclature in speech and paperwork. Activities provided by CPS are intended to achieve the identified goals or objectives as set forth in the consumer's individualized treatment plan. Through these activities, CPSs are able to help consumers regain control over their lives (Sabin & Daniels, 2003). The CPS also serves as a role model, as an example of someone who has overcome mental illness and leads a productive and satisfying life (Solomon, 2004). Certified peer specialists can help move consumers from perceived limitations and assumptions about mental illness into a culture of health and ability. Peer support services, including CPS, share the common values, including the "peer principle" and the "helper principle" (Solomon, 2004). By effectively helping others: (1) the helper feels an enhanced sense of interpersonal competence from making an impact on another's life; (2) the helper feels that she/he has gained as much as they have given to others; (3) the helper receives personalized learning from working with others; and (4) the helper acquires an enhanced sense of self from the social approval received from those helped. With positive feedback and self-affirmation, they are in a better position to help others.

In addition to benefiting those served and those providing services, CPSs may also help in saving costs. Previous research suggests that having peer support decreases hospitalizations and shortens the length of stay, which is the most expensive part of mental health treatment (Chinman et al., 2001). Studies have also shown that having peer support decreases the likelihood of needing to utilize mental health services in the future (Chinman, Weingarten, Stayner, & Davidson, 2001; Klien, Cnaan, & Whitecraft, 1998; Simpson & House, 2002). Simply having a consumer on a case management team yields significantly better outcomes compared to teams with no consumers (Davidson et al., 2006; Felton et al., 1995). In addition, peers are often seen as able to offer more credible and up to date information than professionals (Woodhouse & Vincent, 2006). Peer support may also help consumers counter feelings of loneliness, rejection, discrimination, low self-esteem, and frustration (Deegan, 1992; Solomon, 2004). Additional research is needed to examine similar outcomes and costs associated with CPSs.

Besides the benefits to the mental health care system and to the individuals to whom they provide support, the peer specialists themselves benefit (Gottlieb, 1982; Solomon, 2004). Certified peer specialists experience growth in many areas including: increased confidence in their capabilities, ability to cope with the illness, self-esteem, and sense of empowerment and hope (Solomon, 2004). Feelings of stigma due to psychiatric diagnosis can be overcome with improved self-efficacy gained from working as a CPS (Solomon, 2004). Peer providers can also practice their own recovery, engage in self discovery, build their own support system, learn positive ways to fill time, and engage in professional growth including building job skills and moving forward toward a career goal (Gottlieb, 1982; Solomon, 2004).

9.3 CPS Requirements for Medicaid Eligibility

In order for CPS services to be Medicaid eligible, supervision, care coordination and training requirements must be met. Supervision of CPSs must be provided by a competent mental health professional. The definition of a qualified supervisor and the degree of supervision varies from state to state and is partially based on the competency of the CPS. CPS services must also be coordinated within the mental health consumer's individualized treatment plan focusing on that person's individual recovery goals. CPSs must complete training and certification as defined by the state. CPSs must demonstrate basic competencies necessary to function in the position, showing the ability to support the recovery of others from mental illness. In addition to demonstrating an initial competency, there must be a plan for continuing education (Smith, Centers for Medicaid and Medicare Services, 2007).

CPS activities may vary slightly from state to state and even one setting to another. Despite these differences, in order for CPS services to be Medicaid reimbursable the following requirements must be met:

- Supervision must be provided by "competent mental health professionals"
- Peer support services must be coordinated with the individual's treatment plan so that it focuses on the individual recovery goals
- CPSs must complete training and certification as defined by the state in which they work (Smith, Center for Medicaid and Medicare Services, 2007).

Different states have interpreted these requirements in somewhat different ways.

9.4 History of the Kansas CPS Training Program

In late 2005, an administrator from the Center for Community Support & Research (CCSR) at Wichita State University attended a presentation at the "Alternatives Conference" about CPS services being provided in Georgia through the state Medicaid plan. CCSR was uniquely positioned to connect organized mental health service consumer organizations with Kansas social rehabilitative services (SRS), a plan for developing a CPS program was put forward to the State of Kansas. The following year included preparation and program development with the first CPS program starting in July 2007. Within 1 year, over 100 CPS applicants were trained. In 2008, a continuing education and technical assistance component was added.

CCSR staff and their partners recognized the CPS initiative in Georgia as a successful model and aimed to develop a similar CPS program in Kansas. To begin developing the Kansas CPS Training Program, CCSR staff facilitated a task group that included mental health center CSS Directors, consumer leaders from the Consumer Advisory Council (CAC), a representative of Mental Health Association of the Heartland, a representative from Wyandotte Mental Health, and representation from the University of Kansas (Consumers as Advisors Program) and representatives from CCSR. The task group met with representatives of Appalachian Consulting Group (who had previously created the Georgia CPS program) to review program materials modifying them to incorporate into the Kansas CPS Program. The task group outlined a definition of core CPS competencies and the necessary capacities for CPSs. The task group developed training modules and prepared lessons to address identified competencies. The essential components of the Kansas CPS program are described below in more detail.

9.5 Essential Components of the Kansas CPS Program

Early in the planning process, it was decided that the instructors, testers, and graders should be CPSs themselves. Members of the CPS training development committee successfully completed the Kansas version of the certification exam before conducting any training. Therefore, CPS trainers in Kansas are also CPSs, which helps foster an empowering camaraderie during the training. This, combined with the experiential nature of the training, helps provide opportunities for CPS applicants to experience a sense of empowerment and self-direction.

The Kansas CPS Training uses as groundwork a six-principled Strengths Model and a five-stage Recovery Model, then builds around these frameworks focusing on strengthening relevant skills and making explicit the utility of such skills to the work of CPSs. In helping to prepare CPS training participants to aid other mental health consumers in handling stressors like stigma or negative self-talk, they address their own issues of negative stigma, negative self-talk, or other specific stressors commonly associated with severe mental illness. CPS training participants benefit and learn to relay these skills to the consumers they will be supporting.

9.5.1 Strengths Model

After an overview of training and an orientation to the Kansas CPS Training, CPS training participants are introduced to the six principles of the Strengths Model. These principles include:

- People can recover, reclaim, or transform their life;
- The focus is on the individual strengths rather than deficits;
- The consumer is seen as the director of the helping relationship;
- The relationship is primary and essential;
- The preferred setting for services is in the community;
- The community is an oasis of resources.

Each principle is discussed and examples are provided. Throughout the remainder of training, the Strengths Model principles are recalled by trainers when class discussion is relevant to them as a way of helping CPS applicants recognize where the principles apply in their own lives and how they could apply to CPS work. For a current review and implementation information about integration of the Strengths Model into the mental health arena see Chopra and associates recent (2009) work.

9.5.2 Recovery Model

Additional CPS preparation is provided through the five stages of Recovery (See Table 9.1). Three training modules are dedicated to the Five Stage Recovery Model, which describes five ways that individuals relate to "the disabling power of mental illness." These modules describe the framework as well as the challenges faced and what CPSs and the mental health system can do to help people when they relate to diagnosis in the five following ways:

Table 9.1 Types of assistance provided to peers while working as a CPS and previously

Activities	Current M	SD	Before M	SD
1. Assist a consumer in making independent choices	4.63*	1.22	3.76	1.49
2. Help a consumer work on the objectives of their treatment plan	4.45*	1.44	3.72	1.75
3. Teach strategies to independently manage/overcome any psychiatric symptoms	3.88*	1.59	2.91	1.66
4. Refer consumers to other forms of support	4.06*	1.02	3.46	1.44
5. Share my personal story of recovery with consumers	4.16*	1.22	3.17	1.58
6. Help a consumer gain support from others	4.15*	1.20	3.52	1.26
7. Help consumers develop goals	4.12*	1.44	2.87	1.45
8. Help consumers meet other consumers as well as other member of their community	4.01*	1.50	3.70	1.73
9. Assist a consumer in identifying precursors of triggers that result in functional impairments	4.21*	1.23	3.15	1.33
10. Help consumers find jobs	2.30	1.34	2.33	1.45
Total	4.12*	.89	3.37	1.09

*indicates significant difference ($p < .05$) between Current and Before values
Note: 1 = never; 2 = rarely; 3 = some of the time; 4 = frequently; 5 = very frequently; 6 = all of the time

- Impact of diagnosis: Person is impacted by the diagnosis and what it means to his or her self-definition and ability to act.
- Life is limited: Person finds him or herself comfortable believing that life is limited by the diagnosis.
- Change is possible: Person opens her or his self to the possibility that s/he can affect change in his or her life despite having been diagnosed with severe mental illness.
- Commitment to change: Person commits to the belief that change is possible and opens his or her self to the truth that change requires personal action.
- Actions for change: Person commits to personally acting toward the changes that affect the problems in his or her life.

A mental image of each stage is drawn and two large figures are created on crate-paper displays to explain:

- The idea of each stage,
- The dangers faced in each stage,
- The role of the mental health system in each stage.

The training helps to make clear that the five stages in the Recovery Model are not linear. It is emphasized that once a person leaves Stage 2, they are not exempt from revisiting this stage.

After explaining Strengths and Recovery as a foundation, the training provides specific skills useful in carrying out the activities associated with these two models. CPS applicants are taught to:

- Effectively and appropriately use his or her recovery story to aid others;
- Ask effective questions;
- Identify and combat negative self-talk;
- Identify and enhance features of a mental health center that "communicate" consumer empowerment;
- Redirect consumer dissatisfaction into a commitment to change personal behaviors relating to personal strife.

9.5.3 Testing

Within 6 months following the 5-day training that addresses the above-mentioned topics, CPS applicants drive to a centralized location where a CPS training team member administers a paper and pencil test adapted by the Kansas CPS Testing Committee from multiple-choice and short-answer questions. Tests are scored by multiple graders and a consensus is reached. Those CPS applicants who pass gain the title CPS, those who do not have the opportunity to take part in tutoring sessions conducted by the CPS training team, which present a condensed version of the training.

9.5.4 Technical Support to Mental Health Centers

During the development of the Kansas CPS Training Program, one CPS raised the issue that, "If you don't change systems, then you are basically creating a person who has a changed perception of what a consumer can do, and you are putting them back into a system that hasn't changed." This comment and others like it were the impetus for Technical Support to Mental Health Centers. While still developing, requests for technical support have included aid in implementation as well as clarification about CPS roles, hiring advice, and connecting to resources in other mental health centers.

9.5.5 Research Questions

CPSs represent a relatively new type of support that draws heavily from mutual support. The number of CPSs have grown considerably and are likely to continue to grow as additional states consider funding this type of support for mental health consumers. There is a need to better document the emerging role of CPS. Given the relatively new role of CPS in the mental health system, the current chapter will examine (1) who is trained; (2) the services and activities of CPSs; and (3) support from mental health centers. Answering these questions will help paint a detailed picture of CPS in Kansas. With this information, we can identify areas of success and areas that need improvement in both the training and the assistance that CPSs receive, and in the information and education provided to the mental health centers about CPSs.

9.6 Method

9.6.1 Participants

Between September 2007 and March 2009, 140 people submitted applications for the 5-day CPS basic training program. Completion of the training is a requirement of those who wish to become a CPS in Kansas. Out of the 140 applications, 119 people completed the training (85%) and 111 people agreed to participate in this research (93%). The interviews were open to all people who participated in the training session. The gender composition of CPSs was 69% female ($n = 77$) and 31% male ($n = 34$). The race/ethnicity was 81% Caucasian, 12% African American, 2% Hispanic, and 4% who identified belonging to a racial/ethnic category that was not listed. Average age of CPSs was 48 years old (SD $= 10.88$ years), ranging from 21 to 78 years of age. At the time of the survey, 18% reported they were married ($n = 20$), 21% were divorced ($n = 23$), 27% were single ($n = 30$), and 11% were cohabitating. Thirty-nine percent of participants ($n = 34$) did not have any children, while the 61% who did have children reported a range of 1–7 children. When asked of highest level of education obtained, 16% reported they had graduated high school ($n = 14$), 7% reported receiving a GED ($n = 6$), 6% went to technical school ($n = 5$), 42% had some college ($n = 37$), 22% had graduated college ($n = 20$), and 8% had received a graduate degree ($n = 7$).

9.6.2 Measures

9.6.2.1 Job Activities and Services

A 10-item scale was developed for this research that included the aspects of the CPS job description as defined by the state of Kansas. Participants who were currently working as a CPS were asked to rate how frequently they engaged in each job behavior. Those participants who had worked in the mental health center but in a different position prior to becoming a CPS were asked to respond to the same list and report how often they engaged in the same behaviors during their previous appointment at the mental health center (see Table 9.1 for the 10 job activities). Participants rated these items on a 6-point scale ranging from "not at all" to "all of the time." In addition, open-ended questions asked, "What type of assistance do you provide?" and "Briefly describe what you do in a typical week" to complement the Likert items. The scale has been shown to have a high internal validity score (Cronbach's alpha = 0.85).

9.6.2.2 Workplace Integration

The level of integration into the mental health center was assessed by the Workplace Integration scale, which was developed for this research to assess factors indicating integration into a workplace environment (see Table 9.2 for all Workplace Integration questions). Participants rated how much they agreed with each statement on a 6-point Likert scale, ranging from (1) "strongly disagree" to (6) "strongly agree." The scale demonstrates strong internal consistency (Cronbach's alpha = 0.91).

Table 9.2 Workplace integration scale item means and standard deviations

Question	Mean	SD
1. I look forward to coming to work each day	5.25	1.05
2. My ideas are taken seriously by my coworkers	4.88	1.25
3. People at my work look down on me	5.03[a]	1.23
4. I fit in at the mental health center	5.10	1.11
5. It is difficult to get questions answered	4.39[a]	1.58
6. I am comfortable at the mental health center	5.04	1.24
7. There is little support at my mental health center	5.03[a]	1.34
8. I'm left out of discussions at the mental health center	4.67[a]	1.49
9. My coworkers think highly of me	4.99	0.99
10. My coworkers and I work out problems together	4.92	1.16
11. I am part of a team at the mental health center	5.05	1.25
13. Being a certified peer specialist is stressful	3.49[a]	1.50
14. Most days I feel like I do not know what I am doing at the mental health center	4.72[a]	1.44
15. I am accepted at the mental health center	5.16	1.04
Total	4.84	0.88

[a]Scores have been reversed due to a negatively worded question
Note: 1 = strongly Disagree; 2 = disagree; 3 = neither agree nor disagree; 5 = agree; 6 = strongly agree

9.6.2.3 Job/Mental Health Center Satisfaction

Participants' satisfaction with their employment at the mental health center was determined by responses on the Indiana Job Satisfaction Survey (IJSS; Resnick & Bond, 2001). The 32-item questionnaire was developed specifically for employees who have mental illness. The IJSS is comprised of six subscales: (1) General satisfaction; (2) pay; (3) advancement and security; (4) supervision; (5) coworkers; and (6) how I feel on this job. Questions are answered using a 4-point Likert scale with responses ranging from (1) "Strongly Disagree" to (4) "Strongly Agree" (see Table 9.3 for all IJSS questions). The scale has been shown to have high internal consistency (Cronbach's alpha = 0.90).

9.6.3 Organizational Support

Participants' perceived level of organizational support was measured with a shortened version of the 32-item Survey of Perceived Organizational Support (SPOS; Eisenberger, Huntington, Hutchison, & Sowa, 1986). This survey has been shown to have high internal consistency (Cronbach's alpha = 0.97). Following the recommendation of Rhoades and Eisenberger, the 8-item version of the SPOS was used, "because the original scale is unidimensional and has high internal reliability, the use of shorter versions does not appear problematic" (Rhoades & Eisenberger, 2002 p. 699). See Table 9.4 for all SPOS questions. Unfortunately, only 14 CPSs completed this scale because we did not begin to administer it until late in the data collection process.

9.7 Results

Of the 111 participants, 77% gained employment as a CPS ($n = 85$). Employed participants worked an average of 23 h a week (SD = 11.83) with 93% providing direct services to an average of 15 mental health consumers per week (SD = 15.36, $n = 84$). Of the 94 people who answered the question on previous work at the mental health center, 59% ($n = 55$) of CPSs reported working at their current mental health center in a different position immediately before becoming a CPS, while the other 41% ($n = 39$) did not previously work at their mental health center. Previous positions held by CPSs were most frequently "Mental Health Technician," "Attendant Care," and "Recovery Specialist." Of the 83 who answered the question on how they found out about the CPS position, 29% ($n = 24$) were told by a service provider; 46% ($n = 38$) were told by their current supervisor at the mental health center; 12% ($n = 11$) found out through a job posting in "want ads" ($n = 10$); and the remaining 13% found out through other means, such as friends, spouses, and consumer run organizations. Participants were asked how many jobs they had held in their life, after age 18. The number of jobs reported ranged from 3–50 ($M = 11.65$,

Table 9.3 Indiana Job Satisfaction Scale item means and standard deviations

Question	M	SD
IJSS subscale general satisfaction	3.80	0.29
1. I feel good about this job	3.85	0.44
2. This job is worthwhile	3.88	0.33
3. The working conditions are good	3.79	0.41
4. I want to quit this job	3.79[a]	0.65
5. This job is boring	3.71[a]	0.46
IJSS subscale pay	2.58	0.80
7. The vacation time and other benefits are ok	2.87	1.11
8. I need more money than this job pays	2.39	1.14
9. This job does not provide the medical coverage that I need	2.15[a]	1.12
IJSS subscale advancement and security	3.32	0.57
10. I have a fairly good chance at promotion in this job	2.97	0.94
11. This is a dead end job	3.53[a]	0.75
12. I feel there is a good chance of me losing this job in the near future	3.47[a]	0.71
IJSS subscale supervision	3.71	0.44
13. My supervisor is fair	3.76	0.61
14. My supervisor is hard to please	3.64[a]	0.78
15. My supervisor praises me when I do my job well	3.56	0.82
16. My supervisor is difficult to get along with	3.85[a]	0.36
17. My supervisor recognizes my efforts	3.74	0.51
IJSS subscale coworkers	3.63	0.45
18. My coworkers are easy to get along with	3.62	0.70
19. My coworkers are lazy	3.48[a]	0.76
20. My coworkers are unpleasant	3.79[a]	0.48
21. My coworkers do not like me	3.74[a]	0.57
22. My coworkers help me like this job more	3.42	0.75
23. I have a coworker I can rely on	3.74	0.51
24. I have a coworker I consider a friend	3.62	0.70
IJSS subscale how I feel	3.51	0.45
25. I look forward to coming to work each day	3.68	0.59
26. I often feel tense on the job	2.94[a]	0.92
27. I do not know what is expected of me on this job	3.71[a]	0.52
28. I feel physically worn out at the end of the day	3.09[a]	0.79
29. Working makes me feel like I am needed	3.76	0.61
30. My job keeps me busy	3.68	0.48
31. I get to do a lot of different things on my job	3.65	0.65
32. I am satisfied with my schedule	3.59	0.66
Total	3.88	0.34

[a]Scores have been reversed due to a negatively worded question
Note: 1 = strongly disagree; 2 = disagree; 3 = agree; 4 = strongly agree

SD = 9.17, $n = 87$). The length of their last job before working at the mental health center ranged from less than 1 month to 312 months (26 years) ($M = 31.74$, SD = 55.20, $n = 85$).

Table 9.4 Perceived organizational support scale item means and standard deviations

Questions	M	SD
1. The organization values my contribution to its well–being	6.07	1.44
2. The organization fails to appreciate any extra effort from me	5.93[a]	1.49
3. The organization would ignore any complaint from me	6.00[a]	1.30
4. The organization really cares about my well-being	5.38	2.26
5. Even if I did the best job possible, the organization would fail to notice	6.00[a]	1.57
6. The organization cares about my general satisfaction at work	5.86	1.56
7. The organization shows very little concern for me	6.36[a]	1.15
8. The organization takes pride in my accomplishments at work	6.00	1.04
Total	5.93	1.12

[a]Scores have been reversed due to a negatively worded question
Note: 1 = strongly disagree; 2 = disagree; 3 = slightly disagree; 4 = neutral; 5 = slightly agree; 6 = agree; 7 = strongly agree

9.7.1 Activities of CPS

Those who were working as a CPS ($n = 75$) were asked to report how frequently they provided certain services identified as being CPS activities. The activities performed most frequently were "Help a consumer make independent choices" ($M = 4.63$, $SD = 1.22$), "Help a consumer work on the objectives of their treatment plan" ($M = 4.45$, $SD = 1.44$), and "Share my personal story of recovery with consumers" ($M = 4.16$, $SD = 1.22$). Using the same activity scale CPSs who worked at the mental health center in a different position prior to becoming a CPS were asked how frequently they performed these CPS activities during their previous appointment ($n = 41$). A t test was conducted comparing the mean activity score while working as a CPS ($M = 4.12$, $SD = 0.97$) to the mean activity score during the previous position held at the mental health center ($M = 3.37$, $SD = 1.10$). A significant difference was found, $t(43) = -5.68$, $p < 0.01$, Cohen's $d = 0.97$. This indicates there was a significant change in activities once a mental health center employee changed positions to become a CPS. t tests were conducted to compare the means on each activity. Results are displayed in Table 9.1.

9.7.2 Workplace Integration

To evaluate perceived integration into the workplace, participants answered a 14-item Workplace Integration scale ($n = 80$). Overall mean score on this 6-point scale was 4.84 indicating a moderately high level of integration into the workplace. The highest indicators were "I look forward to coming to work each day" ($M = 5.40$) and "I am accepted at the Mental Health Center" ($M = 5.22$). The lowest indicators were "It is difficult to get questions answered" ($M = 4.39$) and "Being a Certified Peer Specialist is stressful" ($M = 3.49$). Questions that were negatively worded were reverse scored for analysis. Results of the Workplace Integration scale are displayed in Table 9.2.

9.7.3 Job Satisfaction

Overall, the mean for the IJSS was 3.48 (SD = 0.34) indicating a moderate level of satisfaction with the job. Subscale scores are as follows: General satisfaction $M = 3.80$, SD = 0.29; pay $M = 2.58$, SD = 0.80; advancement and security $M = 3.32$, SD = 0.57; supervision $M = 3.71$, SD = 0.44; coworkers $M = 3.63$, SD = 0.45; how I feel $M = 3.51$, SD = 0.45. Full results are displayed in Table 9.3.

9.7.4 Organizational Support

Support available to the CPSs was assessed with the Survey of Perceived Organizational Support (SPOS). Items on the SPOS were answered on a 7-point scale ranging from 1 "strongly disagree" to 7 "strongly agree." The overall mean score on the SPOS was 5.93 (SD = 1.12) indicating a high level of organizational support. Results are displayed in Table 9.4.

9.8 Discussion

The current chapter reviewed the recent history of CPSs in light of mental health self-help, described the Kansas CPS program, and presented initial findings from a larger research project related to the Kansas CPS initiative. The demographic composition of the CPS is similar to that of social workers, counselors, and other community workers on the dimensions of gender, age, race, and education (National Association of Social Workers, 2003; U.S. Department of Labor, 2008). Also, it is worth noticing that although post-high school education is not required of CPSs, the majority (78%) have education beyond a high school diploma. Marital status is similar for both groups for "cohabiting" and "single," though the rates for "married" are lower for CPSs, which is likely a factor of the history with mental illness, being that a higher divorce rate has been associated with those who have a mental illness (Merikangas, 1984). These results suggest that demographically the CPSs are similar to their coworkers. Examination of the work histories of the CPS revealed diverse employment histories. The majority of the CPSs worked in their mental health center in another position prior to becoming a CPS and were recruited by their supervisor or other staff at the mental health center to become a CPS. Coworkers and supervisors were apparently encouraging and showed faith in those consumers with whom they had worked. Prior to this research, it was assumed that mental health centers would primarily hire CPSs without extensive history at the mental health center to avoid potential dual relationships and boundary issues. These results are reassuring in that mental health center staffs are advocating for consumers they knew for these new CPS positions.

The CPS service and activity scale demonstrated that the CPSs are typically performing the activities identified to be central to the role of CPS "frequently." This indicates that the CPSs are adhering to the job description of a CPS in the mental health center. It also shows "good faith" by the mental health centers as they are supportive of these CPS activities. Since many CPSs had a previous position at the mental health center, we examined the extent to which CPSs performed new activities associated with the CPS position or if they still performed activities associated with their previous position. When asked the same activity and service scale, CPSs reported performing the activities substantially less in their previous roles. Some aspects of the CPS position may be similar to other positions in the mental health center such as Attendant Care or Mental Health Technician, but the primary aspects of CPS are significantly different. Activities with the greatest significant change were: assisting a consumer in making independent choices, teaching strategies to independently manage psychiatric symptoms, and helping a consumer to identify precursors or triggers that result in functional impairments.

Additional findings indicate that many CPSs are successfully integrated into the workplace. CPSs frequently experience many indicators of workplace integration, including feeling like part of a team, feeling supported at the mental health center, and feeling like other staff at the mental health center did not look down on them. Given the rapid expansion of CPS, it is encouraging to document this integration into mental health centers' culture.

The Indiana Job Satisfaction Scale provides additional insight into particular aspects of working at mental health centers. Overall satisfaction was high with subscales of general satisfaction, satisfaction with coworkers and satisfaction with supervision with the highest ratings, and satisfaction with pay and satisfaction with advancement and security with the lowest ratings. These findings are consistent with other professional roles. Uncertainty about advancement is understandable given that the CPS position is new to the mental health system with little to no defined advancement opportunities. In addition, approximately 50% of the interviews took place after the national economic crisis in 2008. This crisis may have influenced responses, as potential budget cuts and freezes loomed in the state system. More specifically, some CPSs shared concerns that their position was in jeopardy because it was new and therefore if budget cuts took place, they would be the first to be terminated.

Despite some of these concerns, the results from the Survey of Perceived Organizational Support (SPOS) indicate that CPSs feel that the mental health centers are generally supportive. Findings indicate that CPSs feel supported on all dimensions of organizational support measured by the SPOS. Based on these results, it appears that most mental health professionals care deeply about their work and for those they serve, and it seems they are accepting and supportive of the CPS position as well. It is encouraging that the CPSs feel like they are being supported by the mental health center and there appears to be support for the new role of CPS that has been introduced. Additionally, levels of perceived organizational support have been associated with the propensity to continue working at the organization, and employee's commitment to the organization (Armstrong-Stassen & Templer, 2004; Wayne, Shore, & Linden, 1997). Also, perceived organizational support "leads to fulfillment of employee obligations through attitudes and behaviors that aid the organization" (Wayne, et. al., 1997, p. 105–106). It is important to note that the SPOS was included in a later version of the survey, so only 14 participants had the opportunity to complete it.

While the current chapter outlines the development of and initial findings of a statewide CPS program, much more work is needed to support and examine the development of CPSs. Additional research needs to be conducted with the people served. It is important to understand if and how the people who are receiving CPS services benefit from the peer support. Additionally, the role of CPS is different from that of peer support in other realms due to the fact that the CPS is paid for providing support. Due to the nature of working in the current mental health system, and having to adhere to professional boundaries, the peer support provided through CPSs is often unidirectional. These aspects and how it affects the benefits to those receiving services need to be explored. Further, conducting natural and controlled experiments to formally assess the outcomes related to CPS are needed to move the CPS initiative from a promising to a best practice.

Research with CPS supervisors is also needed. It will be important to understand the perceptions of those in supervisory roles as to the benefit of CPS services. Besides asking questions about the general benefit of having CPSs working in the mental health center, it would be helpful to assess the supervisor's level of understanding of the support and services that a CPS could potentially provide.

9.8.1 Conclusion

CPSs are a relatively recent development in mental health peer support. CPSs are being trained and hired to provide peer support in the Kansas and a growing number of states. CPSs are diverse in age, race, and education, with many of them having at least some college course work. CPSs have started to provide new services and engage in new activities that are unique to the role of a CPS and were not previously offered at mental health centers. Overall, the CPSs show high levels of integration into the workplace, high job satisfaction, and strong perceived organizational support. This type of integration will hopefully help buffer against burnout and job turnover rates. These results are encouraging in that they represent a powerful step in evolving the mental health system into an organizational and therapeutic culture based in recovery. Despite the steps taken, additional research is needed to examine the impact of CPSs on the mental health system and the impact of the mental health system on CPSs.

Acknowledgement The authors wish to thank the Kansas Department of Social and Rehabilitation Services (SRS) for its support throughout the years for this work.

References

Armstrong-Stassen, M., & Templer, A. (2004). What are the important factors in retaining older employees? *Proceedings of the Administrative Sciences Association of Canada*, University of Windsor, 1–13.

Chinman, M. J., Weingarten, R., Stayner, D., & Davidson, L. (2001). Chronicity reconsidered: Improving person-environment fit through a consumer run service. *Community Mental Health Journal, 37*, 215–229.

Chopra, P., Hamilton, B., Castle, D., Smith, J., Mileshkin, C., Deans, M., Wynne, B., Prigg, G., Toomey, N., & Wilson, M. (2009). Implementation of the strengths model at an area mental health service. *Australia's Psychiatry, 17*, 202–206.

Deegan, P. E. (1992) The independent living movement and people with psychiatric disabilities, taking control of our own lives. *Psychosocial Rehabilitation Journal, 15*(3), 3–19.

Davidson, L., Chinman, M., Kloos, B., Weingarten, R., Stayner, D., & Tebes, J. K. (1999). Peer support among individuals with severe mental illness: A review of the evidence. *Clinical Psychology: Science and Practice,6*, 165–187.

Davidson, L., Chinman, M., Sells, D., & Rowe, M. (2006). Peer support among adults with serious mental illness: A report from the field. *Schizophrenia Bulletin, 32*, 443–450.

Eisenberger, R., Huntington, R., Hutchison, S., Sowa, D. (1986). Perceived Organizational Support. *Journal of Applied Psychology, 71*, 500–507.

Felton, C. J., Stastny, P., Shern, D. L., Blanch, A., Donahue, S. A., Knight, E., & Brown, C. (1995). Consumers as peer specialists on intensive case management teams: Impact on client outcomes. *Psychiatric Services, 46*, 1037–1044.

Fricks, L. (2005). Building a Foundation for Recovery: A Community Education Guide on Establishing Medicaid-Funded Peer Support Services and a Trained Peer Workforce. DHHS Pub. No. (SMA) 05-8089. Rockville, MD: Center for Mental Health Services, Substance Abuse and Mental Health Services Administration, 2005.

Gottlieb, B. (1982). Mutual – help groups: Members' views of their benefits and of roles for professionals. In L. Borman, L. Borck, R. Hess & F. Pasquale (Eds.), Helping people to help themselves: Self help and prevention. New York: The Hawthorne Press, Inc.

Klien, A. R., Cnaan, R. A., & Whitecraft, J. (1998). Significance of peer social support with dually diagnosed clients: Findings from a pilot study. *Research on Social Work Practice, 8*, 529–551.

Mental Health Association of Southeastern Pennsylvania (2006, July, 27) National professional organization of people in recovery of psychiatric disability is created. [Press release]. Retrieved from http://www.mhasp.org/presspeer.pdf.

Merikangas, K. R. (1984). Divorce and assertive mating among depressed patients. *American Journal of Psychiatry, 141*, 74–76.

National Association of Social Workers (2003). National Association of Social Workers News, May. Washington, DC: National Association of Social Workers.

Reinhart, C. A., & Grant, E. (2008). Certified peer specialist baseline interview report. Center for Community Support and Research, Wichita, KS: Wichita State University.

Resnick, S. G., & Bond, G. R. (2001). The Indiana job satisfaction scale: Job satisfaction in vocational rehabilitation for people with severe mental illness. *Psychiatric Rehabilitation Journal, 25*, 12–19.

Rhoades, L., & Eisenberger, R. (2002). Perceived organizational support: A review of the literature. *Journal of Applied Psychology, 87*, 698–714.

Sabin, J. E., & Daniels, N. (2003). Strengthening the consumer voice in managed care: VII the Georgia peer specialist program. *Psychiatric Services, 54*, 497–498.

Simpson, E. L., & House, A. O. (2002). Involving users in the delivery and evaluation of mental health services: Systematic review. *British Medical Journal, 325*, 1–5.

Smith, Centers for Medicaid and Medicare Services, August 15, 2007, Personal Communication.

Solomon, P. (2004). Peer support/ Peer provided services underlying processes, benefits, and critical ingredients. *Psychiatric Rehabilitation Journal, 27*, 392–401.

US Department of Health and Human Services (2003). *Emerging new practices in organized peer support.* Rockville, MD: National Technical Assistance Center.
US Department of Labor. (2008). Counselors, social, religious workers & all other. Occupational Outlook Handbook. Retrieved online 04-10-2009 from http://www.ocouha.com/cur/ooh020909.htm.
Wayne, S. J., Shore, L. M., & Liden, R. C. (1997). Perceived organizational support and leader-exchange: A social exchange perspective. *Academy of Management Journal, 40,* 82–111.
White, W. (2000). The history of recovered people as wounded healers: From Native America to the rise of the modern alcoholism movement. *Alcoholism Treatment Quarterly, 18,* 1–22.
Woodhouse, A. & Vincent, A. (2006) Mental health delivery plan - Development of peer specialist roles: A literature scoping exercise. Edinburgh: Scottish Recovery Network and the Scottish Development Centre for Mental Health.

Part IV
MHSH Policy

Chapter 10
Finding and Using Our Voice: How Consumer/Survivor Advocacy is Transforming Mental Health Care

Daniel Fisher and Lauren Spiro

Abstract In the past 30 years, the consumer/survivor movement has been developing a consensus national advocacy voice. This chapter reviews three important components in the development of this strong and unified national consumer/survivor Voice: (a) A consensus by the movement that recovery, wellness, and complete community integration are attainable goals for persons labeled with mental illness in contrast to the traditional negative prognosis of maintenance during a life-long disability.; (b)Training programs in advocacy designed and carried out by consumer/survivors, such as Finding Our Voice.; (c)Building the National Coalition of Mental Health Consumer/Survivor Organizations, which amplifies the voice of consumer/survivors at the state and federal level.

Introduction to the authors. This chapter is written by two authors who found our Voices ("Voice" with capital V is used when we are referring to a person's uniquely personal Voice or that of the consumer/survivor movement) and recovered a meaningful place in the community after being diagnosed with schizophrenia. Dan Fisher became a psychiatrist, founded the National Empowerment Center, was appointed to the White House New Freedom Commission on Mental Health, and was able to use the Voice of the consumer/survivor movement to ensure that the Commission report focused on recovery. Lauren Spiro became a psychologist, a senior manager in a non-profit mental health agency, a CARF (Commission on the Accreditation of Rehabilitation Facilities) surveyor and advisor, and co-founded two non-profit mental health corporations before being hired as the first staff person to represent the national coalition in Washington, DC.

D. Fisher (✉)
National Empowerment Center, Lawrence, MA, USA
e-mail: daniefisher@gmail.com

After long debates, our movement has settled on the self-description, "consumer/survivor." We acknowledge that we have all had an interruption in a major life role, however, "consumer" refers to those still using services and "survivor" refers to those who have survived the mental health system.

10.1 Introduction to the Chapter

This chapter consists of three essential elements in the evolution of the consumer/survivor movement. The first part of the chapter deals with the replacement of the medical model of mental illness with an empowerment paradigm of mental health recovery. On both an individual and collective basis, there has been a historic shift in thinking by a critical mass of persons labeled with mental illness from considering ourselves the object of neuro-chemical forces to being empowered agents who are finding the freedom to begin to creatively and effectively run our own lives. This paradigm has emerged through self-help groups in which mental health consumer/survivors have been sharing our lived experience of personal recovery. These shared recovery experiences clearly contradicted the professionally promoted misconception that people could never recover from a serious "mental illness." The second part of the chapter highlights a training program called "Finding Our Voice." This training informs and inspires consumer/survivor advocates, newly freed from the feeling of being the object of neuro-chemical forces, to gain a Voice in the running of their lives. The third part describes the coming together of empowered advocates who began by forming statewide consumer/survivor-run groups, which developed into a national coalition of consumer/survivor-run statewide organizations. These large-scale groups enable the Voice of consumer/survivors to be amplified at the state and federal levels, positively impacting national policies and legislation affecting everyone's recovery. The unifying theme throughout this chapter is the evolution of the Voice of consumer/survivors. We will trace what qualitative research tells us about the emergence of a person's Voice, and how that Voice enables the person to become the architect of their recovery and their life. In a similar manner, the consumer/survivor movement itself has built a Voice, which has powered its evolution into a force for transforming the mental health system and society into a more humane, inclusive, and respectful place to live.

We will share our experiences of advocacy as well of those of other advocates. The importance of consumers finding our Voice is highlighted by the New Freedom Commission Report, which calls for a recovery-oriented, consumer-driven system. To fulfill this Commission goal, however, there needs to be a greater number of effective, informed consumer advocates. This chapter will trace how individuals and groups of consumers have been finding their Voice and using that Voice over the last 30 years in the United States and around the world to promote a recovery-based system and culture. This feat is particularly remarkable in light of how resistant the traditional system is to such a change.

What do we mean by Voice? Just as an artist needs to find their unique artistic Voice to express their creative work, each person, needs to find their unique life Voice to enable them to create a meaningful life, based on their personal values and principles. When people who have developed a life Voice are in emotional distress, they know how they feel and are able to communicate those feelings to those around them. This skill enables both the person experiencing emotional distress as well as those supporting the person to think effectively about what the person needs, to support the person in making informed decisions, to create reasonable accommodations if needed, and to ensure that conditions arise encouraging the person to resume meaningful roles in his/her life. It is not surprising that people in severe distress hear voices, for it seems that in the absence of hearing one's own Voice, we create substitutes for it. Just as John Nash, in the book *Beautiful Mind* (Nasar, 1999), searched for guidance in random numbers in the newspaper, many of us, in periods of severe distress, have looked outside ourselves for a magical message telling us what to do. Dan was convinced that everyone except him received instructions about what to do each day. He thought the instructions were shoved under everyone else's door each morning. So our life Voice is a reflection of the degree to which we are able to influence the opinions of others and affect the important decisions in our life. Without such a life Voice, we feel compelled to seek guidance for our decisions from outside ourselves.

Master Eckhart, a medieval mystic, captured some of the meaning of Voice when he wrote, "the soul has something in it, a spark of speech that never dies ... which is untouched by space or time" (Evans, 1924). Dan and Lauren feel this understanding resonates with their lived experience. Dan found that even during his 1-month period of muteness, he experienced a spark, an ember inside which continued to be vigilant, yearning for an opportunity to speak, if only he could find a safe, trusting relationship. Lauren, though overwhelmed with 'delusions' for over 6 months always remained keenly aware of a core deep inside her that was whole and intact despite all the madness swirling around her. She yearned for safety, someone with whom she could confide in to help clear up the confusion.

One element of finding one's voice is to recognize it is always inside even though we may not express it. Martin Buber said that this spark or Voice is central to our decisions, "for the genuine spark is effective in the single composure of each genuine decision" (Buber, 1965). Having a Voice, therefore, means we have the power to make decisions and run our own lives.

How do we gain our unique, life Voice? Does the consumer/survivor movement embody a Voice? Relationships are essential to the healthy development of one's Voice. I am because you are. As Fichte said in 1797, "The consciousness of the individual is necessarily accompanied by that of another, of a thou, and only under this condition possible." (as quoted in Buber, 1965, pg. 69). This view also corresponds to the philosophy of Ubuntu, a native South African concept. In Zulu, a saying, which epitomizes Ubuntu is, "a person is a person through other persons." Mental health recovery does not happen in a vacuum and it does not happen "to" us. It happens within us as a result of healing, loving relationships in which we find safety to reveal our genuine Voice.

Why is it so important to us individually and collectively to find and to express our Voice? Because our existence depends upon it. Without our Voice we do not experience our life. We can only go through the motions and observe from afar lives that others are living. We are alienated from our deepest self.

Locked in a seclusion room at the age of 16 with a diagnosis of chronic schizophrenia, Lauren thinks back, was a metaphor of her life at that point. She felt trapped, alone, caged, and desperately wanted to belong, to feel she had a meaningful role in the community. Her heart and values pulled her one way, while the culture around her pulled in the opposite direction – toward conforming to roles and principles that did not reflect her deepest yearnings. She became lost in the void between these two overwhelmingly conflicted worlds that never ceased tearing her in opposite directions. Lacking resources and supports that she could trust to assist her in understanding and reconciling these opposing forces, the tension built until it boiled over. The boiling-over bypassed the usual cognitive channels, and instead came out as "delusions." The content of the "delusions," however, reflected verbatim the very conflict she was trapped in. She needed to feel that her life mattered, that she mattered; she needed meaning and purpose that genuinely reflected her Voice in a world that seemed very irrational. And she could not find it. One night – everything changed. That sleepless night in a 9 × 9 foot white barren cell with bars on the windows, she decided that she could no longer bear the pain and agony (of "schizophrenia") and gave herself permission to end her life – to end the torment. Ironically, that decision led to the opening of a new door. She realized that if one option was death, then it made sense to put every ounce of energy she had to focus on finding a life worth living. To find that life she knew she had to reconstruct herself and stop listening to the endless screaming voices and images in her head. She thought that that would make surviving another day possible, bearable. That night, unbeknownst to her at the time, was the beginning of her road to recovery – the beginning of the journey of discovering who she really was.

Dan had to go to the depths of his existence to decide if his life was worth living. Having been a dutiful son who carried out his family expectations, he found himself at age 24 without any sense of his living for himself. He had achieved much, having obtained his Ph.D. in biochemistry and secured a job at the National Institutes of Mental Health. But he was only living for others. He had no idea how he felt. He was pure thought and no feeling. His heart had stopped talking to him. He was only aware of being too angry to go on as he had gone on. Like Martin Luther he said to himself "this is not I!" His biggest step of recovery was to say to himself, stop acting and just be. To do so he stopped going to the job in the Laboratory of Neurochemistry where he was discovering the chemicals responsible for feelings. The chemicals did not define his feelings. The job was not him. He stopped talking, because the words were always ones he used for others. He even stopped moving because all movements seemed alien, not his own. From this very quiet, self-observing place, he decided he would only emerge when he could express the Voice that was uniquely his own. He was hospitalized in Bethesda Naval Hospital in what was described as a catatonic psychosis. Gradually the lowest ranking aides, the corpsmen reached him through nonverbal communication. But his next step in recovery occurred when he could transfer his anger from a stubborn no to life to a yes. It came when he was trapped in seclusion and vowed that he would humanize the mental health system so that everyone similarly suffering could recover. Then his anger became his passion and purpose. This was his deepest Voice speaking to him. It seems the only way for Dan to be freed from the delusion that others were controlling his life, was for him to truly gain a Voice by which he controlled his own life.

Professors Harrop and Trower of England have concluded that, "the life long experience of being intrusively controlled and of having an alien not an authentic (self-constructed) self, and the concomitant loss of a center of initiative, is likely to cause profound dysfunction in the normal operation of consciousness ... and account for some of the anomalous experiences of psychosis." (Harrop & Trower, 2003, p. 85). In other words, if a person is not able to develop a strong, centered, authentic self they have the types of disturbances of consciousness, which can cause them to lose touch with reality and become psychotic. They propose that development and recovery are facilitated by self-construction through relationships.

10.2 Finding and Using Our Authentic Individual Voice

10.2.1 Empowerment Paradigm of Recovery and Development

One of the essential elements in gaining a Voice is to understand that the traditional, chronic disease model for mental health issues has not been a useful construct for many persons who have recovered from states of severe emotional distress. The disease model is not useful in describing how people are able to recover and develop into highly competent and skilled leaders in the recovery movement and elsewhere.

The chronic disease model conceptualizes mental health issues in the same manner as other medical diseases, such as diabetes. But unlike diabetes, this model considers the person's sense of self to be permanently diseased. This explanation incapacitates the very source of a person's empowerment and agency for their recovery. Perhaps the greatest weakness of the chronic disease model is in its description of the most dramatic form of mental illness, schizophrenia. Dr. Richard Bentall (1990) has pointed out that schizophrenia fits few of the characteristics of a disease because:

1. There is such great variability in the symptoms of schizophrenia
2. Diagnoses of schizophrenia frequently overlap with bipolar disorder or major depression
3. There remains great debate over the causation of schizophrenia
4. The outcome and course of schizophrenia is highly variable and unpredictable
5. There is no treatment found to work for everyone and, in fact, each person needs to play a role in designing their own treatment

These findings have led Dr. Bentall to conclude that schizophrenia is a disease with "no particular symptoms, no particular course, no particular outcome, and no particular treatment." (Bentall, 1990, p. 33).

Despite all this variability, schizophrenia is still widely studied through a narrow disease paradigm. Its onset is typically in late adolescence. In the second World Health Organization study of schizophrenia in nine countries, 83% of persons with schizophrenia had their onset in the age range from 15 to 35 (Jablensky and Cole, 1997). The chronic disease model does little to explain why schizophrenia invariably appears during adolescence. Furthermore, the medical model places agency outside the person. The condition is to be primarily controlled by external agents such as the medication and the doctor, not by the person themselves. The first and second WHO studies also concluded that the rate of recovery from schizophrenia was much higher in the developing countries than in the industrial countries (Jablensky et al., 1992). "Patients in developing countries experienced significantly longer periods of unimpaired functioning in the community, although only 16% of them were on continuous antipsychotic medication (compared to 61% in developed countries)" (Jablensky and Sartorius, 2008.) The chronic disease model is found lacking in light of these finding.

As an alternative to the chronic disease model, NEC has proposed an empowerment paradigm of development and recovery, illustrated in Fig. 10.1, which is discussed in greater detail by Fisher (2008).

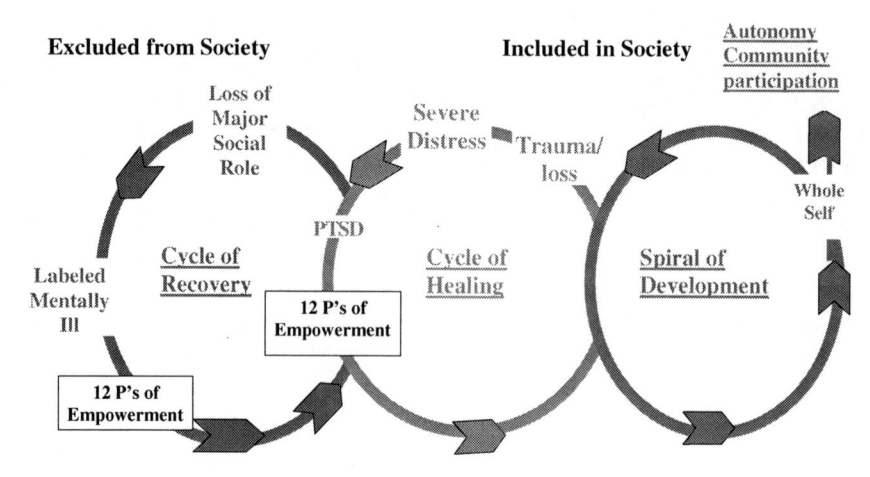

Fig. 10.1 Empowerment paradigm of development, and recovery © 2008 National Empowerment Center

The circle on the right, we call the spiral of development. Though the constraints of using a two dimensional format require us to represent development as a circle, we consider development as a spiral of increasing growth of a person's Voice and Self as they pass into adulthood. This development is nourished by many of the principles of empowerment and wellness (as discussed below) we have found vital to healing from trauma and recovery from what is called "mental illness." Through construction of a strong Voice and a sense of Self, a person is able to establish meaningful relationships, love, and work. Trauma, loss, and insufficient supports, knowledge, and resources may inhibit development and result in severe distress and anger. If the person experiences empowerment and people who believe in them, they can heal and return to their process of development. If they are unable to establish personal, trusting connections, the person feels isolated, powerless, disconnected, and humiliated. Understandably, this often results in a protective strategy of shutting down and their experiencing that their heart no longer speaks to them. In the process of disconnection from one's heart, they are vulnerable to hearing Voices and losing their major social role. At that point they enter the red circle on the left. They are labeled mentally ill and marginalized from society. Then they need to go through recovery to return to their development, which is much more arduous and lengthy.

Harrop and Trower have been developing a similar theory of psychosis. They hypothesize that the self-construction is essential to healthy development. The self-construction depends on a combination of expressions of oneself in the world, which we are calling Voice combined with positive acceptance and understanding by the significant others, we would call people who believe in the deepest you. From this hypothesis, they propose, "The main prediction of this study was that a typical sample of people diagnosed as having schizophrenia [and they are quite critical of this diagnosis] would report emotional episodes which would clearly demonstrate blocks to self-construction" (Harrop & Trower, 2003, p. 96). They go on to do interviews with 21 persons labeled with schizophrenia and show that their hypothesis is validated. In a majority of cases there is a great deal of suppressed anger, which they interpret as the result of blocks in self-construction. A Jungian psychiatrist, Dr. John Weir Perry, came to a similar conclusion. He found that psychosis was part of a person's reorganization of their deepest self such that they could return to their development in a more integrated fashion (Perry, 1974).

Another important support for the connection between lacking Voice and psychosis is the work of Seikkula and Trimble. They propose that psychosis results when people are trapped in monologue. They recommend systems, network therapy to assist persons at their first psychosis in reestablishing dialogue with the significant persons in their life. This approach has been very successful in not only bringing young persons out of psychosis, but also doing so without hospitalization and without long-term disability (Seikkula and Trimble, 2005). Persons are trapped in monologue, as Dan and Lauren were, may be unable to speak with their authentic Voice from their heart.

10.2.2 Developing More Consumer Advocates Through Finding Our Voice Training

When the New Freedom Commission Report (2003) was released in July 2003, the White House gave it little recognition or support, never publicly announced it or advocated for the legislation needed to implements its recommendations. NIMH has similarly distanced itself from the concept of recovery, which is the vision of the report. Given such lack of support at a federal level, it was clear that consumer/survivors, whose very lives were at stake, needed to organize to change the system. There is, however, a drastic shortage of consumer/survivor advocates. Therefore, the most important next step in developing consumer-driven policies is the development of a large number of consumer advocates. The

National Empowerment Center (NEC) has begun piloting such trainings, which are called "Finding Our Voice" training. The training is based on 12 principles of empowerment, which NEC has derived from interviewing of a variety of experienced advocates. The goal of the training is to develop advocates who can amplify their voice to effect change and assist other consumer to develop their Voice.

These 12 principles of empowerment all start with the letter P and are best introduced in a sequence as shown in Fig. 10.2. Following is a brief summary of these principles of empowerment:

Personal Peer Support ⟹ Passion from reactive anger ⟹ Principles of recovery Positive future ⟹

Purpose Meaning Presence ⟹ Planning Goals & Objectives ⟹ Politics Presenting Persistence Persuasion Partnering

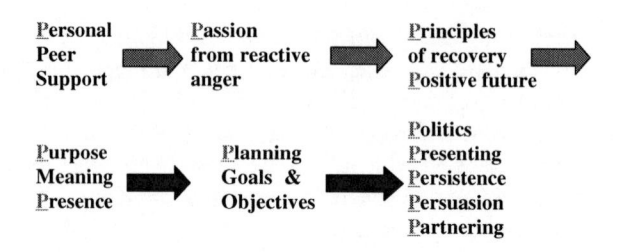

Fig. 10.2 How the 12 Ps of empowerment lead to recovery and transformation

1. *Personal connections*: Perhaps the most important first step in becoming an empowered advocate is to get together with other advocates.
2. *Passion*: It is essential to transform anger and resentment into passion.
3. *Principles of recovery*: Outline a recovery-based system which is consumer-driven and self-determining on the individual and systems levels, centered on peer support and self-help which enables people to achieve full community participation, or social inclusion, through valued roles (e.g., worker, student, parent, tenant, etc.).
4. *Positive view of the future*: Hope needs to reside deeply, insistently inside one's being to inspire oneself and others to hope again.
5. *Purpose*: Many of us have had to find a purpose to anchor and invest in our lives, rather than passively or actively seeking an exit. Empowerment is about finding purpose because having a sense of purpose empowers our life.
6. *Persistence, perseverance, and patience*: Never give up, never quit ... With enough persistence anything can come to be ... what we believe can become reality.
7. *Presence*: Capacity to quickly, positively impact people through pride, poise, and politeness.
8. *Persuasion*: Capacity to get people to see your point of view through discussion.
9. *Practical prioritized advocacy plan which needs to come from a well-prepared participant*: If you are going to change policies you need a concise, prioritized plan, which you can propose.

10. *Public presenting*: Learning how to present your self and your ideas to others is another vital aspect of individual and collective empowerment
11. *Partnering through mediating, and negotiating*
12. *Politics*: Politics is the process by which groups of people make decisions

10.2.3 The Purpose of the Training

The purpose of the training is twofold. First there is the development of the person's individual voice. This means going through the stages of connecting personally to one's self, to the group, to transforming our anger into passion, and to finding purpose. The next phase is to learn about how to work together in a group.

For many consumers this skill has not been well-developed because as discussed previously, we have had an interruption in our development in which we experienced blocks in our self-construction; many of us experienced being trapped in monologue, which has hindered our ability to develop the skills needed to negotiate with others. Thus, participants are taught the skills of engaging in and facilitating dialogue to achieve their goal of learning to collaborate in a group. Then they finish by developing a plan together, and each person makes a presentation to the group.

Following is an outline of the 4 days training:

Day 1: Finding our personal Voice
Module I: Introduction to the program; including creating group comfort zones; introductions are done by all participants and presenters as a warm up exercise, in a circle.
Module II: Personally connecting in small groups.
Module III: Transition to passion from anger and fear; small groups to discuss the meaning of this transition for participants.
Module IV: Review principles of recovery and community building; individual purpose from passion + principles + positive future = Passionate, Principled purpose. Dyads coach each other on getting in touch with their passionate purpose and draft a paragraph on it.

Day 2: Learning to engage in genuine dialogue
Module V: Stages of dialogue; moving from discussion to generative dialogue. In the large group, practice what participants feel are the most important elements of an advocate; clarify the nature of generative dialogue and give feedback to the group on how they are doing in moving from discussion into dialogue.
Module VIa: Personal to political; a facilitator introduces the priorities of the National Coalition of Mental Health Consumer/Survivor Organizations. Then, each small group picks one of the priorities of the National Coalition and develops the plan to address the priority, which they will present on the last day. Small groups begin a dialogue about the subject area they picked. Participants are encouraged to draw on their passionate purpose.

VIb: Local version of the history of the movement; after developing local histories, engage the large group in dialogue about them.

Day 3: How to go from generative dialogue to strategic dialogue
Module VII: Strategic dialogue principles; develop a practical plan through strategic dialogue.
Module VIII: Presenting in public (to large groups); a representative from each group will present the group's plan (5 min each) and then will engage the group in dialogue, ending with feedback from participants and presenters on how well the group presented and dialogued.

Day 4 – Presenting practical plans, feedback, contracts
9 A.M. noon: Continue presentations to the large group.
Module IX: Conclusion; general discussion about contracting as self-employed contractors with your statewide group. Obtain feedback from the group on how to improve the training. Review how to use the training in developing new leaders in their counties. Review materials, manual, when to start making presentations, getting contracts (thus the training also promotes entrepreneurship), business.

10.2.4 Personal Peer Support

The first step in our Finding Our Voice training is to connect the participants with one another on a personal level. This is the essence of peer support. Instinctively, the consumer/survivor movement has learned how vitally important peer support is. By sharing from our deepest truth, we assist one another in our personal and collective evolution by continuously awakening to our completeness as human beings. We evolve in relation to other people. By giving and receiving, sharing and trusting, we become more empowered and aware of interpersonal dynamics. This is essential so we learn and experience that our most important developments are learned in relationships of mutual trust and understanding. Initially this is best accomplished among peers, who because of their experience in the mental health system, share a common bond. Connecting with peers provides further opportunity for the self-construction of a person's Voice. These groups are similar to women's consciousness raising groups. Once the bond has started to form the group is ready to address the issue of how to transform their anger into passion. Initially the training involved teaching the principles of recovery once the peer-support group had bonded. However, piloting the training showed us that the next step needs to be addressing the anger that most people feel as a result of being labeled, hospitalized (which often involves re-traumatization), and marginalized from society. No other learning or planning can effectively take place until peers have had an opportunity to express their anger and move beyond it to passion.

10.2.5 Transforming Reactive Anger into Passionate Advocacy

When individuals are unable to construct their self and find their Voice, they experience a welling up of suppressed anger which often gets expressed in a reactive manner, which in turn impedes successful advocacy. When a consumer/survivor attends a board meeting before they have transformed their anger into passion, they are either very silent or flare out with the anger in a manner that disqualifies their testimony.

Many effective consumer leaders work on deepening their awareness and appreciation of the source of their anger, which is typically rooted in feelings of righteous indignation due to past hurtful or humiliating experiences when their voice was invalidated. Therefore, in our training program for advocates we pay close attention to this issue of how people can be aware of their anger and use it strategically to affect positive change in their community.

As advocates, Cathy and Barry Creighton of Alaska expressed: "angry is something to use – not something to be." In this manner, the energy and the outrage behind their anger is not suppressed but is translated in to a passion, which can then be the source of effective action. Indeed, studies have shown that "people were inclined to easily give up to those who were perceived by them as angry, powerful, and stubborn, rather than soft and submissive" (Tiedens, 2001, p. 86).

It is our belief, that uses of anger may be our greatest challenge as mental health advocates. On an individual or group basis, expressions of anger are important moments of change in awareness and in the conversation. A skilled advocate becomes very adept at using anger to achieve their goals as illustrated in a recent event. Lauren and Dan are part of a cross-disability coalition, Justice For All Action Network (JFAAN, see below), to bring ideas for change to the Obama administration. In a recent teleconference discussion, several members of the group said they were frustrated by the lack of results of their advocacy. Soon there was agreement and the frustration was shared across the group. At that point, a very skilled advocate said, "I think we need to change our tone, and start expressing more anger." In the discussion that followed, there was an interesting debate about when and how much to change our tone and express more anger. Dan marveled at the conversation because he could never recall such a cooperative and strategic discussion of the conscious uses of anger by a group of advocates. Several days later he described the experience to a group of peers who are experienced advocates, and asked "Do we as mental health consumer/survivors face special challenges in our uses of anger not faced by other disability groups?" The other advocates immediately said we do face special challenges (due to discrimination) and as a result we have not developed the skill of effectively using our anger. In this section, we will explore why mental health advocates have unique issues to deal with anger and give some suggestions about what we can do to over come these barriers, which are the result of discrimination.

In many ways, our difficulty with anger stems from what it means to be labeled mentally ill. In this regard, it is useful to look at the origin of the term mental illness. Before medical descriptions of mental illness existed, there were and are many lay expressions of what constitutes mental illness. Perhaps the most revealing is the term madness. In English, the word mad has two meanings. For those of us who have been labeled mentally ill, we are considered in less clinical circles as being mad meaning crazy. We were at times called madmen. But if you have not been labeled as a crazy person, being described as mad can mean you are angry. Normal people get mad and they are not diagnosed. They are listened to. A peer of ours captured this distinction very well. She said she worked within a department of mental health and noticed that her colleagues were frequently getting angry at each other and about their work. When they expressed their anger there was no clamping down on their behavior. In fact, it seemed the norm, for them. However, when she expressed her anger, there were stern looks of censure. Her unlabeled colleagues would inquire in patronizing tones, "Are you feeling alright?" "Perhaps you are having a breakdown?" "It would be a good idea to see if you need more medication." Thus, it seems that there are two very different uses of anger and attitudes toward persons expressing anger. People who have not been labeled can express anger as a day-to-day part of their life without being told that they must not be feeling well. Now there are exceptions, which also are revealing. For instance, women are not given as much freedom in their expression of anger as men. In fact, women who express anger too frequently or too loudly are given the B–h label. In mental health circles, people who express anger are given another B label: borderline. In fact, supervisors frequently told Dan, during his training, that the best way to know that you were dealing with a borderline (invariably a woman) was if they made you feel angry. It also is frowned upon for an employee to express too much anger toward a supervisor. In the days of slavery, an angry slave was uppity and at risk of punishment. So anger is closely related to issues of power. Peer support then is extremely valuable because we are the freest to express our anger with peers where the power is equal. All other relationships involve power imbalances, where we as consumers are in a lower power position. It is usually risky to express anger in a relationship where you have less power. Yet, expressing anger we saw is a way to gain power.

10.2.6 What Do Experienced Advocates Say About Using Anger?

To gain a deeper understanding of this issue, we elicited feedback from experienced consumer/survivor advocates:

Barry and Cathy Creighton of Alaska: "Culturally, anger is not an easy subject. There is a semi-conscious religious stigma that anger is not Christian. (A saint would never use it.) That makes anger a very concentrated word. So we have found that one of the first steps is to broaden the word anger to be just one of the many colors on the palette of emotions. Next, bring in another word, 'listening' – a skill and an art that our newly elected President has demonstrated enormous capacity for."

"Advocacy implies that one is speaking to a political group or cultural prejudice. In that, one would want to listen very carefully and openly to the thought patterns and even prejudices and emotions of those you are addressing. One needs to grok [grok is the concept of deeply understanding a situation and comes from the book,

Stranger in a Strange Land by Robert Heinlen] who and what you are talking to. Then it becomes possible to use the entire palette of emotions – all the way from anger to compassion – effectively. In this respect, the amounts used of any particular emotion are a critical part of the dance between the advocates and who they are addressing."

"We have done this successfully with the Alaska legislature. In the process of addressing possible political change, we have used anger at some of the stigmas in our culture to enroll legislators in helping us bring about incremental change."

Crystal D. Choate of Alaska: "I have let my anger motivate me to gain more knowledge and do more research so that I can speak with a clear voice, firmly and calmly. Words sometimes have more meaning when you put them on paper, then I can re-adjust thoughts so they are not so angry."

Kamaree Altafer of Alaska: "If I take the time to break the anger down, it's other things that I'm feeling. In the beginning of my recovery, my anger was more frustration and hopelessness. In talking about professionals, I could not find anyone that would listen to what I was saying. If I didn't follow their agenda, they didn't want to work with me. The impression was that they didn't know what to do because of my dual diagnosis issues, stuff like that. I think the break for me was getting someone that would work WITH me. If I were to say how I used my anger, it would be persistence. Now that I am recovered, I use my anger, which I continue to feel is more frustration than anything, as a tool to drive my helping others along in recovery. I cannot stay angry and stay healthy. Anger leads to negativity and bitterness."

Jim Gottstein of Alaska:"Most of the time when consumers use anger in advocacy it is not only ineffective, but counterproductive and even dangerous since it is labeled a symptom. I think anger is most often effective for those with power over the person against whom the anger is expressed. That's not always the case of course."

Mike Wood of Iowa: ". . . anger crops up when I begin to take the actions or lack of actions of others personally. I have a fairly sophisticated filtration system, but occasionally anger tilts toward rage. I begin writing poison pen e-mails, make phone calls and otherwise lessen my short and long-term effectiveness as an advocate."

" I believe on the lower end of the anger scale, I can be effective. Dissension, frustration, discomfort in group settings seem to focus attention on the unresolved issues. Those people to whom we wish to reach are usually very uncomfortable with our anger. I think it shuts them down rather than activating them."

" My anger is usually suppressed. That leaves frustration. This may take a toll on me, but provides a better position to deliver a message. When I remain angry, I get all twitchy and it is sort of ugly. The suppression method was learned early from family."

"I have been researching some and have found a 1969 book by James C Coleman titled *Psychology and Effective Behavior*. One sentence reads, 'In many situations anger and hostility are normal reactions that may lead to constructive action.' And then, 'Anger and hostility aroused by autocratic and unjust treatment of oneself or others may be used constructively in working for social reforms'."

Debbie Whittle quotes Kenny Logans as saying his "anger fuels his truth."

Heather Peck of Virginia: "Holding onto anger is like picking up a burning coal to throw at the object of my anger all the while deeply burning myself" according to the Buddha as quoted by Thich Nhat Hahn. "I am powerless over the thoughts, words, and actions of others. I am responsible for the focus of my thoughts, words, and deeds." "Feeling anger informs me that I have been unfair to myself or another person has spoken or acted in a way that I perceive is unfair."

Molly Cisco of Wisconsin: "The use of anger is most effective when a conscious decision has been made to use this strategy among many to be considered. It is important to stick to strategy no matter your emotions. I have used my anger effectively, for example, in writing letters to editors, testifying before policy making bodies and teaching advocacy to others. When used well, people listen. If anger is used as just raw emotion, you risk losing your credibility and your issue. So use anger wisely."

Amy Shipman of South Dakota: "When I am part of an advocacy group, and we are able to achieve even a modest goal, I feel some of the anger seep out of me."

From these examples there are certain conclusions we can draw about anger and advocacy:

1) Raw anger interferes with advocacy.
2) Anger is a healthy reaction; it reflects a passionate desire to affect positive change to get our needs met.
3) Expressing and working out one's anger and frustration ahead of time can be a motivator of social change.
4) Anger is most effective when we feel we can use it rather than be it.
5) Being part of an advocacy group gives individuals more power which itself decreases frustration and anger.
6) Advocacy is much more important when practiced as part of a group because the cohesion of the group allows one to transform anger to passion more readily and one can effect more change when part of a group which further reduces anger and frustration.
7) If we do not learn to let go of our anger, it eats away at us and destroys our ability to positively contribute to developing a cooperative and cohesive community.

Drawing on the developmental model, we can consider the progression of an advocate as learning that "angry is something to use – not something to be." To Dan, this has meant to develop a greater sense of who he is. In his early years of advocacy he felt his anger so intensely that there was little opportunity to observe either his own reactions to the anger or to other peoples' reactions. He would be dismissed as overly biased toward consumers and no middle ground could be found. A good example was his advocacy for a consumer who was hospitalized in a mute state. He had made an agreement with her that she would not be forcibly medicated as long as she did not harm herself or others. She kept her end of the bargain, but the hospital staff wanted Dan to forcibly medicate her anyway. After several days, he lost the showdown with the supervisors, partly because his outrage made negotiation and broader advocacy impossible. It also did not help that he was a psychiatric resident (a relatively low status position in the psychiatric hierarchy) at the time.

Recently Lauren found herself challenged to effectively express her anger and communicate her concern about misleading the public and fueling discrimination. She had been part of a panel of experts on a TV show covering the topic of forced treatment. She felt that the consumer/survivor perspective was not well-represented. Because of the nature of her job and the topic that needed addressing, she asked others for feedback. Several advocates quickly became passionately involved, and together sculpted the letter, which literally and figuratively expressed our collective Voice. Below are some excerpts:

"I am writing to express my disappointment concerning the fact that the panel (for a television show) did not actually constitute a dialogue. The word 'dialogue' implies that more than one opinion is well represented. . . ."

"There are at least two perspectives on the issue of forced treatment. Some believe that it can be lifesaving – and that position was given a disproportionate percentage of attention during the taping. Others believe that forced intervention is, by definition, traumatizing and counterproductive. I am hoping that the final version of the program addresses this imbalance by including more information about the need for choice and self-determination in regard to mental health treatment, and the short- and long-term damage inflicted by the use of force and coercion. . . ."

"Because of the pervasive abrogation of individuals' civil rights – even a person accused of serious criminal behavior is given greater legal protection and due process than a person diagnosed with mental illness – these issues are not being properly considered by the courts" (Gottstein, 2008; Perlin, 2005; Morris, 2005).

Lauren is inspired by the righteous indignation, courage, passion, and tenacity that have brought the consumer/survivor movement this far. We will not be silenced. We are building our national Voice and awakening to a renewed sense of meaning, purpose, and belonging. We will continue to learn from our experiences, share our knowledge and become wiser about harnessing our passion. Lauren is confident that we are moving closer to an inclusive world community, where human differences are respected and diversity is honored. When she goes into stillness and hears the "violin strings playing in the gentle breezes," the cries of those whose voice was not heard, and carries them with the love and support so apparent today – this is the wind under her wings.

With education, support, and experience we will continue to develop the art of using anger instead of being angry. Harnessing that passion will open doors and accelerate our movement.

10.3 Finding and Using Our Authentic Collective Voice

This section will focus on the national organizing we have done to use our Voice to influence local and federal policy. The authors have also been involved in statewide organizing. The NEC published a book on this topic called "Voices of Transformation." This resource is based on the NEC's surveying the experiences of consumer-run, statewide advocacy organizations in Maryland, Vermont, California, and Ohio over the last 25 years. It has also been helpful in organizing consumers in other states to form new groups, including those Iowa, South Dakota, and Oregon.

10.3.1 Forming and Using a National Voice of Consumer/Survivors

The National Coalition of Mental Health Consumer Survivor Organizations (NCMHCSO) was built on the foundation laid by the courageous work of those who started the mental health consumer/survivor movement in the early 1970's. Those early leaders were people labeled with mental illness, who were inspired by people who were finding strength, courage, and power by joining together to work for human and civil rights. The visionary leaders of the consumer/survivor movement understood the only way to gain rights and independence was to come together and unite in a common cause. Through meetings in churches, apartments, and basements, we discovered the power of sharing our stories, of *being heard and of being understood*, instead of the idea that our labels defined us. We discovered we could shift into a vision of leading independent lives where we become authors rather than victims in our lives. Following in the footsteps of this early leadership, hundreds of self-help groups, consumer-run initiatives, and statewide consumer organizations formed all over the country. These groups have had some success in influencing policy and practices on the local level. Despite this, we had, until 2006, been unable to form a single, national organization, which could gain recognition and influence on a national level. In order to effect change at the national level, we needed to have a united national consumer/survivor voice. Leaders of other national groups in Washington, DC, elected officials, and the media have been searching for our united consumer voice. Without such a group to directly represent us, family groups or organizations of providers have been "speaking" for us and we have protested this misrepresentation. We have proclaimed, "Nothing about us without us."

Today consumers and survivors are uniting nationally as never before. Our movement has gained the experience, wisdom, and maturity to realize that it is time to see beyond our differences to the greater struggles urgently at hand. In May 2006, a series of teleconferences began to be held with representatives of major consumer/survivor groups from a number of statewide, consumer-run organizations and three national federally funded Technical Assistance Centers (CONTAC, Self-help Clearinghouse, and NEC). The formation of this national coalition was built on passion forged from collective anger. The final outrage was an essay written by Dr. Sally Satel, a highly placed psychiatrist in the Bush administration who criticized the ten components of recovery developed by SAMHSA. The psychiatrist particularly criticized self-determination, saying that persons with mental illness could never be self-determining. She also called for the dissolution of SAMHSA. From this groundswell of outrage, the coalition crafted a mission, a statement of purpose and formed a Steering Committee, whose bios are on our website, www.ncmhcso.org. The fundamental principle of the coalition is self-determination. The Steering

Committee hired a Director of Public Policy, Lauren Spiro, and we opened an office in Washington, DC. The Steering Committee developed a set of membership criteria, for admitting statewide consumer-run organizations or Technical Assistance (TA) Centers as members:

1. The group be genuinely consumer/survivor run, meaning that the majority of the board and the staff are consumer/survivors.
2. The organization be involved with consumer/survivors statewide or in a significant region of their state and that the organizations agree to be in regular communication with their networks and ensure that they are inclusive and representative of their state.
3. The organization's board approve in writing the mission and statement of purpose of the coalition.
4. The organization agrees to work out differences among themselves and any other member organizations in a collaborative fashion.
5. The organization advocate that the voice of consumer/survivors be central to decision making at all levels.

Currently, there are 31 member states, and efforts are underway by the Coalition and the TA Centers to organize statewide consumer organizations in the other states not yet represented.

We have conducted three annual open face-to-face meetings, typically having over 200 consumer/survivor participants. Our first annual meeting was held in Portland, Oregon and was an opportunity to announce the formation of the coalition and answer questions from across the country. Our second meeting, held in October 2007, in St. Louis, MO, was primarily used to develop a set of priority public policy issues. Our third annual meeting was held in October 2008 in Buffalo, New York where we fine-tuned our public policy priorities, heard from a state that has been very successful in securing state funds and shared some of our accomplishments in the past year. We reaffirmed that our top priority is adequate funding to ensure sustainability of consumer/survivor-run networks in every state.

10.3.2 Major Accomplishments of NCMHCSO During 2007–2008

I. September 2007: The Coalition expanded its CD Series: "Voices of Hope and Recovery: Our Stories, Our Lives" to 12 extraordinary stories to educate and inspire. These are personal stories of recovery by leaders and others involved in the consumer/survivor movement. These stories – honest, gut-wrenching, and triumphant – demonstrate the power of the human spirit to prevail.
II. September 2007: The coalition secured a contract to create a history exhibit of the mental health consumer/survivor movement. The coalition formed an advisory committee that selected the artifacts for the exhibit, which were collected from across the United States.

III. November 2007 and July 2008: The coalition co-sponsored two Presidential Forums. During that forum, the National Coalition, along with more than 20 other national disability rights organizations, co-hosted a *Presidential Candidates' Forum: A National Forum on Equality, Opportunity and Access*, in Manchester, New Hampshire. This historic, day-long event featured presidential primary candidates speaking on disability issues and answering questions from the audience. There were over 500 people and over 30 television cameras with Ted Kennedy, Jr. moderating when the first speaker, Senator Hillary Rodham Clinton, electrified the room. The second forum occurred in Columbus, Ohio, July 26, 2008. This Forum featured the 2008 Presidential Candidates. John McCain and Senator Harkin, who served as the surrogate for Barak Obama, presented their visions for the future of disability policy in America.

IV. March 2008: At the Sante Fe (NM) Summit, Lauren Spiro introduced the coalition to the audience and invited them to work with consumer/survivors in their state to develop or strengthen a statewide consumer/survivor network. Participants in the session on the National Healthcare Address included among others, Tommy G. Thompson, former Health and Human Services (HHS) secretary and four-term governor of Wisconsin. The 3-day Summit ended with participants sharing the actions they would take. Lauren said "the most important thing is that I will continue to advocate that people with the lived experience of recovery and their families will be at the head table. We will continue to move towards eliminating the oppressive policies, practices and attitudes that contribute to spiraling healthcare costs, unnecessary suffering, and premature death.

V. July 2008: Press release by the Coalition: WASHINGTON, D.C. " *Mummies of the Insane" Galvanizes National Coalition of People with Psychiatric Histories*. "A national coalition of people who have psychiatric histories is demanding an end to the 'sideshow' exhibition of two mummified female cadavers, whose bodies were sold in 1888 by the West Virginia Hospital for the Insane to an amateur scientist."

VI. June 2008: The National Coalition began developing Emotional CPR (eCPR), a peer-developed educational program for the general public designed to teach individuals to assist people through an emotional crisis by three simple steps of C = Connecting, P = emPowering, and R = Revitalizing. eCPR is based on the principles of trauma-informed care, counseling after disasters, peer support for recovery from mental health problems, emotional intelligence, suicide prevention, and cultural attunement.

VII. September 2008: The Coalition conducted its first grant funded organizing effort which took place in Washington, DC on September 16, 2008. One hundred and fifty participants from diverse communities, working together, from diverse communities formulated recommendations to transform mental health care in the Washington, DC Metropolitan Region. This is a step toward ensuring that our voice is heard and that together we work toward improving the system of care so that it does a better job in meeting the real needs of people.

VIII. September 2008: Coalition received a contract to produce materials about speaking from our heart with our advocacy voice and changing the world. We did a conference workshop, have a webcast scheduled, and a manual in development.
IX. December 2008: President-elect Barack Obama's transition team invited representatives from the coalition to meet and discuss our policy priorities. These meetings were made possible through the coalition working collaboratively with other disability groups. Through collaboration, the coalitions' Voice has grown much stronger.
X. December 2008: Press release: WASHINGTON, DC, *Tragedies Underscore Crisis in U.S. Public Mental Health System: National Advocacy Organization Demands Reforms*, "In the wake of the deaths of two persons in public psychiatric institutions – highlighting a pattern of abuse and neglect of those who have psychiatric disabilities – a national coalition of such individuals is calling on the incoming Obama administration and the nation's top mental health officials to institute widespread, substantive reforms in America's mental health treatment system. These would include raising standards and regulatory expectations, and identifying and funding pilot programs to demonstrate best practices in psychiatric emergency, inpatient and community-based care."

"'The death of Steven Sabock, a 50-year-old man diagnosed with bipolar disorder who died on April 29 in a North Carolina state psychiatric institution after he had choked on medication – while, nearby, hospital employees, ignoring his plight, entertained themselves with cards and TV – is just one example of the dangerous dysfunction of the public mental health system,' said Dan Fisher, M.D., Ph.D., of the National Coalition of Mental Health Consumer/Survivor Organizations (NCMHCSO)." In response to a similar death of a consumer in the waiting room of a New York hospital, supporter organization, NYAPRS held hearings throughout New York state to seek solutions. These hearings highlighted the need for alternatives to psychiatric hospitalization such as warmlines and peer-run crisis respite.
XI. Most recently, we helped secure for FY 09 just under one million dollars from congress to fund, through the Substance Abuse Mental Health Services Administration/Center for Mental Health Services, 12 additional consumer-run statewide networks bringing the total of networks funded to 32.

Though we are pleased with what we have accomplished in a short period of time we look forward to building more statewide networks and a stronger national coalition. We have found the common ground that unites us in the values of human and civil rights and our passion for recovery. We are building our infrastructure and accelerating the progress of our movement, which provides the vehicle for having the consumer/survivor voice heard so that we can impact decisions on policy, regulation, evaluation, training, funding, services, and other areas that influence our lives. We are increasing our effectiveness by working in partnership with organizations such as the Judge David L. Bazelon Center for Mental Health Law, the

American Association of Persons with Disabilities, and other person-led national disability organizations.

10.3.3 International Organizing

In August 2007, in St. Catherines, Canada, Dan assisted in the formation of an international coalition of national consumer/survivor organizations. This coalition's name is Interrelate (www.interrelate.info) which reflects the value the group places on relating deeply, as equals. The group consists of representatives from Australia, Canada, England, Ireland, New Zealand, Scotland, and the United States. Interrelate plans to participate in the next International Initiative on Mental Health Leadership to be held in Australia in March 2009. The mission of the group is, "to inspire hope and strengthen the capacity of people with mental health issues to lead in the creation of national and international policies, which achieve recovery and well-being." Connecting with each other and sharing our experiences gives greater courage to each of the members of the group. Through the formation of Interrelate we truly know that the recovery well-being, and protect of human rights.

10.4 Conclusion

Consumer/survivors have made remarkable progress in organizing at the local, state, national, and the international levels. Each level inspires and reinforces the further development of the others levels. Continued progress will require that peer support keep up with advocacy development. Our leaders often have just enough energy and skills to gain a voice but still need to attend to an equal complement of peer support to sustain these gains. Often a person's first involvement with the consumer/survivor movement is as a consumer who wants additional support rather than systems change. Gradually, through peer support, consumers get in touch with their anger toward a system and a society, which has marginalized them. They learn that they are neither isolated nor passive victims of societal misunderstanding and discrimination. When this outrage can be forged into passion for change, peers transition into advocates and survivors. Other disability groups are further along in the development of their empowered, advocacy Voice and serve as models for us in their use of political strategy to affect systems change. It will be increasingly important to learn to collaborate with other disability organizations led by persons with disabilities as well as the larger community of disability organizations.

The National Coalition of Mental Health Consumer/Survivor Organizations has begun to build these connections at a national level. Three examples of strong national disability groups led by persons with disabilities are the American Association of Persons with Disabilities (AAPD), National Council of Independent Living Centers (NCIL), and ADAPT, a nationwide grassroots organization of people with disabilities. AAPD was founded by legendary disability leaders, Justin

Dart and Fred Fay. They both were excellent at reaching out to leaders in the consumer/survivor movement. As a result the NCMHCSO has entered into a national cross-disability network organized by AAPD consisting of NCIL, ADAPT, and nine other national disability groups run by persons with disabilities, called Justice For All Action Network or JFAAN. As a result of being part of JFAAN, NCMHCSO has been invited to two meetings with senior policy officials from the Obama White House. We are using our voices to enter into respectful dialogue with these allies in this historic struggle to humanize post-industrial society.

References

Bentall, R. P. (1990). *Reconstructing schizophrenia*. London: Routledge.
Buber, M. (1965). *Between man and man*. New York: Collier Books.
Evans, C. de B. (trans.). (1924). *Meister Eckhart*, by Franz Pfeiffer, 2 vols. London: Watkins.
Fisher D. (2008). Promoting recovery. In: T. Stickley & T. Basset (Eds.), *Learning about mental health practice*. Chichester: Wiley.
Gottstein, J. (2008). Involuntary commitment and forced psychiatric drugging in the trial courts: Rights violations as a matter of course. *Alaska Law Review, 25*, 51–53.
Harrop, C., & Trower, P. (2003). *Why does schizophrenia develop at late adolescence?* London: Wiley
Jablensky, A., & Cole, S. W. (1997). Is the earlier age of onset of schizophrenia in males a confounding variable? *British Journal of Psychiatry, 170*, 234–240.
Jablensky, A., Sartorius, N., Ernberg, G., Anker, M., Korten, A., Cooper, J. E., Day, R., & Bertelsen, A. (1992). *Schizophrenia: Manifestations, incidence and course in different cultures. A World Health Organization ten-country study*. Psychological Medicine Monograph Supplement 20. Cambridge: Cambridge University Press.
Jablensky, A. Sartorius, N. (2008). What did the WHO studies really find? *Schizophrenia Bulletin, 151*:1745–1701.
Morris, G. H. (2005). Pursuing justice for the mentally disabled. University of San Diego School of Law, *31*, 1–33.
Nasar, S. (1999). *A beautiful mind*. New York: Simon and Shuster.
New Freedom Commission on Mental Health (2003). *Achieving the promise: Transforming mental health care in America*. Rockville, MD: Substance Abuse and Mental Health Services Administration. Retrieved from www.mentalhealthcommission.gov
Perlin, M. (2005). And my best friend, my doctor/Won't even say what it is I've got: The role and significance of counsel in right to refuse treatment cases. *San Diego Law. Review, 42*, 735–756.
Perry, J. W. (1974). *Far Side of Madness*. Putnam, CT: Spring Publications.
Seikkula, J., & Trimble, D. (2005). Healing elements of therapeutic conversation: Dialogue as an embodiment of love. *Family Process, 44*, 461–475.
Tiedens, L. Z. (2001). Anger and advancement versus sadness and subjugation: The effect of negative emotion expressions on social status conferral. *Journal of Personality and Social Psychology, 80*, 86–94.

Chapter 11
How Governments and Other Funding Sources Can Facilitate Self-Help Research and Services

Crystal R. Blyler, Risa Fox, and Neal B. Brown

Abstract Despite the inherent grassroots nature of self-help, there is much that governments and other funding sources can do to facilitate the development and provision of self-help services and research. Through persistent attention to self-help concepts, provision of resources, and attention to emerging trends that might provide future opportunities, governments and other funders can be valuable partners for pushing the field of self-help research and services in new directions. This chapter provides examples of the types of activities in which governments and other funding sources can engage to facilitate and support self-help research and services. A number of ideas regarding potential sources of funding for self-help researchers and service providers are presented and future directions for self-help research and services are discussed. By supporting self-help on the national stage, we believe that the efforts of the federal Community Support Program has contributed to the growth of self-help over the past 30 years.

11.1 How Governments and Other Funding Sources Can Facilitate Self-Help Research and Services

Due to the inherent nature of self-help, self-help services develop through the initiative of individuals tackling their own difficulties and seeking to support peers with similar experiences. Despite the grassroots origins of self-help initiatives, however, governments and other funding sources can facilitate the development of self-help and the conduct of related research and evaluation in a variety of ways. In the United States, the federal Community Support Program (CSP), currently housed as a branch

---

C.R. Blyler (✉)
SAMHSA Center for Mental Health Services, Rockville, MD, USA
e-mail: crystal.blyler@samhsa.hhs.gov

The views expressed in this chapter are those of the authors and do not necessarily represent the opinions of the Substance Abuse and Mental Health Services Administration or its Center for Mental Health Services.

of the Substance Abuse and Mental Health Services Administration (SAMHSA) Center for Mental Health Services (CMHS), has supported mental health self-help efforts for the past 30 years. Based on our experience, this chapter provides examples of the types of activities in which governments and other funding sources can engage to facilitate and support self-help research and services. A number of ideas regarding potential sources of funding for self-help researchers and service providers are also presented, and the chapter closes with a discussion of how we see the field of self-help research and services evolving over the next 5–10 years.

Although our experience is grounded in our work as part of a federal agency in the United States, the chapter is intended to inform all types and levels of government (international, federal, state, local, organizational), as well as other funding sources such as private foundations. In addition, the chapter aims to help researchers and service providers to understand the role that governments and other funders have, do, and can play in their work. As the saying goes, money talks. Funding sources are often seen as simple distributors of money to people in the field who use it to move their own ideas forward. However, governments and other funders have considerable discretion to determine how the money is spent. The ways in which they choose to spend not only the money, but also their time and other resources, give funders considerable influence to shape how the field progresses.

11.2 Defining Self-Help

A strict definition of self-help focuses exclusively on "the act or an instance of providing for or helping oneself without dependence on others" (Webster's New Collegiate Dictionary, 1981, G. & C. Merriam Company, Springfield, MA). Within the mental health field, however, self-help is often defined in terms that emphasize peer support rather than self-reliance, as described by the Surgeon General (U.S. Department of Health and Human Services, 1999): "People with a shared condition who come together can help themselves and each other to cope" (p. 289). This definition suggests that peer groups focus on coping with the mental illness itself rather than on gaining independence. Van Tosh and del Vecchio (CMHS, 2001a) blend the concepts of peer support and self-reliance in defining self-help as "the process whereby individuals who share a common condition or interest assist themselves rather than relying on the assistance of others" (p. 4).

Based on what we have learned from consumers involved in federal initiatives, this chapter expands upon these definitions to include *any act or activity in which consumers help themselves or other consumers to achieve their own goals*. Within this definition, the term consumer is broadly defined as a person who currently receives mental health services, has received them in the past, or is eligible to receive them but chooses not to. Although our work has focused primarily on consumers of publicly funded mental health services, many of the suggestions contained in this chapter are applicable to the more general population. Using an inclusive definition, our concept of self-help support goes beyond peer support to include a wide array of services that help individuals to achieve independence. Under our broad concept fall such diverse services as self-determination models of funding mental health services; services that help consumers to attain and sustain independent employment and housing; and services that help consumers to know and protect their rights. Not coincidentally, more and more self-help organizations are addressing these service areas, not only through advocacy but also by delivering such services directly (CMHS, 2001).

11.3 The Federal Community Support Program

The federal Community Support Program (CSP) was launched in 1977 with a mission to improve services for "adult psychiatric patients whose disabilities are severe and persistent but for whom long-term skilled or semi-skilled nursing care is inappropriate" (Turner & Ten Hoor, 1978, p. 319). From its inception, consumers were involved in developing guidelines for the Community Support Systems (CSS) that CSP promoted, and the national plan that initially guided CSP's work included "mutual and self-help" among its suggested service system principles (Steering Committee on the Chronically Mentally Ill, 1981, p. 2–45). The steering committee for the national plan further specified that "the Department should support research and evaluation of self-help, patient-run, and parent-run alternative programs" (p. ES-14). CSP continued to develop and promote the CSS model throughout the 1980s (National Institute of Mental Health, 1987), and its guiding principles continued to include self-determination and consumer involvement "in all aspects of planning and delivering services" (Stroul, 1988, p. 7). Peer support and self-help continued to be included among the "essential components that are needed to provide adequate services and support" (p. 8).

Originally housed within the National Institute of Mental Health, CSP became a branch of the Center for Mental Health Services (CMHS) when the Substance Abuse and Mental Health Services Administration (SAMHSA) was formed in 1992 (42 USC 290aa). With original CSP staff members among its personnel and principles underlying CSP ingrained in the organizational culture, the CSP branch and CMHS as a whole continued to support and expand upon self-help-related initiatives into the 1990s. In 2009, we continue to seek ways to develop, support, and promote self-help, peer support, and consumer-driven services. Two of the authors (R.F. and N.B.B.) have been with CSP since the late 1970s, and this chapter summarizes our experiences in supporting self-help initiatives across the decades.

11.4 Ways that Funders Can Facilitate Self-Help

11.4.1 Involve Consumers in Everything You Do.

The first step in supporting self-help is involving consumers in everything you do (International Association of Psychosocial Rehabilitation Services, 1998; National Association of State Mental Health Program Directors, 1989). Consumers began to develop self-help alternatives prior to the creation of CSP (Chamberlin, 1978). As the originators of self-help approaches, consumers involved in the development of CSP advocated for self-help alternatives to be included in the model Community Support System (Turner & TenHoor, 1978). Without consumers in the room, self-help approaches are often forgotten as mental health service providers focus on the professional supports for which they are responsible. When self-help approaches are considered, the consumers who develop and benefit from self-help are essential for providing knowledge and expertise regarding the feasibility, desirability, usefulness, and logistical details of implementation, sustainability, and evaluation.

The national plan that guided CSP's initial activities discussed the leadership role of the federal government in involving consumers in planning and, in response, included liaison representatives from consumer organizations on the National Mental Health Advisory Council (Steering Committee on the Chronically Mentally Ill, 1981). Governments and other funders have many opportunities to support consumer involvement in both their own work and in the work of those with whom they collaborate or whom they fund. Such opportunities include involving consumers in setting priorities for services and research; involving consumers as principal investigators and project directors, and as research and program staff; hiring consumers within their own organizations; specifying requirements, including monetary requirements, for consumer roles in grants and contracts; including consumers on peer review panels for grants, contracts, and publications; measuring grant and contract performance related to consumer involvement; and supporting the development of consumer leadership.

11.4.1.1 Involve Consumers in Setting Priorities for Services and Research

Governments and other funders can involve consumers in setting priorities for services and research through all of the means available to them for gathering stakeholder input. In order to ensure meaningful consumer involvement, special efforts should be made to ensure that consumer voices are heard. Conducting or funding ad-hoc focus groups and surveys can provide means to sample opinions from a wide array of diverse consumers regarding issues of current significance. Over a 4-month period in 2001, for example, the CMHS-funded Recovery Outcomes Systems Indicators (ROSI) project gathered input from 115 consumers through ten focus groups held in nine states regarding what helps and what hinders their recovery (Onken, Dumont, Ridgway, Dornan, & Ralph, 2002). These data were used to develop an instrument for measuring both the recovery-orientation of mental health services and systems and individual recovery. Widespread use of the Internet provides increasing opportunities for both formal and informal collection of consumer input.

In addition to ad-hoc gatherings and surveys, funders may establish standing processes and procedures for gathering consumer input and feedback regarding priorities for services and research. One way that CMHS has done this is by regularly hosting caucuses at annual conferences that draw national audiences, such as Mental Health America's annual conference and the CMHS-funded Alternatives conference. In addition, CMHS' Consumer Affairs Program regularly holds regional meetings around the nation. In 2000, CMHS established a subcommittee on Consumer/Survivor Issues, comprised of people who have experienced mental illness, treatment, and recovery, that reports to the legislatively mandated National Advisory Council in order to "provide experiential knowledge in seeking federal improvement of the public mental health system" (CMHS, 2002, p. 1).

In addition to establishing consumer input and feedback mechanisms for their own work, the United States has promoted consumer involvement in setting priorities for state and local jurisdictions. The Mental Health Planning Act of 1986 (Publ. L. 99–660) required consumer involvement at every stage of developing and implementing state comprehensive mental health plans, as well as requiring states to establish Mental Health Planning Councils to advise them on the development of their mental health services plans. In support of federal guidelines stating that "the rights, wishes, and needs of...consumers are paramount in planning and operating the mental health system" (National Institute of Mental Health, 1987, p. 11), at least four states (Arizona, Arkansas, Maryland, and Colorado) used CSP Statewide Systems Improvement Grants awarded from 1987 to 1989 to create strong consumer and family components of their statewide community service systems (Mulkern, 1995). To further strengthen the involvement of consumers in state planning, the 3-year State Service System Improvement grants that CSP awarded in 1990–1991 were specifically designed to

> demonstrate and evaluate service system improvement strategies that integrate consumers and family members into the planning and provision of mental health and support services at state and local levels. (Mulkern, 1995, p. 35)

Since 1992, legislation has mandated the use of Mental Health Planning Councils that include consumers and families in order for states to receive Community Mental Health Service Block Grant funding (42 USC 300x). Through Mental Health Transformation State Incentive Grants (CMHS, 2005a), CMHS extended the requirement for consumer involvement in the formulation and implementation of state comprehensive mental health plans through mandatory inclusion of consumers on the Transformation Working Groups that guide such plans.

Although perhaps less common, involvement of consumers in setting research priorities is as critical as their involvement in setting service priorities. Del Vecchio and Blyler (2009) described crucial differences between consumers and researchers in terms of desired outcomes and priorities for research. Consumer involvement in research, as in services, often redirects evaluation efforts toward self-help-related concepts such as recovery, peer support, self-determination, and consumer-operated services. When asked to suggest priorities for CMHS during a consumer/survivor planning meeting that CMHS convened in 1995, for example, consumers recommended that CMHS fund a demonstration program on the cost-effectiveness of self-help services (CMHS, 1996b). In response, beginning in 1998, CMHS made $20 million available to fund the Consumer-Operated Services Program multisite research initiative, which evaluated the effectiveness of consumer-operated services over a 4-year period (CMHS, 1998; Rogers et al., 2007).

Oftentimes, initial consumer involvement in a more limited capacity stimulates ideas for ways in which consumers can become more involved in research in the future. Such was the case, for example, with CMHS' Consumer/Survivor Research and Policy Work Group: "Starting from a focus group on mental health outcomes, initiated in June 1992..., by its second meeting in July, the Workgroup expanded its focus to include formulation of policy research, including a national consumer-/survivor-driven research agenda....By their third meeting (October 1–2, 1992), ...not only did they want to participate on grant review groups, but they wanted to determine criteria for grant review...for consumer/survivor involvement of grants. They also wanted input determining the content of [grant and contract solicitations]" (McLean, 1994, pp. 12–13). The Work Group went on to participate with CMHS' Mental Health Statistics Improvement Project in the development of a managed care report card for mental health and substance abuse (Manderscheid & Henderson, 1995).

11.4.1.2 Involve Consumers as Principal Investigators and Project Directors, and as Research and Program Staff

One way to ensure that consumer voices are heard in setting priorities for services and research is to involve consumers as principal investigators and project directors, and as research and program staff (Campbell, Ralph, & Glover, 1993; Danley & Ellison, 1999; Wallcraft, Schrank, & Amering, M., 2009). A 2003 survey of consumer research activities in states found that consumers involved in research and evaluation were interested in reviewing the evidence regarding consumer-operated and recovery-oriented services, measuring recovery, and evaluating a variety of consumer-operated services (Weaver, 2003). Early CSP service and research demonstration grants involved consumers not only as project advisors but as program and evaluation designers, executive directors and service providers in the programs being demonstrated, peer counselors, evaluators, data collection interviewers, disseminators of research and program information, and employers of other evaluators (McLean, 1994; Mulkern, 1995). Consumers held similar roles in the Consumer-Operated Services Program (CMHS, 1998) and other CMHS multisite research initiatives conducted in the late 1990s (e.g., the Women and Violence multisite initiative, Prescott, 2001). Consumers have also directed and/or been involved in conducting numerous state-funded projects, such as California's Well-being Project (Campbell & Schraiber, 1989), development of Ohio's Mental Health Consumer Outcomes System (http://mentalhealth.ohio.gov/what-we-do/protect-and-monitor/consumer-outcomes/history/index.shtml, accessed 4/5/09), and projects in Massachusetts (conducted through Consumer Quality Initiatives, Inc., Roxbury) and Maryland (through On Our Own of Maryland, Inc., Baltimore).

Providing mentoring and specific funding support for consumer involvement in research can help ensure meaningful consumer participation. A 2003 survey found that although 56% of informants stated that consumers led research and evaluation activities in their state, professional researchers or evaluators typically worked side by side as mentors (Weaver, 2003). As a federal example, the CMHS-funded

Evaluation Technical Assistance Center operated by the Human Services Research Institute provided collaboration, mentoring, and support to the consumer-governed Kentucky Center for Mental Health Studies, Inc. to evaluate the CMHS-funded Consumer and Consumer Supporter National Technical Assistance Centers in 2001 and 2002 (Kentucky Center for Mental Health Studies, 2001, 2002). This same partnership created a Consumer Evaluator Network to provide small grants to support consumers involved in research (Weaver, 2003).

11.4.1.3 Hire Consumers Within Your Own Organization

Just as employing consumers within research and service systems can facilitate self-help efforts, consumers employed within positions within governments and funding organizations can also help to move self-help efforts forward. Early efforts of CSP led to the establishment of Offices of Consumer Affairs within the states (McLean, 2003). Twenty-six states had such offices in place in 1993 (Campbell et al., 1993) when the National Association of State Mental Health Program Directors established the National Association of Consumer/Survivor Mental Health Administrators (NACSMHA; CMHS, 1996b). By 2000, nearly 40 state mental health authorities had such offices (Van Tosh, Ralph, & Campbell, 2000). The latest NACSMHA roster reveals that 49 states, the District of Columbia, and Puerto Rico hire consumers in state offices (accessed online at http://www.nasmhpd.org/nacsmha.cfm, 4/4/09). At the federal level, CMHS hired its first Consumer Affairs Specialist in 1995 (CMHS, 2001) and added a second Consumer Affairs Specialist in 1996 (CMHS, 1996a). Today, the CMHS Consumer Affairs staff encompasses five full-time positions plus internships. Although Campbell (1998) found no significant relationship between presence or absence of Offices of Consumer Affairs and the number of consumer programs funded by state mental health authorities, the Offices were significantly associated with provision of state mental health authority resources for conference support and technical assistance. In addition, the Offices were significantly associated with consumer involvement in state, local, and internal review boards; direct hire of consumers/survivors for services evaluation activities; and consumer involvement with state mental health authorities through participation in focus groups and public forums. Within CMHS, the Consumer Affairs staff has served to bring self-help concepts and approaches to bear across the programs of all of the organization's divisions, as well as individually or jointly sponsoring specific projects emphasizing self-help (e.g., the Consumer-Operated Services Program multisite research initiative, the development of the National Consensus Statement on Mental Health Recovery, and projects on self-determination and shared decision making).

Employment of consumers within research and service systems is not limited to positions within Offices of Consumer Affairs or other consumer-specific positions, such as peer specialists. Consumers bring valuable perspectives related to self-help concepts to any mental health service or research position. Within CMHS, federal hiring authorities that exist to expedite hiring of people with psychiatric disabilities (e.g., Schedule A, 5 CFR 213.3102u) provide access to a high quality, largely untapped labor pool with experience and expertise that is directly relevant to the work that we do. Use of this authority has resulted in multiple successful hires. Similar hiring authorities or policies may be available to other levels of government and funding organizations. Consumers hired into general project officer roles within CMHS have emphasized the importance of fostering self-help approaches in their work on such diverse subject areas as trauma-informed care, employment support services, criminal justice involvement, services for older adults, and mental health systems transformation.

11.4.1.4 Specify Requirements (Including Monetary) for Consumer Roles in All Grants and Contracts

Because a substantial portion of the work of governments and other funders is completed through grants and contracts, specifying requirements for consumer roles within these funding vehicles is essential (e.g., Guidelines for Consumer and Family Participation, SAMHSA, 2009). Review criteria that include evaluation of the applicant or offerer's plan for consumer participation in the work proposed can help to ensure that awardees will meet the stated requirements. The contract solicitation for the evaluation of the CMHS Mental Health Transformation State Incentive Grant program, for example, specified the following review criterion worth 20% of the total score:

> The proposal will be evaluated based on the demonstrated understanding of mental health consumers and family members as sources of experience and expertise critical to the success of transformation. The proposal should demonstrate and document a clear commitment to involving consumers and family members in all aspects of the evaluation, including design and conduct phases, as well as interpretation and presentation of results. The proposal should demonstrate experience with and a proven capability for identifying, recruiting, hiring, convening, and adequately compensating mental health consumers at a national level. (Solicitation No. 280-06-0148, May 16, 2006, p. 9)

Grant and contract awards must be specific in requiring adequate compensation for consumers' work, and budgets should be examined to ensure that funds are designated for this purpose. Specifications for the transformation grant evaluation contract, for example, included

> The Contractor shall reimburse consumers and family members involved in designing and conducting the cross-site evaluation for their time and expenses....The Contractor shall arrange and pay for travel, lodging, per diem, [and] consultant fees...for...members of the consumer workgroup....The Contractor shall arrange and pay for any necessary teleconferences. (p. 15)

When funding is specifically designated to self-help organizations, requirements to ensure genuine consumer composition of applicants within the solicitations have proven beneficial. Applicants for CMHS grants for National Consumer Technical Assistance Centers, for example, must certify and provide proof of the following:

- The applicant is an organization that is controlled and managed by consumers and dedicated to the improvement of mental health services.

- The applicant organization has a Board of Directors comprising more than 50% consumers.
- The applicant organization has been in operation as a legal entity for a minimum of 1 year.
- The Internal Revenue Service has issued the applicant organization tax-exempt status.
- The consumer Board of Directors has been in operation for more than 1 year.
- The applicant organization will take an active role in the fiscal management and oversight of the project and will be legally, fiscally, administratively, and programmatically responsible for the grant and has not submitted a "pass through," "umbrella," or "cover letter" application (CMHS, 2007a, pp. 33–34).

Similar certification and documentation must be submitted by applicants for CMHS Statewide Consumer Network Grants (CMHS, 2009b).

11.4.1.5 Include Consumers on Peer Review Panels for Grants, Contracts, and Publications

As in other roles, consumers who participate on peer review panels provide unique expertise for judging the feasibility, importance, usefulness, acceptability, and validity of approaches related to self-help. When solicitations and publications specifically target self-help organizations and/or specifically focus on self-help and related concepts, the unique expertise of consumer reviewers is especially critical. Over the past two decades, CMHS grants specifically targeting consumers have been reviewed by all-consumer panels. Some technical assistance has been provided to ensure that all reviewers understand the process and have the necessary skills.

11.4.1.6 Measure Grant and Contract Performance Related to Consumer Involvement

In addition to establishing requirements and rigorously assessing plans and proposals, ongoing evaluation of project performance is essential for ensuring that expected consumer involvement actually occurs. For the Mental Health Transformation State Incentive Grant program, CMHS included the number of consumers who are members of statewide consumer networks as a core indicator of improvements made through transformation to mental health system accountability (CMHS, 2005a). To assess consumer involvement in the transformation process itself, consumer focus groups and interviews are being conducted in each state by independent cross-site evaluation teams that include consumer and family consultants (CMHS, 2009a). A wide variety of other measures can also be considered by funders, such as number of consumers participating in various ways, percentage of participants who are consumers, consumer satisfaction with their roles, and process measures assessing the impact of consumer involvement on project activities. Involving consumers in selecting performance measures and in collecting and interpreting the resulting data will help to ensure that the results accurately represent consumer involvement in the project.

11.4.1.7 Support the Development of Consumer Leadership

Supporting the development of consumer leadership will help ensure the ready availability of diverse consumers who are prepared to apply their expertise and skills to self-help and related endeavors. Consumers vary in their perspectives and, like anyone, have limited time and resources. Seeking out and helping to expand the pool of consumers prepared to become involved in the mental health services and research fields is, therefore, crucial.

CMHS has long facilitated consumer involvement in public mental health discussions through grants that support development of statewide consumer networks (CMHS, 2009b). Grants that CMHS awarded to states in the early 1990s supported the initial adoption of Leadership Academies designed to teach the basic skills necessary for consumers to become effective leaders in grassroots advocacy organizations (Hess, Clapper, Hoekstra, & Gibison, 2001; Stringfellow & Muscari, 2003). The Idaho Bureau of Mental Health used CMHS grant funds to form a new organization, the Idaho Leadership Academy, and hired consultants who adapted advocacy training materials previously developed for people with physical disabilities (Balcazar & Seekins, 1993) for use by mental health consumers (Sabin & Daniels, 2002). Together with the hired consultants, the Idaho Consumer Advocacy Coalition, the Idaho Alliance for the Mentally Ill, and the Shoshone Bannock Tribal Health and Human Services first implemented Leadership Academy workshops between 1993 and 1995 (Hess et al., 2001; Sabin & Daniels, 2002). Outcomes reported from Idaho showed that participation in Leadership Academies resulted in the development of self-help programs addressing crisis respite care, advocacy against stigma and for consumer rights, strengthened relationships with law enforcement, tasks forces for the prevention of suicides, and consumer-run drop-in centers (Hess et al., 2001).

When one of Idaho's consultants, Robert Hess, took a position with the West Virginia Office of Behavioral Health Services in 1994, he joined with the West Virginia Mental Health Consumers' Association and the West Virginia Alliance for the Mentally Ill to explore ways in which the state could strengthen consumer and family participation in oversight of the mental health system. Impressed with the results reported for Idaho, the group used CMHS grant funds to implement the West Virginia Leadership Academy in 1995 (Sabin & Daniels, 2002; Stringfellow & Muscari, 2003). Through CMHS grants awarded to the West Virginia Mental Health Consumers Association to operate the Consumer Organization and Networking Technical Assistance Center (CONTAC) from 1998 through 2007, the Leadership Academy has evolved into a nationwide vehicle for training consumers in advocacy skills such as identification of issues of concern in their communities and development of strategic action plans from the perspective of a variety of groups; expressing opinions in a clear, positive, and assertive manner, both orally and in writing; working with the media; fund-raising; conducting effective meetings; teaching advocacy and leadership skills to others; developing local advocacy groups and online networks; and collecting data to assess the impact of their leadership on the local, state, and national levels.

Recently, CMHS has provided additional support for the development of consumer leadership by funding Leadership Institutes (http://www.attcnetwork.org/explore/priorityareas/wfd/lead/institute.asp, accessed 6/7/10) that provide individual training in core leadership competencies and pair consumers with mentors of their choice to work with them on leadership projects over a 6-month period. Leadership Institutes differ somewhat from Leadership Academies in that they were originally adapted for leaders in the substance abuse treatment field and take a broad approach to developing core competencies thought to be applicable for leadership in any field, such as conflict management, resilience, problem solving, political savvy, and human resources management. In 2006, for example, CMHS sponsored a Leadership Institute in which consumer and non-consumer leaders involved in the Mental Health Transformation State Incentive Grant program were trained together using an identical curriculum. Another approach that funders might consider would be to provide training grants, such as those that CMHS provides through its Minority Fellowship Program (CMHS, 2008), to increase the number of consumer mental health professionals.

11.4.2 Directly Fund Self-Help Services and Research

Of course, involving consumers in everything you do is only the first step in facilitating self-help services and research. Ideally, governments and other funders will directly fund these activities. In the federal system, states remain primarily responsible for the funding of direct services, including self-help. Nevertheless, the federal government and other funders can push the field forward by funding demonstration programs and development grants. In 1984, with support from four Foundations, consumer-run demonstrations began operating in the San Francisco Bay Area (Parrish, 1990). Two years later, CSP awarded 3-year grants to states for local service demonstrations related to homelessness, services for older adults, and young adults with co-occurring mental health and substance abuse problems (Mulkern, 1995). Some of the states used these grants to fund consumer-run service programs, while others included roles for consumers as service delivery providers or volunteer peer counselors. During the same time period, CSP awarded more than 40 three-year grants to improve statewide community service systems for adults with severe and persistent mental illness (Mulkern, 1995). At least one state, Utah, used these funds to provide a number of mini-grants to help consumer self-help groups to develop sources of funding for ongoing support.

From 1988 to 1992, CSP initiated a grant program to support local consumer-operated service demonstration projects, the first of their kind to be supported by a federal agency in the United States (CMHS, 2001). Fourteen states received 3-year grants totaling $5 million (CMHS, 2001; Mulkern, 1995). Funds supported a number of self-help-related activities including drop-in centers, business enterprises, Offices of Consumer Affairs, peer support groups, outreach and food for consumers who were homeless, and public education (CMHS, 2001). In 1991, CSP awarded 3-year grants to 21 states to

> demonstrate and evaluate service system improvement strategies that integrate consumers and family members into the planning and provision of mental health and support services at state and local levels....Most of these projects provided various types of administrative and organizational development support to existing consumer and family groups. (Mulkern, 1995, pp. 35–36)

Activities supported by these grants included organizing self-help and support groups across the state; developing newsletters and disseminating other types of material; developing teleconferencing networks; designing membership campaigns, including some focused on increasing participation from minority groups; developing consumer-run services, especially to provide housing and vocational rehabilitation; training consumers and family members how to run and sustain organizations; developing training packets, anti-stigma campaigns, and other public relations materials to educate mental health professionals, legislators, and the public; and developing ways to involve consumers and family members as evaluators of mental health services.

Promotion of self-help services through demonstrations and development grants is not, of course, limited to federal funding. From 1982 to 1990, for example, Michigan funded twenty-five consumer-run demonstrations (Mowbray & Tan, 1993; Parrish, 1990). Similarly, in 1989 Pennsylvania funded the development of consumer drop-in centers throughout the state (Kaufmann, Ward-Colasante, & Farmer, 1993). Following the leadership of CSP's 1988 to 1992 consumer-operated service demonstrations (McLean, 2003), by 1993, 36 states and territories directly funded at least one consumer project, and 280 consumer-run organizations received public mental health funds (Campbell et al., 1993).

The history of federal support for self-help research mirrors that for services. The first CSP funding for self-help research was provided in 1982 when nearly $1 million were designated for CSP-related research; projects on Evaluating Self-help Organizations and a Self-help Groups Resource Book were included among the 26 funded projects (Stroul, 1984). From 1989 to 1991, CSP awarded 3-year research demonstration grants to evaluate case management, crisis intervention, and psychosocial rehabilitation services (Brown, 1989). Although only one of the 23 grants was awarded directly to consumers, 9 included substantial consumer involvement, including in the delivery of case management, companion, crisis, and vocational rehabilitation services (Mulkern, 1995). Three of the demonstrations (CA, ME, and PA) compared consumer case management to traditional case management, one evaluated consumer case management for people who were homeless (MO), and one evaluated a consumer crisis intervention (KY; Brown, 1989). In 1992, CSP funded research centers in Michigan and California specifically focused on self-help research (CMHS, 2001). Under the auspices of SAMHSA, in 1998 CSP embarked on the first ever multisite randomized controlled trial of consumer-operated services

(CMHS, 1998; Del Vecchio & Blyler, 2009). CMHS is currently using results from the trial (e.g., Rogers et al., 2007) to develop an evidence-based practice toolkit for implementing consumer-operated services. Through a 2004 grant announcement jointly funded with CMHS, the National Institute of Mental Health (NIMH) also awarded a grant to the Kansas Department of Social and Rehabilitation Services to conduct a 3-year study regarding the implementation of consumer-operated services as an evidence-based practice (NIMH, 2004). Successful solicitation, award, and completion of such self-help research activities rests on close adherence to the guidelines for consumer involvement described above.

11.4.3 Provide Technical Assistance and Training

Beyond directly funding self-help services and research, governments and other funders can significantly influence the direction of the field through technical assistance and training mechanisms. At the most basic level, funders can educate and inform consumers about what is happening within the larger fields of mental health services and research. The early CSP program convened a series of Learning Community Conferences (Turner & TenHoor, 1978) that included consumers among the participants (Mulkern, 1995; Parrish, 1991). In addition to national conferences, consumers were important participants in regional conferences (Stroul, 1984). Today, CMHS' Consumer Affairs Program provides scholarships that support the attendance of individual consumers at various national meetings. Early on, CSP produced a newsletter, *Community Support Network News*, to keep all stakeholders informed (Stroul, 1984) and since 1996, CMHS' Consumer Affairs Program has continued the tradition by widely distributing an electronic *Consumer Affairs Bulletin* to consumers and other stakeholders across the nation.

In addition to providing educational opportunities for consumers, funders can advance self-help services and research by providing opportunities for consumers to talk to each other. This was especially important during the early years of CSP when "the mentally disabled ha[d] yet to organize as an effective interest group" (Turner & Ten Hoor, 1978, p. 325). "This suggest[ed] the need for a process to convene and nurture such a constituency – a coalition of concern – within each state and community" (p. 326). The initial national plan that followed the creation of CSP recommended that

> the federal government should provide assistance in developing a variety of mechanisms to enable advocates to meet in order to compare notes about latest developments in the field and to provide mutual support in conducting their advocacy activities. (Steering Committee on the Chronically Mentally Ill, 1981, p. 2–126)

In response, Boston University convened national monthly teleconferences of consumer leaders in the early 1980s on behalf of CSP (CMHS, 2001). Peer group discussions that took place during CSP Learning Community Conferences led to adoption of consumer self-help efforts as a priority for the future (Stroul, 1984). In support of state level organizing, CSP has funded grants to consumers for the past decade to develop statewide networks (CMHS, 2009b). The communication among consumers generated by such networks has facilitated the development of self-help support services in states across the nation.

In 1985, CSP sponsored the first annual national *Alternatives* conference organized by and for consumers. Four hundred people attended the first conference (http://www.onourownmd.org/history.html, accessed 3/15/09). The twenty-first *Alternatives* conference was held in 2007 and included 720 registered participants, including 37 scholarship recipients. Participants

> heard 128 speakers present more than 60 workshops, nearly 20 institutes and six plenary sessions. Evening events included nearly two dozen caucuses, and 30 exhibit tables offered a range of information about programs around the country. (http://www.mhselfhelp.org/news/view.php?news_id=263, accessed 3/15/09)

These conferences

> provide a forum for consumers from all over the nation to meet, exchange information and ideas, and provide and receive technical assistance on peer support and peer-operated services along with other relevant topics, such as self-help, protection and advocacy issues, empowerment and recovery. The conferences also provide information on best practices in mental health and support services. The knowledge gained through attending these conferences helps consumers advocate for effective treatments and services, and improve service systems. (http://mentalhealth.samhsa.gov/cmhs/communitysupport/consumers/alternatives.asp, accessed 3/15/09)

Another helpful action that funders can take is to create materials for providing technical assistance and training to consumers and other stakeholders specifically about self-help and related concepts, including information about self-help research. Examples include CSP's provision of funding to the California Network of Mental Health Clients to produce *Reaching Across: Mental Health Clients Helping Each Other* (Zinman, Harp, & Budd, 1987), a seminal technical assistance manual still in use; CMHS' development of the *National Consensus Statement on Mental Health Recovery* (CMHS, 2005b); and CMHS' current efforts to produce an evidence-based practice toolkit for implementing consumer-operated service programs. First funded in 1992, the CMHS National Consumer Technical Assistance Centers have been a source for producing a wealth of such materials as well as for providing training and consultation to individual consumers and self-help organizations (CMHS, 2001, 2007a). Consultation regarding the fundamentals of business development, such as the Wichita State University Center for the Community Support and Research, as provided in Kansas since 1989 (www.ccsr.wichita.edu, accessed 4/26/09) can be particularly helpful for developing self-help organizations.

11.4.4 Use Your Stage and Lend Your Clout to Self-Help Services and Research

Governments and other funders are often uniquely positioned to know about activities occurring among diverse stakeholders across vast geographic regions. Funders can take advantage of this position to identify and promote models for others to follow. One way to do this is to fund the creation of self-help clearinghouses. CSP first funded the National Mental Health Consumer Self-Help Clearinghouse in 1988 (CMHS, 2001). Still funded by CSP within CMHS, the Clearinghouse now hosts an online Directory of Consumer-Driven Services that includes listings for over 250 organizations (http://www.cdsdirectory.org, accessed 4/4/09). Another way to hold up models and lend clout to self-help services and research is to utilize the public speaking and convening powers of individuals of stature. Substantial credibility was gained for self-help approaches when the U.S. Surgeon General C. Everett Koop brought together nearly 200 leaders in the self-help movement in 1987 to develop specific recommendations aimed at expanding and strengthening the role of self-help groups in protecting and enhancing the nation's health (U.S. Department of Health and Human Services, 1988).

In addition to individuals of stature, documents of stature can also be influential. Several such documents have been cited throughout this chapter. In 1989, for example, the National Association of State Mental Health Program Directors (NASMHPD) released their *Position Statement on Consumer Contributions to Mental Health Service Delivery Systems*. Among other points, the statement asserted that

> client-operated self-help and mutual support services should be available in each locality as alternatives and adjuncts to existing mental health service delivery systems. State financial support should be provided to ensure their viability and independence. (NASMHPD, 1989)

The International Association of Psychosocial Rehabilitation Services' (IAPSRS') *Consumer Policy Guidelines for the IAPSRS Board, Committees, Chapters and Central Office* acknowledged and supported the inclusion of consumer practitioners and consumer-run organizations among their membership and governing bodies (IAPSRS, 1998). More recently, the President's New Freedom Commission on Mental Health (2003) validated self-help services and research by acknowledging consumer-run services and consumer-service providers and citing research that shows that they "can broaden access to peer support, engage more individuals in traditional mental health services, and serve as a resource in the recovery of people with a psychiatric diagnosis" (p. 37).

11.4.5 Liaison with Non-mental Health Agencies and Organizations Regarding Self-Help and Related Concepts

The community support system model recognizes that consumers have a range of needs that cannot all be met by the mental health system operating in isolation (Stroul, 1984, 1988; Turner & TenHoor, 1978). Governments and other funders can support self-help efforts by serving as liaisons to agencies and organizations that address such diverse subjects as health, employment, education, income supports, housing, transportation, aging, youth development, disability, criminal justice, protection and advocacy, voter empowerment, physical fitness, recreation, the arts, parenting, domestic violence, public education, cultural competence, workforce development, information technology, business and organizational development, research, community development, social services, and so forth. Linkages can be forged in order to identify resources that supplement those provided by mental health systems in helping individual consumers to meet their goals; identify resources to support the work of self-help organizations; reduce barriers that impede self-help efforts; and facilitate direct communication between partner agencies or organizations and mental health service consumers, including through hiring of consumers within partner agencies and organizations. The nature of interagency collaboration can include direct sharing of information with one another; facilitating introductions and meetings among diverse groups; joint production and delivery of materials, training, technical assistance, and communication of messages of importance; and interagency agreements to jointly fund grants of mutual interest.

The earliest CSP efforts focused on interagency work with the Rehabilitative Services Administration (RSA) and Housing and Urban Development (HUD; Stroul, 1984; Turner & TenHoor, 1978). A 1978 cooperative agreement between RSA and CSP led to joint funding of two research and training centers, at Boston University and the University of California at Los Angeles, to address the rehabilitation of "the mentally disabled" (Stroul, 1984). Today, CMHS continues to co-fund two Rehabilitation Research and Training Centers (RRTC) with the National Institute on Disability and Rehabilitation Research (NIDRR). The Boston University RRTC, continuously funded since its inception, focuses its current efforts on Recovery and Recovery-Oriented Psychiatric Rehabilitation for Persons with Long-Term Mental Illness. The second RRTC, now located at the University of Illinois at Chicago, focuses on consumer-driven services, recovery self-management models, self-directed health care financing mechanisms, peer services, consumer-operated programs, return-to-work services, financial asset development, and preparing consumers for research careers. The RRTCs have been leaders in the field of self-help services and research for the past 30 years. CSP's early interactions with HUD have also had long-term repercussions, as the CMHS Homeless Programs Branch continues its strong relationship with HUD today. The principles of CSP continue to guide this work, and support for self-help, peer support, and support for self-employment are included among the recommended services to be provided to consumers who are homeless (CMHS, 2003a, 2003b).

One of the critical roles that governments and other funders can play in supporting self-help research through interagency work is to bring consumers, service providers (including consumer-providers), and researchers (including consumer-researchers) together to discuss the interplay of research and services in the self-help arena. From their earliest days, CSP made special efforts to bring these groups together through the Learning Community Conferences and Project Directors' meetings in order to "increase the likelihood that research will be relevant and meaningful to the field" (Stroul, 1984, p. 46). Since joining SAMHSA, CSP has continued to make special efforts to bring these groups together through collaboration with NIMH. From 2006 to 2008, for example, CMHS and NIMH jointly sponsored a series of science and service meetings in four regions of the country so that researchers, policy-makers, administrators, service providers, and consumers could work together to develop state plans focused on integrating research and practice.

In addition to serving as self-help liaisons to relevant agencies and organizations, governments and other funders can provide grants or contracts that bring self-help concepts to interagency work occurring within various communities. One program that was successful in this regard was the Community Action Grant Program that CMHS funded from 1997 through 2003. One-year $150,000 grants were awarded to support consensus building among state and community groups regarding adoption of exemplary mental health practices. Among the grants awarded, nine communities adopted consumer Leadership Academies, two adopted peer-led Wellness Recovery Action Planning (Copeland, 2002), and one adopted peer-supported housing (http://mentalhealth.samhsa.gov/cmhs/CommunitySupport/other_programs/grantees.asp, accessed 4/27/09).

Another rich source of collaboration potential is between funders and academia, professional associations, and accrediting and licensing bodies. Such collaborations can encourage research on self-help, ensure that professionals are adequately trained regarding self-help-related concepts, and create programs to train consumers in how to implement and evaluate self-help and related programs. One product of the CMHS-NIDRR RRTC at the University of Illinois at Chicago, for example, is an innovative academic curricular transformation effort that incorporates principles of recovery and evidence-based practice into university instruction in the medical, social, and behavioral sciences (http://www.cmhsrp.uic.edu/nrtc/, accessed 5/25/09). With the support of CMHS and others, consumers are also instigating college and university collaborations to create innovative educational programs such as the Community Support Specialist Program that provides mental health technician certification to consumers in Maine (http://www.mcd.org/domestic/cssp.htm, accessed 5/25/09).

11.5 Summary

In sum, governments and other funders are uniquely positioned to see and understand what is happening across the geographic and political spectrum and to raise emerging trends, needs, and best practices up so that all may see them. Funders can synthesize information from a wide variety of sources, model the behavior they want to see in the field, widely disseminate information, and provide financial and performance-based incentives to support activities that are responsive to consumer priorities. Numerous examples have been provided to illustrate how these strategies can be used specifically to support self-help research and services. Using this tactical arsenal, governments and other funders can make substantial contributions to moving self-help research and services forward.

11.6 Potential Sources of Funding for Self-Help Research and Services

11.6.1 CMHS and NIMH

The first and most obvious sources of funding for mental health self-help services and research are CMHS and NIMH, respectively. The largest portion of CMHS funding is distributed through the Community Mental Health Services Block Grant Program to the states. Block grant dollars have few restrictions, and their flexibility allows states to use them for many innovative purposes, including support for self-help and related initiatives.

In addition to Block Grant funding, each year CMHS offers discretionary grants for a variety of targeted purposes related to mental health service provision, typically with a small portion of the funds set aside for program evaluation. These grants are time-limited (generally fewer than 3–5 years) and are awarded on a competitive basis. Self-help organizations or researchers seeking grants must fit within the specifications described in individual grant announcements.

Contracts to provide technical assistance, develop materials, organize meetings, or conduct analyses or evaluations may also be awarded, most often through a list of pre-qualified companies known as Indefinite Delivery Indefinite Quantity (IDIQ) contractors, or through small businesses. Self-help organizations or researchers typically must serve as subcontractors or consultants to qualified businesses in order to receive contract funding. CMHS does not have standing grant or contract announcements but, rather, funding opportunities vary from year to year. Those interested in CMHS funding, therefore, must keep an eye on the SAMHSA Web site (http://www.samhsa.gov), the *Federal Register*, and/or *Federal Business Opportunities*.

The *Federal Register* and *Federal Business Opportunities* are the single points of entry for federal grant and contract funding, respectively, and are therefore vital resources for those seeking funding from a variety of federal agencies. In addition to competitive grants and contracts, funding may be awarded on a noncompetitive basis under certain circumstances. Most commonly, non-competitive grants are designated through Congressional appropriations. Such grants are commonly referred to as earmarks and are obtained by constituents forming direct relationships with their Congressional representatives. Sole-source contracts can sometimes be awarded to organizations that submit specific unsolicited proposals if the agency is interested and can justify that the proposal is unique and meets criteria for non-competitive award. Although federal agencies vary in the manner and degree to which the different funding mechanisms are utilized, these descriptions of competitive and non-competitive grants and contracts form the core of most federal funding.

In contrast to CMHS' agency-directed funding, the bulk of NIMH funding supports investigator-initiated research grant awards through standing Program Announcements; technical merit is determined by standing Initial Review Groups (IRGs). The priorities of the Services Research and Clinical Epidemiology Branch most often offer the best fit with self-help-related proposals. Obtaining funding through NIMH's competitive process can take 2–3 years, typically requiring multiple revisions and resubmissions before an award is granted. The standards for theory, methodology, and academic qualifications are high, which may present significant barriers for self-help research that may be based on hard-to-specify concepts and messy real-world applications. The fundamental value of choice, for example, may be at odds with the gold standard of the randomized controlled trial, making it difficult for self-help proposals to compete against more scientifically rigorous applications.

Occasionally NIMH will set aside a portion of funding for a specific time-limited purpose that is advertised through Requests for Applications (RFAs, for grants) or Requests for Proposals (RFPs, for contracts). Under the right circumstances, self-help proposals may be better able to compete for funding under RFAs or RFPs, as ad-hoc IRGs are formed and may be given special instructions that even the playing field. An example is the State Implementation of Evidence-Based Practices: Bridging Science and Service grants (RFA-MH-05-004) that CMHS co-funded with NIMH in 2002 and 2004. The announcement was written specifically for state applicants, and a number of specifications were made to ensure meaningful review of this unique set of applicants. The ad-hoc IRG, for example, comprised not only researchers but also system administrators, technical assistance and training specialists, service providers, and primary consumers. Instructions were provided to the reviewers regarding how to evaluate the qualifications of state personnel and how to consider the priorities and methodologies of the proposals. This targeted RFA resulted in many high quality proposals from states, including a successful application regarding the implementation of consumer-operated services.

11.6.2 Beyond Mental Health

Through our interagency work over the years, we have become aware of a wide variety of potential funding sources that might be considered by self-help organizations and researchers. As mental health services and research become increasingly integrated into the mainstream (Frank & Glied, 2006; New Freedom Commission on Mental Health, 2003), individuals and organizations should expand the search for funding beyond mental health-specific resources. In addition to direct funding, mainstream organizations might provide other resources that could be useful to self-help efforts, such as technical assistance, access for making influential policy changes, etc. Although we present information about potential sources of which we are aware from our national perspective, we encourage readers to seek out similar sources at the state, local, and organizational levels, as well as from national and local philanthropic foundations. Goldstrom et al. (2006a) found that consumer organizations typically obtain their funding from a variety of sources including grants, contracts, donations, fund-raising activities, affiliated organizations, services or products sold, and membership fees.

11.6.3 Healthcare Resources

The focus on mental health allows self-help to be couched within the terms of general health. As such, self-help researchers and service providers may be eligible for funding from a wide variety of health-related sources. At the federal level, SAMHSA has partnered in various ways with the Center for Medicaid Services, the Health Resources and Services Administration, the Maternal and Child Health Bureau, the Department of Veteran's Affairs, the Indian Health Service, the Centers for Disease Control, and the Agency for Healthcare Research and Quality. Each of these agencies provides funding that might be applicable to mental health self-help efforts. The Center for Medicaid Services, for example, allows Medicaid reimbursement for peer specialists and conducts various demonstration projects that encourage innovation in healthcare delivery. The Health Resources and Services Administration funds federally Qualified Health Centers, which are becoming of increasing interest as the nation strives to better integrate mental health and primary care. Two federal Web sites are now available to simplify searching for funding across multiple agencies: http://www.usa.gov offers a single portal to all government agencies for any audience, while http://www.grants.gov focuses specifically on grant funding.

11.6.4 Disability Resources

Self-help efforts related to serious mental illness or psychiatric disability may be eligible for funding from a wide variety of disability-related sources. The Department of Education's Office of Special Education and Rehabilitative Services is one of the nation's leaders in funding disability services and research. Relevant subunits and programs within the Department of Education include the National Institute on Disability and Rehabilitation Research, the Rehabilitation Services Administration (for self-help activities related to employment), and the Office of Special Education Programs (for activities related to young people). The Centers for Independent Living, funded by the Rehabilitation Services Administration, provide self-help services to people with all types of disabilities, including psychiatric disabilities. Mandated by the Rehabilitation Act, these Centers have an ongoing funding stream and special access to resources from various federal agencies. Mental health self-help efforts can benefit through partnering with such Centers.

Other federal agencies that support disability work that may be relevant to mental health self-help focused on employment include the Social Security Administration (SSA) and the Department of Labor. The SSA Office of Employment Support Programs manages the Ticket to Work and Work Incentive Planning and Assistance programs, both of which accept self-help organizations as service providers. Through other disability offices, SSA also supports demonstration programs (such as the Mental Health Treatment Study, projects on youth transition, and the now concluded State Partnership Initiative) that offer opportunities for self-help involvement. Disability-specific initiatives at the Department of Labor are led by the Office of Disability Employment Policy, most often in collaboration with the Employment and Training Administration. These collaborations focus on efforts to ensure the inclusion of people with disabilities, including psychiatric disabilities, in mainstream employment efforts such as the One-Stop Career Centers, Workforce Investment Boards, apprenticeships, workforce training, and employment initiatives targeting veterans.

In addition to http://www.usa.gov and http://www.grants.gov, http://www.disability.gov provides linkages to disability resources across the federal government.

11.6.5 Other Sector-Specific Resources

The services provided by self-help organizations vary widely, and self-help organizations should consider any sources of funding available to support their topics of interest. Specialized funding sources exist for such areas as housing, transportation, criminal justice, trauma, women's issues, public education, civil rights, parenting, arts, information technology, aging, community development, education, cultural diversity, substance abuse, youth development, poverty. In addition to federal agencies, an enormous number of local and national philanthropic organizations offer grants for these diverse purposes. Directories of philanthropic foundation support are available from public libraries and through the Internet.

11.6.6 Workforce Development Resources

In addition to resources to support specific content areas of interest, self-help organizations and researchers may benefit from general workforce development resources. Grants offered by the Department of Labor or Small Business Administration, for example, may be used to develop self-help businesses, organizations, and personnel. Grants targeting development of the healthcare or human services workforces may be particularly relevant for self-help organizations.

11.7 Emerging Trends and Priorities for Self-Help Services and Research

11.7.1 New Service Trends in Need of Research

The self-help service field has grown tremendously over the past 30 years. Unfortunately, self-help research has not kept pace. The self-help service developments in need of research, therefore, are vast. Nevertheless, self-help services are continuing to expand and change. In keeping with the New Freedom Commission's (2003) emphasis on coordinating mental health services across agencies, for example, consumer organizations are increasingly seeking ways to bring self-help concepts to the attention of non-mental health partners, such as the criminal justice system and employment initiatives. Research on the best ways to accomplish this goal would be welcomed. In a related vein, self-help organizations are exploring the best ways to serve different populations of consumers, such as those with criminal justice backgrounds, co-occurring mental health and substance use problems, trauma histories, and diverse cultural backgrounds. While substantial mental health services research has been directed toward the best ways for professionals to serve these populations, particular efforts are needed to determine how they might best be served within a self-help context.

Another concept that has taken on renewed importance since publication of the New Freedom Commission's final report (2003) is the concept of consumer-*driven* care. This concept expands significantly upon previous concepts of consumer-*directed*, *-guided*, *-oriented*, or *-involved* care. Consumers are no longer to be supplemental advisors but rather, as stated by the CMHS National Advisory Council's Subcommittee on Consumer/Survivor Issues (2007b), "Consumer-driven means mental health consumers have the primary decision-making role regarding the mental health and related care that is offered and received" (p. 1). This is true not only for one's own care, but also collectively "in determining all aspects of care for consumers in the community, state, and nation....from planning to implementation to evaluation to research to defining and determining outcomes" (p. 1). This concept launches self-help principles into the forefront and raises numerous research questions about the nature of relationships among consumers and the professionals with whom they work (or, based on the new concept of consumer-driven care, who work for them).

Similar questions about how consumers and professionals are to relate to one another are raised by growing interest in models of self-determination, self-directed care, advanced directives, shared decision making, and peer support specialists. Self-determination and self-directed care models take consumer-driven care to the level of having each consumer decide for him or herself how to allocate public resources allotted to them, rather than having professionals determine how dollars are spent for an individual's care. Advanced directives are becoming more popular as consumers strive to predetermine the care they will receive should they become incapacitated. Recognizing the value of both professional experience and training as well as consumer experience and preferences, shared decision-making models are being developed to guide the individual relationships of consumers with those providing them with services. Developments in each of these areas are ripe for both process and outcome research. In addition, the booming peer support specialist movement (Sabin & Daniels, 2003; National Association of Peer Specialists, http://www.naops.org, accessed 6/7/10) has raised a variety of issues calling for research, such as the best means to train and credential peer providers, as well as organizational issues regarding confidentiality, staff relations, and cost-effectiveness.

As self-help organizations have proliferated, consumers are increasingly recognizing and seeking information and support regarding business development.

Both nonprofit and for-profit business information are needed to inform both consumer-run organizations and individual consumers interested in self-employment and entrepreneurship. Although substantial research has demonstrated the effectiveness of professionally run supported employment programs, very little has addressed how to support consumers in independent business ventures. A newly emerging area of related interest is the development of financial literacy and asset development and accumulation. As consumers look toward increasingly independent living, they are seeking ways to better manage their resources in order to accumulate savings that might be used for large purchases such as homes, automobiles, and businesses, or as cushions for possible future hard times. At present, self-help organizations and their supporters are searching among financial resources that are currently available to the general population of people with low incomes or people with disabilities. Self-help research can assist by bringing the academic literature on various financial strategies to bear and by demonstrating their effectiveness for people with serious mental illnesses.

11.7.2 Other Research Areas to Address

Numerous opportunities for self-help research exist beyond those created by the newly emerging trends described above. Perhaps most important is the need for validation and use of consumer-developed measurement instruments that assess self-help concepts of importance to consumers. Most notable among such measures are those assessing individual recovery and recovery-orientation of services and systems (del Vecchio & Blyler, 2009). Although numerous recovery measurement tools have been developed in recent years (Campbell-Orde, Chamberlin, Carpenter, & Leff, 2005; Evaluation Center at Human Services Research Institute, 2007), efforts to further establish the psychometric properties of such measures would be welcomed. Research demonstrating the recovery-orientation of professional as well as self-help services and their effect on individual recovery, as consumers define it, is also necessary to validate rampant claims being made about services supporting recovery (del Vecchio & Blyler, 2009, pp. 106-109). In addition to recovery measures, consumers should be involved in developing instruments to measure other concepts that are important to them, such as coercion (see, e.g., the "Vicki Scale," del Vecchio & Blyler, 2009, p. 105). Significant for self-help specifically would be additional work on measures to document, describe, and quantify program adherence to self-help principles, such as the *Fidelity Assessment Common Ingredients Tool (FACIT)* developed through the CMHS Consumer-Operated Services Program (Johnsen, Teague, & Herr, 2005).

Although the FACIT quantifies key elements thought to be common to self-help organizations, self-help programs vary considerably from one another in types of services offered. A wealth of research opportunities exist for documenting the unique effects of programs focusing on such diverse services as housing and employment supports, statewide consumer networking, hospital-to-community bridger programs, crisis services, trauma services, peer support groups, etc. A critical question asked at the policy level about all services is how much they cost and what is gained for the money spent; cost-effectiveness, cost-benefit, and cost-savings studies, therefore, would contribute meaningfully to pushing the self-help field forward. Finally, efforts should be made by the research field to support the training and development of researchers who are themselves consumers. The unique perspectives of people with lived experience have been and will continue to be invaluable in demonstrating the most important aspects of self-help.

11.8 Conclusion

Although direct funding of self-help services and research would be preferable, even with limited dollars to contribute, governments and other funders can have a significant influence on the direction of the field. Strategic use of resources to continually bring attention to self-help efforts can help to lay the groundwork that allows self-help to thrive. By supporting self-help on the national stage, we believe that federal efforts have contributed to the growth of self-help over the past 30 years. As stated by one author,

> Through contacts at the CMHS and mutual writing of CSP grant applications, consumer leaders came to know mental health program directors of their states. By the end of 1989, every director or commissioner signed the NASMHPD Position Paper on Consumer Contributions to Mental Health Service Delivery, which affirmed consumers' unique contributions to program formation and evaluation and in educating mental health professionals in their perspectives. (McLean, 2003, fifth page of print-out from unnumbered online manuscript)

In 1993, 36 states and territories directly funded at least one consumer project, and 280 consumer-run organizations received public mental health funds (Campbell et al., 1993). By 2002, a national survey found 7467 mutual support groups, self-help organizations, and consumer-operated services programs across the nation, greatly eclipsing the number of traditional mental health organizations (4546); self-help organizations reported a total of over a million members (Goldstrom et al., 2006b). A further indication of the growth is the founding of the National Association of Peer Specialists in 2004 (http://www.naops.org, accessed 4/4/09), and the National Coalition of Mental Health Consumer/Survivor Organizations in May 2006, a meta-association comprised 34 statewide and regional consumer organizations and 4 national technical assistance centers (http://www.ncmhcso.org, accessed 4/4/09).

On the research front, we are most pleased to see the growth in consumer involvement in research (Wallcraft et al., 2009) and the development of instruments to measure consumer-defined outcomes, particularly those related to recovery. Less than a decade ago, a review of the literature yielded a limited collection of instruments that measured only certain aspects of recovery and/or content related to, but not synonymous with recovery, such as empowerment or hope (Ralph, Kidder, & Phillips, 2000). By 2005, however, numerous endeavors to measure the broader concept of recovery had ensued, and Campbell-Orde, Chamberlin, Carpenter, and Leff collected nine instruments for measuring individual recovery in a Compendium of Recovery Measures; in addition, four instruments were found that measure recovery-promoting environments. Two years later, two additional instruments measuring recovery-promoting environments were identified (Evaluation Center at Human Services Research Institute, 2007).

Through persistent attention to self-help concepts, provision of resources, and attention to emerging trends that might provide future opportunities, governments and other funders can be valuable partners for pushing the field of self-help research and services in new directions. Self-help organizations and researchers can help to focus attention on the importance of self-help by partnering with funding organizations and continually advocating for initiatives that target self-help concepts. Governments and other funders can respond by looking for opportunities to support self-help across all of their initiatives. By doing so over several decades, the federal Community Support Program has shown that together, we can make a difference.

References

Balcazar, F., & Seekins, T. (1993). *Consumer involvement in community advocacy organizations* (Vols. 1–4). Boise, ID: Idaho Department of Health and Welfare, Bureau of Mental Health.

Brown, N. B. (1989, Oct). *Community support and rehabilitation developments in the United States.* Presentation to the 2nd World Congress on Psychosocial Rehabilitation, Barcelona, Spain.

Campbell, J. (1998). *Technical assistance needs of consumer/survivor and family stakeholder groups within state mental health agencies.* Alexandria, VA: National Technical Assistance Center for State Mental Health Planning, National Association of State Mental Health Program Directors.

Campbell, J., & Schraiber, R. (1989). *In pursuit of wellness: The well-being project: Mental health clients speak for themselves.* Sacramento, CA: California Department of Mental Health.

Campbell, J., Ralph, R., & Glover, R. (1993, Oct.). From lab rat to researcher: History, models, and policy implications of consumer/survivor involvement in research. *Proceedings of the 4th Annual National Conference on State Mental Health Agency Services Research and Program Evaluation*, pp. 138–147. Rockville, MD: Substance Abuse and Mental Health Services Administration and National Institute of Mental Health, U.S. Department of Health and Human Services.

Campbell-Orde, T., Chamberlin, J., Carpenter, J., & Leff, H. S. (2005). *Measuring the promise: A compendium of recovery measures: Vol. II* (Publication No. 55). Cambridge, MA: Human Services Research Institute.

Center for Mental Health Services (2009a). *Mental health transformation state incentive grant cross-site evaluation plan.* Rockville, MD: Substance Abuse and Mental Health Services Administration.

Center for Mental Health Services (2009b). *Statewide consumer network grant* (Request for Applications No. SM-09-014). Rockville, MD: Substance Abuse and Mental Health Services Administration.

Center for Mental Health Services (2008). *Minority fellowship program.* (Announcement No. SM-08-006). Rockville, MD: Substance Abuse and Mental Health Services Administration.

Center for Mental Health Services (2007a). *Grants for national consumer and consumer supporter technical assistance centers* (Announcement No. SM-07-003). Rockville, MD: Substance Abuse and Mental Health Services Administration.

Center for Mental Health Services (2007b). *Principles of consumer-driven care*. Rockville, MD: Substance Abuse and Mental Health Services Administration. Retrieved from http://download.ncadi.samhsa.gov/ken/msword/Final_Consumer_Driven_1-8-2007.doc, 6/7/10.

Center for Mental Health Services (2005a). *Cooperative agreements for mental health transformation state incentive grants* (Request for Applications No. SM-05-009). Rockville, MD: Substance Abuse and Mental Health Services Administration.

Center for Mental Health Services (2005b). *National consensus statement on mental health recovery (Publ. No. SMA05-4129) [Brochure]*. Rockville, MD: Substance Abuse and Mental Health Services Administration.

Center for Mental Health Services (2003a). *Blueprint for change: Ending chronic homelessness for persons with serious mental illnesses and co-occurring substance use disorders* (DHHS Pub. No. SMA-04-3870). Rockville, MD: Substance Abuse and Mental Health Services Administration.

Center for Mental Health Services (2003b). *Work as a priority: A resource for employing people who have a serious mental illness and who are homeless* (DHHS Pub. No. SMA 03-3834). Rockville, MD: Substance Abuse and Mental Health Services Administration.

Center for Mental Health Services (2002). *National Advisory Council Subcommittee on Consumer/Survivor issues briefing paper*. Rockville, MD: Substance Abuse and Mental Health Services Administration.

Center for Mental Health Services (2001). *Consumer/Survivor-operated Self-Help Programs: A Technical Report*. (DHHS Publication No. (SMA) 01-3510). Rockville, MD: Substance Abuse and Mental Health Services Administration.

Center for Mental Health Services (1998). *Cooperative agreements to evaluate consumer-operated human service programs for persons with serious mental illness* (Guidance for Applicants No. SM 98-004). Rockville, MD: Substance Abuse and Mental Health Services Administration.

Center for Mental Health Services (1996a). Consumer affairs staff grows. *Consumer Affairs Bulletin, 1*(1). Rockville, MD: Substance Abuse and Mental Health Services Administration. Retrieved from http://mentalhealth.samhsa.gov/publications/allpubs/CMH96-5012/cabvo01.asp, 6/7/10.

Center for Mental Health Services (1996b). *July 1995 Consumer/Survivor planning meeting report*. Rockville, MD: Substance Abuse and Mental Health Services Administration.

Chamberlin, J. (1978). *On our own: Patient-controlled alternatives to the mental health system*. New York: McGraw-Hill.

Copeland, M. E. (2002). Wellness recovery action plan: A system for monitoring, reducing and eliminating uncomfortable or dangerous physical symptoms and emotional feelings. *Occupational Therapy in Mental Health, 17*, 127–150.

Danley, K., & Ellison, M. L. (1999). *Handbook for participatory action researchers*. Boston, MA: Center for Psychiatric Rehabilitation, Boston University.

del Vecchio, P. & Blyler, C. R. (2009, June). Identifying critical outcomes and setting priorities for mental health services research. In J. Wallcraft, B. Schrank, & M. Amering (Eds.), *Handbook of Service User Involvement in Mental Health Research*, pp. 99–112, Chichester: Wiley.

Evaluation Center at Human Services Research Institute (2007). *Addendum to measuring the promise: A compendium of recovery measures, (*Vol II). Cambridge, MA: Evaluation Center at Human Services Research Institute.

Frank, R. G. & Glied, S. A. (2006). *Better but not well*. Baltimore, MD: Johns Hopkins U. Pr.

Goldstrom, I. D., Campbell, J., Rogers, J. A., Lambert, D. B., Blacklow, B., Henderson, M. J., & Manderscheid, R. W. (2006a). Mental health consumer organizations: A national picture (Ch. 21). In R. W. Manderscheid & J. T. Berry (Eds.), *Mental Health, United States, 2004*, pp. 247–255. Rockville, MD: Center for Mental Health Services, Substance Abuse and Mental Health Services Administration.

Goldstrom, I. D., Campbell, J., Rogers, J. A., Lambert, D. B., Blacklow, B., Henderson, M. J., & Manderscheid, R. W. (2006b). National estimates for mental health mutual support groups, self-help organizations, and consumer-operated services. *Administration and Policy in Mental Health and Mental Health Services Research, 33*, 92–103.

Hess, R. E., Clapper, C. R., Hoekstra, K., & Gibison, F. P. (2001). Empowerment effects of teaching leadership skills to adults with a severe mental illness and their families. *Psychiatric Rehabilitation Journal, 24*, 257–265.

International Association of Psychosocial Rehabilitation Services (1998). *IAPSRS Consumer Policy Guidelines*. Columbia, MD: IAPSRS.

Johnsen, M., Teague, G., & Herr, E. M. (2005). Common ingredients as a fidelity measure for peer-run programs (Ch. 11). In S. Clay (Ed.), *On Our Own, Together*, pp. 213–238, Nashville, TN: Vanderbilt U. Pr.

Kaufmann, C. L., Ward-Colasante, C., & Farmer, J. (1993). Development and evaluation of drop-in centers operated by mental health consumers. *Hospital and Community Psychiatry, 44*, 675–678.

Kentucky Center for Mental Health Studies (2001). *Report on the consumer and consumer supporter National technical assistance centers funded by the center for Mental Health Services, Substance Abuse and Mental Health Services Administration: An Evaluation of the Centers' Activities for the Month of April 2001*. Cambridge, MA: Human Services Research Institute, Evaluation Center at HSRI.

Kentucky Center for Mental Health Studies (2002). *Assessing the promise: An evaluation of the work of the consumer and consumer supporter National technical assistance centers funded by the Center for Mental Health Services, Substance Abuse and Mental Health Services Administration*. Cambridge, MA: Human Services Research Institute, Evaluation Center at HSRI.

Manderscheid, R. W. & Henderson, M. J. (1995). *Speaking with a common language: Past, present and future of data standards for managed behavioral healthcare*. Rockville, MD: Center for Mental Health Services, Substance Abuse and Mental Health Services Administration.

McLean, A. (1994). *Role of consumers in mental health services research and evaluation: Report and concept paper (No. 92MF03814201D)*. Rockville, MD: Center for Mental Health Services, Substance Abuse and Mental Health Services Administration.

McLean, A. (2003). "Recovering" consumers and a broken mental health system in the United States: Ongoing challenges for consumers/survivors and the New Freedom Commission on Mental Health. *International Journal of Psychosocial Rehabilitation, 8*, 47–68.

Mowbray, C. T., & Tan, C. (1993). Consumer-operated drop-in centers: Evaluation of operations and impact. *Journal of Mental Health Administration, 20*, 8–19.

Mulkern, V. (1995). *Community support program: A model for Federal state partnership* (Monograph). Washington, DC: Mental Health Policy Resource Center.

National Association of State Mental Health Program Directors. (1989). *Position statement on consumer contributions to mental health service delivery systems*. Alexandria, VA: National Association of State Mental Health Program Directors.

National Institute of Mental Health (2004). *State implementation of evidence-based practices II – Bridging Science and Service* (Request for Applications No. RFA-MH-05-004). Bethesda, MD: National Institute of Mental Health.

National Institute of Mental Health (1987, Oct). *Toward a model plan for a comprehensive community-based mental health system*. (Administrative Document). Rockville, MD: Alcohol, Drug Abuse, and Mental Health Administration, U.S. Dept of Health and Human Services.

New Freedom Commission on Mental Health (2003). *Achieving the promise: Transforming mental health care in America. Final report* (DHHS Pub. No. SMA-03-3832). Rockville, MD: Substance Abuse and Mental Health Services Administration.

Onken, S. J., Dumont, J. M., Ridgway, P., Dornan, D. H., and Ralph, R. O. (2002). *Mental health recovery: What helps and what hinders? A national research project for the development of recovery facilitating system performance indicators*. Alexandria, VA: National Association of State Mental Health Program Directors National Technical Assistance Center for State Mental Health Planning.

Parrish, J. (1990). *Effectiveness of Self-Help Alternatives*. Unpublished manuscript.

Parrish, J. (1991). CSP: Program of firsts. *Innovations & Research in Clinical Services, Community Support, and Rehabilitation, 1*(1), 8–9.

Prescott, L. (2001). *Consumer/Survivor/Recovering Women: Guide for partnerships in collaboration*. Delmar, NY: Policy Research Associates.

Ralph, R. O., Kidder, K., & Phillips, D. (2000). *Can we measure recovery? A compendium of recovery and recovery-related instruments* (Publication No. 43). Cambridge, MA: Human Services Research Institute.

Rogers, E. S., Teague, G. B., Lichenstein, C., Campbell, J., Lyass, A., Chen, R., & Banks, S. (2007). Effects of participation in consumer-operated service programs on both personal and organizationally mediated empowerment: Results of multisite study. *Journal of Rehabilitation Research and Development, 44*, 785–800.

Sabin, J., & Daniels, N. (2003). Managed care: Strengthening the consumer voice in managed care: VII. The Georgia peer specialist program. *Psychiatric Services, 54*, 497–498.

Sabin, J. E., & Daniels, N. (2002). Managed care: Strengthening the consumer voice in managed care: IV. The Leadership Academy Program. *Psychiatric Services, 53*, 405–411.

Steering Committee on the Chronically Mentally Ill (1981). *Toward a National Plan for the Chronically Mentally Ill* [DHHS Publ. No. (ADM) 81-1077]. Washington, DC: U.S. Department of Health and Human Services.

Stringfellow, J. W., & Muscari, K. D. (2003). Program of support for consumer participation in systems change: The West Virginia Leadership Academy. *Journal of Disability Policy Studies, 14*(3), 142–147.

Stroul, B. A. (1988). *Community support systems for persons with Long-term mental illness: Questions and answers*. Rockville, MD: Community Support Program, National Institute of Mental Health.

Stroul, B. A. (1984). *Toward community support systems for the mentally disabled: The NIMH Community Support Program*. Rockville, MD: National Institute of Mental Health.

Substance Abuse and Mental Health Services Administration (2009). *Guidelines for consumer and family participation*. Retrieved from http://www.samhsa.gov/Grants/guide_family.aspx, 6/7/10.

Turner, J. C. & TenHoor, W. J. (1978). NIMH community support program: Pilot approach to a needed social reform. *Schizophrenia Bulletin, 4*(3), 319–344.

U.S. Department of Health and Human Services (1999). *Mental health: A report of the surgeon general*. Rockville, MD: U.S. Department of Health and Human Services, Substance Abuse and Mental Health Services Administration, Center for Mental Health Services, National Institutes of Health, National Institute of Mental Health.

U.S. Department of Health and Human Services (1988). *Surgeon general workshop on self-help and public health, University of California, Los Angeles, CA, September 20–22, 1987*. Rockville, MD: Health Resources and Services Administration, Bureau of Maternal and Child Health and Resource Development.

Van Tosh, L., Ralph, R. O., & Campbell, J. (2000). Rise of consumerism. *Psychiatric Rehabilitation Skills, 4*(3), 383–409.

Wallcraft, J., Schrank, B., & Amering, M. (Eds.) (2009). *Handbook of service user involvement in mental health research*. Chichester: Wiley.

Weaver, P. (2003). *Consumer research activities in the states*. Cambridge, MA: Human Services Research Institute, Evaluation Center at HSRI.

Zinman, S., Harp, H. T., & Budd, S. (1987). *Reaching across: Mental health clients helping each other*. Sacramento, CA: California Network of Mental Health Clients.

Part V
Technical Assistance

Chapter 12
Consumer and Consumer-Supporter National Technical Assistance Centers: Helping the Consumer Movement Grow and Transform Systems

Susan Rogers

Abstract There are currently four federally funded consumer and consumer-supporter national technical assistance centers (TACs) that serve current and former recipients of mental health services throughout the United States. These TACs were created to meet the needs of what is now known as the mental health consumer/survivor movement. They are funded by the Substance Abuse and Mental Health Services Administration (SAMHSA), Center for Mental Health Services (CMHS), of the U.S. Department of Health and Human Services. The centers support mental health consumer empowerment by fostering self-help/recovery-oriented approaches in the planning, delivery, and evaluation of mental health services and in promoting system transformation, as well as providing other information about mental health, upon request, to consumers and others. The consumers they serve are involved in a movement for social justice that has its roots in the 1970s and that has evolved to include an array of consumer-run services and supports in nearly every state. This chapter covers the centers' history, goals and objectives; the challenges and barriers they face; and how they find solutions to those challenges and barriers. It includes interviews with leaders of the TACs as well as some of the individuals and group leaders they have served, and with the TACs' government project officer.

There are four federally funded consumer and consumer-supporter national Technical Assistance Centers (TACs), which serve current and former recipients of mental health services throughout the United States.[1] These TACs were created to meet the needs of what is now known as the mental health consumer/survivor

---

S. Rogers (✉)
National Mental Health Consumers' Self-Help Clearinghouse, Philadelphia, PA, USA
e-mail: srogers@mhasp.org

[1] A fifth national technical assistance center, operating under the auspices of the Depression and Bipolar Support Alliance, was funded for the first time in the 2007 SAMHSA grant cycle but has since relinquished its grant.

movement.[2] This chapter covers the history of the centers, their goals and objectives, and the challenges and barriers they face, as well as how they find solutions to those challenges and barriers. It incorporates interviews with leaders of the TACs as well as the TACs' government project officer and with some of the individuals they have served. The goal of this chapter is to demonstrate the vital importance of the TACs to consumer-operated services and to individual consumers around the country, as well as the work the TACs do to combat the discrimination and stigma associated with psychiatric disabilities, and to promote wellness and recovery.

In the early 1970s, many people diagnosed with mental illnesses were coming out of psychiatric institutions outraged by the treatment they had received, which was frequently involuntary (Whitaker, 2002). Focused on reclaiming control over their own lives, some of these individuals, in a few cities around the country, began to support each other in a movement for social justice. People started organizing self-help and advocacy groups with the goals of fighting for their rights and against forced treatment, ending the discrimination and stigma associated with mental disorders, and designing and implementing peer-run services that offered choice and self-determination as alternatives to the traditional mental health system (Chamberlin, 1978). Many of these early groups had names such as Insane Liberation Front and the Network Against Psychiatric Assault. The individuals involved in such groups considered the mental health system destructive and disempowering (Campbell, 2005).

By the late 1970s, the movement had evolved to encompass a variety of viewpoints. According to a history of the consumer/survivor movement[3] on the National Mental Health Consumers' Self-Help Clearinghouse Web site:

By 1980, individuals who considered themselves consumers of mental health services had begun to organize self-help/advocacy groups and peer-run services. While sharing some of the goals of the earlier movement groups, consumer groups did not seek to abolish the traditional mental health system, which they believed was necessary. Instead, they wanted to reform it. Consumer groups encouraged their members to learn as much as possible about the mental health system so that they could gain access to the best services and treatments available.

Recipients of mental health services demanded control over their own treatment and began to have an influence on the public mental health system. Whether they considered themselves consumers or survivors, movement activists demanded a voice in mental health policy-making: a "seat at the table." Increasingly, they gained access to mental health policy-making and advisory committees. In addition, the number of peer-run services – drop-in centers, employment services, residences, and others – increased. Many of these services incorporated and received 501(c)(3) (tax-exempt) status. Many received funding from federal, state, and local agencies. Studies found that peer-run services were effective, and cost-effective [Campbell, 2005].

---

[2] There are a number of words and phrases that describe people who have been diagnosed with mental illnesses. The default term in this chapter is "consumer," but other words and phrases will also be used.
[3] Ibid.

Fast forward to 2009: There are currently four national technical assistance centers funded by the Substance Abuse and Mental Health Services Administration (SAMHSA), Center for Mental Health Services (CMHS), of the U.S. Department of Health and Human Services. These centers support consumer empowerment by fostering self-help/recovery-oriented approaches in the planning, delivery, and evaluation of mental health services and in promoting system transformation, as well as providing other information about mental health upon request to consumers and others.

I am the director of the National Mental Health Consumers' Self-Help Clearinghouse, previously its director of special projects, and have helped staff the Clearinghouse since its founding in 1986. To write this chapter, I interviewed at least one key leader at each of the centers, as well as the centers' government project officer and a few individuals who had been served by some of the centers, in order to provide a reasonably comprehensive portrait of the work of these organizations.

I conducted the interviews by telephone in November and December 2008, with follow-up contact with everyone via e-mail in 2009 to confirm quote accuracy. I interviewed the following individuals (alphabetically): Lynn Borton, chief operating officer, National Alliance on Mental Illness (NAMI); Christa Andrade Burkett, technical assistance coordinator, National Mental Health Consumers' Self-Help Clearinghouse; Daniel Fisher, M.D., Ph.D., executive director, National Empowerment Center; Risa Fox, M.S., L.C.S.W., public health advisor, Center for Mental Health Services, Substance Abuse and Mental Health Services Administration; Stephen Kiosk, M.Div., L.P.C., director, NAMI's STAR (Support, Technical Assistance, and Resource) Center, and former director of Mental Health America's National Consumer Supporter Technical Assistance Center (NCSTAC); Jim McNulty, former director, NAMI's STAR Center; Kathy Muscari, Ph.D., executive director, Consumer Organization and Networking Technical Assistance Center (CONTAC); Joseph Rogers, executive director, National Mental Health Consumers' Self-Help Clearinghouse; Dianne Dorlester Shenton, former director of NCSTAC and now development director of On Our Own of Maryland; Jim Simbeck, a consumer leader in South Dakota; and Vincent Rivas, a peer counselor in New York City.[4] I reached out to other individuals via e-mail and received e-mail responses.

I started with a list of questions:

- In what ways, if any, is your center different from the other TACs?
- What are some key successes of your center?

---

[4]I have also quoted from an e-mail dated February 27, 2009, 7:54 p.m., that I received from Carole Glover, CEO and president of Meaningful Minds, the statewide consumer organization in Louisiana; an e-mail dated February 4, 2009, 12:01 p.m., that I received from Bart Dunn, then a consumer leader in Delaware (now deceased); an e-mail dated April 7, 2009, 2:51 p.m., that I received from Kate Gaston, vice president of affiliate affairs at Mental Health America, and an e-mail dated March 2, 2009, 1:23 p.m., that I received from Mark Salzer, Ph.D.

- What are the challenges and barriers your center faces in doing its work?
- How do you balance advocacy with the requirements of a federal grant?
- Can you talk about the work with your two states? (In addition to their other initiatives, each of the TACs is working intensively with two states, respectively, that CMHS determined to be in need of help in order to foster the consumer movement in those states.)
- Can you connect me with some people you have helped?

I asked those who had been served by the centers to tell me something about the services they had received, and their feelings about those services. In addition, I interviewed the TACs' government project officer, Risa Fox, M.S., L.C.S.W. "The TACs, along with the statewide consumer network programs, are unique," explained Fox, "in that only consumer or consumer supporter organizations are eligible to apply [for funding], and are directly funded for the purpose of strengthening the capacity of consumers and consumer supporters to assist in the transformation of the mental health system by fostering a recovery-oriented, consumer-/family-driven system of care."

Fox, a public health advisor at the Center for Mental Health Services, notes that there is a critical need for consumer- and family-driven approaches to transform mental health care in the United States: "The TACs are a fundamental means for SAMHSA to provide leadership to meet this crucial need."

The TACs engage in systems transformation efforts and a range of other projects to promote consumer empowerment. They also provide information and referral services to consumers and others around the country (SAMHSA, n.d.). In addition, as noted above, each of the TACs is working intensively with two states, respectively, chosen by CMHS in order to foster the consumer movement in those states. The consumer-run TACs also alternate in organizing the national Alternatives conference, an annual forum for consumers to network and to exchange information and ideas.

Currently, the two federally funded consumer-run centers are the National Empowerment Center (NEC) Technical Assistance Center (TAC) and the National Mental Health Consumers' Self-Help Clearinghouse; the latter operates under the auspices of the Mental Health Association of Southeastern Pennsylvania (MHASP). The two federally funded consumer-supporter centers are Mental Health America's National Consumer Supporter Technical Assistance Center (NCSTAC) and the STAR (Support, Technical Assistance, and Resource) Center, operating under the auspices of NAMI (National Alliance on Mental Illness). Another center – the Consumer Organization and Networking Technical Assistance Center (CONTAC), operated by the West Virginia Mental Health Consumers' Association – was funded by SAMHSA from 1998 through 2007 and continues to be involved in the TAC network and to serve as a national technical assistance center, but is not a current recipient of a federal grant.

12.1 History

In 1986, Joseph Rogers, a national consumer movement leader, saw the need for a consumer-run national technical assistance center to support the burgeoning movement. To address this need, he created the National Mental Health Consumers' Self-Help Clearinghouse (known as the Clearinghouse) as a division of Project SHARE (Self-Help and Advocacy Resource Exchange), which Rogers founded in 1984 as a consumer-run self-help and advocacy organization based at the Mental Health Association of Southeastern Pennsylvania in Philadelphia. The Clearinghouse, staffed by Project SHARE, handled calls from people from all over the country looking for information on starting and maintaining self-help groups as well as general information about mental health.

The Clearinghouse received its first funding from the National Institute of Mental Health (NIMH) Community Support Program through the Boston University Center for Psychosocial (now Psychiatric) Rehabilitation. In 1992, the Clearinghouse was awarded a three-year ($250,000-a-year) national technical assistance grant from the federal Substance Abuse and Mental Health Services Administration, Center for Mental Health Services' Community Support Program Section to fuel an expansion of its services. "After an eight-year struggle, Project SHARE has won a major victory," Joseph Rogers told MHASP's newsletter, *Lines of Communication* (Rogers, 1992). Federal funds for the grant became available as a result of an ambitious MHASP advocacy effort, led by MHASP's then director of public policy, Mary Hurtig, with officials at NIMH and elsewhere in the federal government.

Neal Brown, now chief of CMHS's Community Support Programs Branch, Division of Service Systems Improvement, was an early and enthusiastic champion of the consumer/survivor movement, and was instrumental in the successful effort to fund the Clearinghouse. Federal officials such as Brown were so pleased with the Clearinghouse's efforts that they decided to offer funding for two such centers, on a competitive grant basis. "We're very excited about this opportunity," Brown, then chief of the Community Support Section at the National Institute of Mental Health, told the MHASP newsletter.[5] "I personally think it's a chance to provide information and assistance to a broad group of consumers and ex-patients around the country. We're fortunate to have two very excellent groups involved in this activity, and we look forward to close collaboration and some helpful assistance for consumers around the country."

The other national technical assistance center funded by NIMH at that time was the National Empowerment Project (now the National Empowerment Center Technical Assistance Center). The National Empowerment Project was co-founded/-directed by Dan Fisher, M.D., Ph.D., a psychiatrist and psychiatric survivor, and Laurie Ahern, also a psychiatric survivor (and now president of Mental

---

[5] Ibid.

Disability Rights International). In 1998, a third consumer-run national technical assistance center was awarded a federal grant: CONTAC (Consumer Organization and Networking Technical Assistance Center), then headed by Larry Belcher, with Kathy Muscari as his second in command. (Muscari now runs CONTAC.) Subsequently, CMHS decided to also fund two consumer-supporter national TACs: NAMI's STAR Center and Mental Health America's NCSTAC.

All of the individuals who currently have roles in TAC management have first-hand experience with psychiatric disorders. Joseph Rogers and Dan Fisher had been deeply involved in the consumer/survivor movement for decades; some others were relative newcomers. "I had plenty of experience being a consumer but had not previously been involved in the consumer movement," said Dianne Dorlester Shenton, who until 2008 directed NCSTAC. "But, following a serious and devastating episode of major depression right around 1999, after many, many months of being unwell, I got well and came out the other side; and I decided it was time to make a career switch to using my background in non-profit management to work in mental health. My personal experience and my passion for progressive social issues and social service issues have led that to be a very good fit."

12.2 Networking and Grassroots Growth

The consumer-run and consumer-supporter national technical assistance centers have played a major role in helping consumers across the country network with each other and in helping the movement grow. "In a diverse movement that is almost doggedly grassroots in nature, helping people come together and share and network and even create community on a national basis has at times been difficult. One mechanism for this effort has been the national technical assistance centers," said Clearinghouse executive director Joseph Rogers. "So, even beyond the concrete technical assistance – which is quite substantial and runs the gamut from creating and disseminating curriculums, manuals and periodicals; conducting conference workshops, Webcasts, and on-site trainings; and helping statewide consumer groups get organized; to answering individuals' personal requests for help – we have also felt that an important role was just to get people together so that they could, in essence, provide technical assistance to each other. If you are running a small self-help/mutual support program in a small town, nothing is better than to have a chance to meet with someone from a similar small town, even if it's across the country, to talk about the issues and problems and celebrate the victories," he said.

"That's one reason the Alternatives conference has played such an important role in the movement," Rogers continued. "I've heard it called the Woodstock of the mental health consumer movement in that we bring people together to celebrate and create a sense of community and movement." Jim McNulty, former director of the STAR Center, added, "We go to meetings like Alternatives and you see the dots connect."

12.3 Alternatives Conferences

The first Alternatives conference – an annual national conference created by and for consumers – was organized in 1985 by On Our Own of Baltimore, an early consumer-run self-help organization. Now, the consumer-run TACs take turns organizing the conferences. According to conference literature, "Each conference offers in-depth technical assistance on peer-delivered services and self-help/recovery methods. Topics include starting peer-run programs, developing personal resources, and the latest social services research. Beyond the exchange of knowledge and networking, Alternatives offers a rich social, artistic, and healing environment. What consumers learn helps them improve their lives as well as advocate for system transformation." Said an attendee at Alternatives 2008, "The greatest gift I received was the motivation and inspiration to reevaluate my own definition of wellness and what contribution I can make."

The theme of Alternatives 2008, which was organized by the National Empowerment Center TAC, was "Creating Community Through Active Citizenship." The 703 conference attendees participated in 101 workshops, three institutes, 17 caucuses, and other events, as well as plenary presentations. The workshops and institutes were organized under five topic headings: Living as Change Agents, Embracing Differences: Cultural Competency and Beyond, Creating Personal and Community Wellness, Engaging in the Arts, and the History of Our Movement.

The Alternatives 2007 conference, organized by the Clearinghouse, was similarly large and similarly well received. Of the 97 respondents (about 13% of conference attendees) completing the Alternatives 2007 evaluation form, 100% wrote that they learned new ways to be involved in creating policy and/or delivering services, new treatment options, new recovery possibilities for themselves and others, and new information skills they can use in their work. Ninety-nine percent indicated that they learned new ways to support others; and 98% learned new cultural perspectives and how to be a part of transforming the system.

12.4 Information and Referral

A basic component of the TACs' mission is to provide information. Clearinghouse technical assistance coordinator Christa Andrade Burkett plays a significant part in fulfilling that mission. "I build relationships," Burkett explained. "People write, e-mail, call, explain their situation, and I try to send them what they need," she said. "I feel really good about the impact of what I do," Burkett continued. "I speak to several people on a daily basis who I feel I have helped with either a specific problem or just added to their knowledge. I have sent many people information to start consumer support/advocacy groups. I've pointed people in the right direction to funding, given them information on grant and proposal writing, and really equipped them with the tools to do effective advocacy for themselves and others."

One individual whom Burkett has helped is Vincent Rivas, who until early 2009 was a peer counselor at Opportunity Self-Help Center in Corona, N.Y., where he worked for seven years. "The advocacy training I got from the Clearinghouse, it was like a Christmas present in my mailbox," he said. "The Clearinghouse opened a lot of doors for me." Rivas shared materials he has received from the Clearinghouse with the consumers at the Opportunity Self-Help Center. "The consumers were able to apply what Christa had given me," he said.

The Clearinghouse has also created a Consumer-Driven Services Directory,[6] the purpose of which is to provide consumers, researchers, administrators, service providers, and others with a comprehensive central resource for information on national and local consumer-driven programs.

12.5 Statewide Organizing

As one of the requirements of the 2007 grant cycle, each of the TACs chose two states that CMHS determined to be in need of help to organize their statewide networks. Iowa and South Dakota were assigned to the NEC TAC, Delaware and North Carolina to the Clearinghouse, Montana and Nevada to NCSTAC, and Arizona and Rhode Island to the STAR Center. The consumer networks in these states range from those that have established tax-exempt status, a board, and a Web site to states that are just starting to organize. The technical assistance involves an invitation for the consumer leaders to take on more responsibility over time. "I have found that the challenge for any group is to gather enough folks together, to go through a bonding process and come out with equal and mutual respect and esteem such that they are able to comfortably share leadership, assign tasks, focus on their identified strategies, and then choose someone to be the 'leader' of the process from within their ranks," wrote Kate Gaston, Mental Health America's vice president for affiliate services.

When Stephen Kiosk, then NCSTAC director, worked in Montana, he had been communicating with key leaders on a regular – usually weekly – basis, providing consistent support through phone calls and e-mails. "Providing encouragement and coaching assisted the consumer leaders in breaking down the various goals and tasks into smaller, more manageable action steps, which helped consumers avoid feeling overwhelmed," Kiosk said.

The National Empowerment Center TAC is working in Iowa and South Dakota. The consumer organizations in the two states are in different stages of development. Iowa's statewide network, Iowa Advocates for Mental Health Recovery, has a

---

[6]The National Mental Health Consumers' Self-Help Clearinghouse welcomes all programs in which consumers play a significant role in leadership and operation to apply for inclusion in its Directory of Consumer-Driven Services. The directory, accessible at http://www.cdsdirectory.org, is searchable by location, type of organization, and targeted clientele, and serves as a free resource for consumers, program administrators and researchers.

501(c)(3), has sponsored two statewide conferences on recovery from dual diagnosis or co-occurring disorders (substance abuse and mental health), and has received a couple of small grants, according to Fisher. "The challenge there," he explained, "was in bringing together leaders who had not worked together. The best core leaders often are the leaders who put the group first – and they're not always the existing leadership. We've helped form a statewide group of core leadership and then invited in some of the already existing leaders."

Fisher said that South Dakota posed a bigger challenge than Iowa because they only had one longstanding consumer/survivor leader: Jim Simbeck, whom Fisher described as "holding the torch for 20 years." Simbeck said that, after an initial "cold shoulder" from the state mental health authority in response to a request to use block grant dollars to create a statewide organization, state officials became more receptive after NEC stepped in, and they began to "work towards a better consumer inclusion." The organizing group chose the name South Dakota United for Hope and Recovery, developed a vision and a mission statement, and sent two of its leaders to the Alternatives conference. Simbeck credits NEC with "helping me personally as a consumer leader to where I can mentor other consumer leaders."

In Delaware, the Clearinghouse is assisting the statewide organizing committee for the Consumer Recovery Advocacy Coalition of Delaware (C.R.A.C.D.) in its efforts to recruit more members; engage in strategic planning; develop a brochure, a Web site, and a speakers' bureau; and provide input into Delaware's Division of Substance Abuse and Mental Health practices, procedures, programs, and policy. The Clearinghouse is sponsoring regular meetings in each of Delaware's three counties in order to further develop the statewide group. "The people at the Clearinghouse are knowledgeable and enthusiastic, and are motivating and directing us on how to be of more help to people with mental and/or substance abuse illnesses in Delaware," Bart Dunn, a leader of the C.R.A.C.D., wrote in an e-mail. *(Author's note: Bart Dunn has since died.)*

The TACs also provide technical assistance to states other than those with which they are working intensively. For example, aside from its work in Delaware and North Carolina, in the past year the Clearinghouse has provided technical assistance to consumer organizations in such states as Montana, Kansas, and Oregon. In Oregon, the Clearinghouse helped create a curriculum to train peer specialists and provided on-site training as the curriculum was piloted. Feedback to Joseph Rogers from Meghan Caughey, peer wellness coordinator of Benton County, who had created the curriculum, read: "Wow – you really rocked Oregon! Thank you so much for your generosity and wisdom. . . .I know that I and everyone else who you taught received some very precious tools and we will put them to use in the upcoming years of our work."

The NEC TAC is also working in Oregon as well as in Idaho. And CONTAC worked with a group in Maine on formalizing their organization and developing their vision and mission, Kathy Muscari said. The group became the Advocacy Initiative of Maine. Within a year, they had almost 100 graduates of the Leadership Academy and got their first grant – several hundred thousand dollars, according to Muscari.

"NCSTAC worked intensively with eight organizations over a three-year period, providing a combination of funds, resources, technical assistance, on-site training and consultation," said Dianne Shenton, whose professional background is in non-profit management and development.

Leadership development is a key focus of the TACs in all the states, and all of the TACs were able to take advantage of an opportunity, made available by CMHS, to arrange for key consumer leaders of their target states to participate in a week-long leadership training, with follow up, offered by the Danya Institute (www.danyainstitute.org).

12.6 Challenges of Statewide Organizing

All of the TACs report challenges and lessons learned in working with their respective states. "Statewide organizing is difficult," said Joseph Rogers of the Clearinghouse. "In even the smallest state, like Delaware, we have found that getting unity across the state is pretty hard, if not almost impossible. For example, Delaware has only three counties, but each county is unique and celebrates its differences."

In Delaware, as with many states, the statewide organization is located in the capital and, if it has grassroots efforts, they tend to be centered around people from the immediate area surrounding the capital. So the Clearinghouse is working on developing local groups that would be branches of the statewide organization, similar to organizations that have state chapters and local branches of those chapters. "The hope is that the local groups would continue to identify and support the statewide group," Rogers said. "This is an experiment." He noted that most statewide consumer groups don't have the resources to maintain contacts across the state through outreach and networking, and "our movement is an extremely grassroots movement. If people identify with a group, it's usually their local group, where they get the most support and know the leadership personally." In Delaware, the Clearinghouse is holding regularly scheduled statewide teleconferences so that people can stay involved in what's happening statewide without having to travel to the state capital or some other central location as frequently.

In a presentation on April 15, 2009, at a conference on self-determination organized by the University of Illinois at Chicago (UIC), representatives of the TACs addressed the challenges they faced in statewide organizing, along with lessons learned.

The challenges named by the NEC TAC included lack of funding and support for a statewide consumer-run organization, finding appropriate leadership, and doing outreach in rural areas. Lessons learned included being persistent and creative in obtaining buy-in and support, piggybacking on-site trips with other speaking engagements, and seeking and cultivating leadership from "not-so-obvious" people.

Among the challenges cited by NCSTAC during the UIC presentation were the difficulties involved in working with huge, "frontier" states – Montana and Nevada – 2,500 miles from NCSTAC's home base; scattered populations; no metropolis; small state capitals; bi-annual or short-term legislatures; a lack of healthcare funding; a lack of communication infrastructure, computer, and Internet savvy or access; a "behind the times" state government in terms of the inclusion and participation of consumers; and the idea that consumers are "users" that may still pervade the culture – a "frontier" culture that discourages accepting a helping hand. Among the lessons NCSTAC reported were focusing on achieving two to three objectives in the first two years; making sure that the TAC acts as a consultant, not a member of the team, so that it is not seen as the "leader" or the entity whose opinion matters most; and supporting the "folks in the room" in becoming their own team/leaders. "In Montana, the group confronted and changed the health of the leadership," according to the NCSTAC presenter, Kate Gaston of Mental Health America.

In Rhode Island, reported Stephen Kiosk of the STAR Center, the challenges included the fact that the state has a highly developed provider system and that consumer-run organizations are not seen as essential to systems of care. In addition, "self-empowerment" is not widely perceived as a recovery goal there. The STAR Center noted that, in Arizona, which has many consumer-run organizations, various such organizations seem to work separately. In addition, immigration issues are a challenge in regard to building trust and participation, and there are few mental health services in rural and tribal areas. Kiosk noted that it was important to have honest and direct conversations about what is needed and wanted as well as what kinds of technical assistance are available, along with consistent e-mail and phone contact as well as site visits. Self-assessments were far more helpful than the TAC's pointing out deficiencies. The STAR Center also highlighted the importance of patience, persistence, and creativity.

However, despite obstacles, all of the TACs report successes in aiding the development of statewide consumer groups.

12.7 Cultural Diversity

One of the challenges the consumer/survivor movement faces is how to attract more people of color, and all of the TACs have worked to promote cultural diversity within the movement. The 2004 TAC evaluation noted, "From the start, the TACs have made a concerted effort to reach out to minority groups." (KCMHS, 2006, p. 47).

Among the efforts of the Clearinghouse to pursue this goal is its sponsorship of the first organizing meeting of a national organization of people of color as part of Alternatives '92, in Philadelphia, and another meeting of the group at Alternatives '94, in Anaheim, California. In addition, several years ago, the Clearinghouse convened a meeting of African American women leaders at Fellowship Farm, a retreat center in Pottstown, Pennsylvania.

NAMI's STAR Center specializes in cultural competence and outreach into diverse communities. Lynn Borton, NAMI's chief operating officer, explained that this was "both because there's a crying need for it and because NAMI has actually done some good work in this area and we felt we had a lot to offer." The STAR Center has presented a Leadership Academy in Spanish in Arizona, one of the two states with which it is working closely. Although Jim McNulty, who at the time directed the STAR Center, and STAR Center project coordinator Carmen Argueta both speak fluent Spanish, McNulty said, "we worked through the Recovery Empowerment Network (REN), a Maricopa County-based, peer-run organization, because they were intimately acquainted with conditions in the Phoenix area. There was substantial ongoing police activity targeting undocumented individuals (also sweeping up folks with documents), helping create conditions that made the Latino community in Arizona suspicious of outsiders, and afraid to work closely with individuals and groups that they did not already know," he said. McNulty added that REN trains extensively using the Leadership Academy model, and Rosa Navarro, one of the managers at REN and also a fluent Spanish speaker, had participated in a pilot of the Spanish-language Leadership Academy a year earlier, in California.

"By leveraging REN's local connections and relationships with the Latino community, the STAR Center was able to assist in beginning the process of inclusion of the Latino community into the mental health delivery system in Maricopa County, an area that is close to majority Latino," McNulty continued. The Latino community in Maricopa is historically underrepresented in the mental health community, as providers, advocates, and recipients of service. "This Leadership Academy gives more ability to do its outreach work, and bring more balance to the system," he said.

McNulty said that many consumer leaders want to assume that "simply because we share a common experience around mental health problems, that means that we share the same values, aspirations and culture. For some populations that doesn't work, so the question is how to be inclusive of them." Toward this end, the STAR Center organized three days of open cultural dialogues during Alternatives 2008 and created summary reports of the dialogues. A key question asked during the dialogues was how to make the movement and its leadership more representative and inclusive, and more empowering to all communities. Working with the University of Illinois at Chicago, the STAR Center has developed a cultural competence assessment tool for consumer-operated groups and services.

All the TACs agree that reaching out to members of diverse cultures who have psychiatric disabilities is key to their respective missions and visions, and all the centers continue to do this work.

12.8 Advocacy

The organizations that operate the consumer-run and consumer-supporter TACs have erected firewalls to cordon off their federally funded activities from the rest of their operations. This allows them to engage in the kind of advocacy that would otherwise be prohibited because of federal grant requirements.

Fisher noted that the issue is not clear-cut. "It's in our grant to organize people to have a voice. As long as the voice we're promoting is not a partisan voice and not strictly political – we don't have them influence a particular political position – then part of being a citizen is being able to educate legislators and decision makers. As an organization ourselves, and also with the groups we work with, we help them understand that. Other aspects of advocacy we do independently."

Because of the distinct separation between Clearinghouse TAC activities and the Mental Health Association of Southeastern Pennsylvania (MHASP), under whose auspices the Clearinghouse operates, when Joseph Rogers received a draft of "Mental Health: A Report of the Surgeon General" (1999) he was able to advocate for revised language in the section about electroconvulsive therapy (ECT). The draft language claimed that ECT was "safe and effective," although "not a single scientific research study was cited in support of that or any other claim," according to Linda Andre, who heads the Committee for Truth in Psychiatry, which advocates for truly informed consent around ECT. Rogers was a member of a CMHS panel charged with reviewing the report; and so, Andre (2009) wrote in her new book, *Doctors of Deception*, he "was able to see a draft of the ECT section [and] he leaked the four paragraphs to the public. Thanks to the advocacy community and to Rogers's ability to generate media coverage, a firestorm broke out" (Andre, 2009, p. 236). This included coverage of the controversy in the New York Times (Goode, 1999, Oct. 6) and, eventually, an improvement in the report's language, albeit a modest one (Andre, 2009).

Again relying on the distinction between the Clearinghouse technical assistance center and MHASP, Rogers and MHASP's then director of public policy, Mary Hurtig, were able to repeatedly advocate with the Congressional Appropriations Committee to ensure that Congress continue funding the TACs. For example, as a result of their efforts, the following language was inserted in the CMHS section of House Report 108-10, Fiscal Year 2003: "The conference agreement provides $2,000,000 above the request to continue the current level of funding for the consumer and consumer-supporter national technical assistance centers as proposed by the Senate. The conferees direct CMHS to support multi-year grants to five such national technical assistance centers." Similar language was in previous and subsequent years' conference reports.

Since 2006, the National Coalition of Mental Health Consumer/Survivor Organizations has taken up the gauntlet to help the TACs' funding continue. The National Coalition was founded and is coordinated by the National Empowerment Center; 32 statewide consumer-/survivor-run organizations are members. The efforts of the Coalition membership to keep the TACs going are critical. "Each year, we have to renew our efforts to educate legislators about the importance of what we do," Fisher said.

Mindful of the need to keep advocacy separate from technical assistance center activities, Fisher noted that "we've divided the NEC into three divisions so it's not just a technical assistance center. The technical assistance center is funded by the federal government and in those activities we don't do advocacy. We bring people together and we have statewide organizing. But then we have two other divisions, one of which is education and training – that's one where we actually give talks and sell some products as a supplement to the federal grant. Then the third one is networking and coalition building, and in that one we help organize the states that are not part of our federal grant, like Oregon, and we're working now in Idaho – states that have no one assigned to them. That's the division under which we've helped form this national coalition, with foundation money rather than the core federal grant."

It is clear that the TACs' advocacy is needed to maintain federal funding to continue their work, as well as to promote the cause of social justice; and all the TACs are careful to avoid violating federal policy in order to be able to continue to do such work.

12.9 Responding to Crises

An example of how the TACs step up to the plate is their response to Hurricanes Katrina and Rita in 2005. In the aftermath of Katrina, which wreaked devastation on New Orleans and surrounding areas, NEC convened a committee of local and national experts, including TAC representatives, on peer support and consumer leadership. The committee, Louisiana CORK (Consumers Organizing for Recovery after Katrina), developed a curriculum, presented several two- to three-day trainings, and did a Webcast on teaching other consumer groups how to prepare for or respond to a disaster, employing a combination of psychological first aid and peer support. "Consumers are very good at this kind of support because we look for strengths, not weaknesses, and we want to bring people together to help each other," Dan Fisher said.

On September 19, 2005 – within three weeks after Katrina – the Clearinghouse/Mental Health Association of Southeastern Pennsylvania, coordinating with Texas Mental Health Consumers, the statewide consumer group, flew a Clearinghouse/MHASP team to Texas to meet with people in areas around the state with a high concentration of those who fled before the storm or survived its devastation (PRNewswire, 2005, Sept. 19). The goal was to help those evacuees and to provide training in how to mobilize Texas volunteers – especially people who can provide peer support – to offer hope and aid to the evacuees. The training was based on lessons learned after 9/11 when MHASP, in collaboration with the University of Pennsylvania, helped develop a guide to facilitating recovery among individuals affected by traumatic events that have a community impact (Salzer, 2003).

At the same time, NEC traveled to Louisiana. "We did a three-day training three weeks after the first hurricane," recalled Fisher. "We assisted the consumer group there, Meaningful Minds of Louisiana, in developing a much stronger core." The NEC helped the group apply to FEMA (Federal Emergency Management Agency) for a grant, with help from consumer leaders such as LaVerne Miller, who had done similar work after 9/11 in New York, and Kay Rote, who had done such work in Oklahoma after the bombing of the federal building. "They were able to get FEMA funding to continue training and placing peers on teams," Fisher said.

"Another thing we did in Louisiana was to strengthen their leadership and their ability to be taken seriously by the Department of Mental Health there," Fisher continued. "They had to really get a place at the table, and having national leaders come in is a very important model to get the attention of local departments of mental health."

Dianne Dorlester Shenton, who until 2008 directed NCSTAC, delivered on-site technical assistance to Meaningful Minds, along with Fisher and others. Shenton said she worked very intensively with their board, teaching them how to function as a board, understanding roles and responsibilities. "Because of the hurricane, they ended up being thrust forward much quicker than anticipated because the need was so great to connect with any support, especially peer-to-peer support. So their programmatic support happened very rapidly, even before they had a solid infrastructure in place," she explained.

"At the start, they were a group of committed and passionate consumer advocates," said Shenton. Afterward, she said, they had "a few hundred thousand a year, they had a director and two paid staff and they were training peer-support specialists. They were working in partnership with the state, especially in the disaster recovery mode to do outreach to people with mental health needs."

Carole Glover, Meaningful Minds' CEO and president, is grateful. "The impact on Meaningful Minds from Dan and the [National] Empowerment Center has been the life blood that sustains us and gives us the stability we have today," Glover reported. "Before the hurricanes, the word 'recovery' was not spoken from the lips of the professionals or my peers. That is why during the training immediately after Hurricane Katrina that was done by Dan or others that came with him, there were 'high fives,' tears and laughter of joy because of the hope the training brought. Without the [National] Empowerment Center and Dan, our organization would not be in existence today." Glover also reported that NCSTAC and Dianne Shenton were "awesome in that the funds [NCSTAC provided] helped with infrastructure to help us with the Board of Directors' responsibilities, day-to-day activities and support."

Responding to crises, whether caused by natural or manmade disasters (or a combination of the two), is something that the TACs feel a natural calling to do. This may be because a large number of people diagnosed with mental illnesses – as TAC leaders and staff have been – are trauma survivors, so working with trauma survivors is a natural fit for them (Missouri Institute of Mental Health, 2002).

12.10 Barriers

Among the barriers to the work of the TACs are the stigma and discrimination associated with mental disorders. "There are providers and professionals who really still adhere to the maintenance model, family members who are afraid that their sons or daughters [who have psychiatric disabilities] will not be safe if they take risks or make changes in their lives," Fisher said. "Further, there is the public perception that we not only don't recover but are somehow dangerous. Those are some of the larger barriers. They not only affect our core funding, they affect our sustainability," he said. Peer support has developed a track record in helping people recover and get off Social Security, but "the traditional system is itself worried about being financed so it holds tightly to existing programs and it's hard to get new ones funded," Fisher said. "We're the new kids on the block. Foundations in many ways are often as traditional as the government."

Fisher believes that consumer-run entities face a lot of the same challenges that new enterprises and small businesses face. "Many of us have not had the training to be a small business," he said. "There are a lot of skills to learn in terms of accounting and leadership development. We're having to learn a lot of things all at one time to survive."

One challenge the TACs share is how to leverage their resources to have the greatest impact. "I was actually glad to see us go to the two target states, as opposed to just the nationwide focus," McNulty said. "Our grants are not huge, and doing technical assistance on the national front was really more than you could expect to see results with. Here we have, at least in part, a defined scope of action, two states, and we're working on defining the outcome measures. All things being equal, we should be able to see change on a smaller scale more easily."

Geography poses an additional challenge. For example, CONTAC is based in a rural state, "where there is a lot of economic hardship and communication and transportation difficulty," said Muscari, and "we found these to be common themes in many other states."

Another challenge is to draw consumers back into their role as advocates. Jim McNulty said, "One of the things that were amazing to me – and I saw this when I took a job with the state of Rhode Island as director of the Office of Consumer and Family Affairs – [was that] these guys had, more or less, become providers of services, and advocacy fell by the wayside. The problem was that, when they hit bad times in the last year, no one knew how to go back in and shake the tree to at least keep some money going."

Conversely, some consumer groups see organizational challenges as stemming from their status as consumers. Dianne Shenton said that when any of the organizations NCSTAC was working with were having such challenges, such as in the area of board/staff relations, "consumers were kind of quick to assume that it was because they were a consumer organization that they were having these challenges. It was a big educational effort to help them see that those were just normal challenges in the life of a non-profit." She said she worked to help them move beyond the "learned helplessness" that may have become ingrained in people who have been part of the mental health system. "It was really rewarding to see them all realize that they can use their passion and frustration and experiences to help build the organization in a positive way and, just because they are now acknowledging and learning business aspects, it doesn't detract from the mission and the reason they're all there."

In sum, all of the TACs, as well as their constituents, have to battle stigma and discrimination, along with many of the same obstacles that confront the general public when they attempt to create new initiatives, such as a dearth of business and leadership skills as well as financial resources, not to mention the challenges posed by geography. In addition, sometimes staff of peer-run services may lose their connection to their roots as advocates and become complacent. Others may exhibit "learned helplessness." The TACS work to overcome all of these challenges.

12.11 Special Projects

Each of the TACs has developed special projects to promote consumer empowerment. For example, CONTAC has its Leadership Academy (Sabin & Daniels, 2002), which Kathy Muscari describes "as a series of lessons about civic participation and collective self-determination that help people identify issues, particularly around making their communities better places to live, helping make the system more responsive to individual needs."

The Clearinghouse's Freedom Self-Advocacy Curriculum teaches self-advocacy skills to consumers. Besides a dozen technical assistance manuals on such subjects as systems advocacy, serving effectively on boards and committees, and consumer-run services and businesses, the Clearinghouse also publishes a monthly e-newsletter called the Key Update – news and notes on mental health issues – and another periodical called the Key Assistance Report (KAR), which offers in-depth analysis on selected topics, such as supported housing, spirituality, wellness, and program sustainability.

The NEC TAC has developed a program called e-CPR (Emotional Connection, emPowerment, Revitalization). "It was the consumer response to Mental Health First Aid [www.mhfa.com.au], which did not involve consumers in its development," Fisher said. "We're developing this as a skill and a confidence builder so that everybody can help with each other's recovery and prevent emotional difficulties and crises from reaching such a point that people have to be hospitalized or more severely labeled." Among NEC's other initiatives are the PACE (Personal Assistance in Community Existence) model, an empowerment model of recovery and development; a manual on statewide organizing called *Voices of Transformation*; and the Finding Our Voice training. Dan Fisher describes Finding Our Voice as being "about how people make the transition from being a consumer and a victim to being an agent and a leader, both in their own life and the lives of others."

NCSTAC published a series of publications on topics – such as grant-writing and fundraising – that were geared specifically to consumer-run non-profits. "Sometimes I would get calls from various groups who really just needed to know how to apply for their 501(c)(3)," Shenton said. "We put out a publication on that (NCSTAC, n.d.). I reviewed a lot of IRS applications for people and helped them craft or revise their bylaws."

The West Virginia Mental Health Consumers' Association has used a tool NCSTAC designed – a research and assessment tool to look at both the qualitative and quantitative characteristics of a community, county, state, and city. It assesses service delivery as well as financing mechanisms, strengths, barriers, and consumer preferences. Shenton said, "It provides a very thorough assessment of everything about the delivery system so that when consumers are advocating for systems change, they have some real data; they have a very systematic, organized way to approach and prioritize how they're advocating for change and what changes need to be made."

12.12 Collaboration

In an effort to encourage collaboration within the consumer/survivor movement, the Clearinghouse sponsored and organized the first National Summit of Mental Health Consumers and Survivors, in Portland, Oregon, in August 1999 (NSMHCS, 1999). The summit, organized with the help of the Oregon Office of Consumer Technical Assistance and co-sponsored by consumer/survivor groups from around the country, aimed to develop consensus around the issues of greatest concern to consumers and survivors and create action plans for future work. The unifying principle was the construction of a platform from which the movement would be able to influence the national debate.

In the last 10 years, a greater spirit of collaboration has evolved within the movement. For example, the organizations that oversee the consumer-run TACs – the National Empowerment Center and the National Mental Health Consumers' Self-Help Clearinghouse/Mental Health Association of Southeastern Pennsylvania – collaborate in the National Coalition for Mental Health Recovery (www.ncmhr.org), previously the National Coalition of Mental Health Consumer/Survivor Organizations.

When Dan Fisher served on the President's New Freedom Commission on Mental Health, he cast a wide net within the movement to ensure that consumer/survivor viewpoints were heard. His efforts had an impact on the Commission's (2003) report – *Achieving the Promise: Transforming Mental Health Care in America* – which reflects a recovery orientation.

All of the TACs routinely refer people to the other TACs. "We have no hesitancy in recommending the other national technical assistance centers as very capable of providing areas of support that perhaps we are not as experienced in, and I think that team approach has helped strengthen the states too," said Muscari.

The TACs also collaborate with other organizations and work to bring other groups together. For example, in the mid-1990s, when Medicaid was switching in most states from fee-for-service to Medicaid-managed care, the Clearinghouse, along with the National Mental Health Association (now Mental Health America), NAMI, the Bazelon Center for Mental Health Law, the National Depressive and Manic-Depressive Association (now the Depression and Bipolar Support Alliance), and other members of the ad hoc National Managed Care Consortium, played a major role in bringing people together to understand the emerging managed care system, explore its impact, and help create a blueprint for action.

In another collaboration, when the Protection and Advocacy for Individuals with Mental Illness (PAIMI) Act became law in 1986, "we helped consumers understand the PAIMI Act and helped network them through caucuses and conferences around how they could become active members of protection and advocacy agencies with an emphasis on real consumer involvement in P&As [protection and advocacy agencies] across the country," Joseph Rogers said. Rogers also served on the congressionally appointed Task Force on the Rights and Empowerment of Americans with Disabilities, which was instrumental in the passage of the Americans with Disabilities Act, a landmark piece of civil rights legislation, in 1990.

In 2006, the Clearinghouse convened a group of stakeholders and experts from around the United States to create a new national trade association to promote the emerging profession of certified peer specialist. The organization has since blended with the National Association of Peer Specialists, whose 2008 national conference in Philadelphia the Clearinghouse helped organize. "Besides providing technical assistance, the Clearinghouse is an instrument for networking and bringing people together," Rogers said.

The Clearinghouse also partners with the University of Pennsylvania in the UPenn Collaborative on Community Integration, a national rehabilitation research and training center devoted to promoting community integration for individuals with psychiatric disabilities, funded by the National Institute on Disability and Rehabilitation Research. One initiative that the Clearinghouse/MHASP collaborated in involved legislative advocacy about child custody issues for parents who have psychiatric disabilities. These efforts "have managed to make inroads in increasing awareness and changing or removing discriminatory language that determines that a mental illness/disability is grounds for not providing reasonable efforts to preserve or reunify a family" (Kaplan et al., 2009).

"The Clearinghouse provides essential leadership and direction in the University of Pennsylvania Collaborative on Community Integration," writes Mark Salzer, Ph.D., who heads the UPenn Collaborative. "Consumer voices and visions drive the research questions, research procedures, interpretation of results, as well as to whom and how the findings are disseminated. This level of partnership underlies the quality and relevance of our work."

All of these collaborative efforts create an impact that is greater than the sum of its parts.

12.13 TACs' Effectiveness

A recent evaluation, by the Kentucky Center for Mental Health Studies (2006), validated the TACs' effectiveness and impact. The evaluation determined that the TACs help individuals with mental health disabilities play a critical role in the mental health arena and work toward their recovery. "Overall," the report stated, "the TACs continue to be productive leaders and partners in transforming America's mental health system given the service they render to consumers, family members, and the public. The 2004 evaluation has only underscored their value and the essential nature of their work on behalf of persons with serious mental illness, 'some of America's most disenfranchised citizens' (Assessing the Promise, 2004, p. 63)." The evaluation continued, "Hopefully, their work will lead consumers to reach for dreams that only recovery can bring – the recovery valued by designers and developers of America's transformed mental health system – recovery that saves and changes lives" (KCMHC, 2006, p. 52).[7]

12.14 Recommendations and a "Wish List"

In their presentation at the UIC self-determination conference in April 2009, representatives of the TACs explored ways that the Center for Mental Health Services and the Centers for Medicare & Medicaid Services (CMS) could help the consumer/survivor movement. These suggestions included expanding self-directed care, peer specialist, and peer-support services; using the Federal Executive Steering Committee and the Federal Partners Senior Workgroup to increase consumer interaction with different federal agencies, including the Social Security Administration, CMS, and others; and disseminating emerging best practices, such as crisis alternatives. The "wish list" it presented at the conference (see Table 12.1) included promoting self-determination, involving "a shift to a system of care that puts treatment planning squarely in the hands of service recipients, and that includes their meaningful involvement in mental health services policy, planning, training (including peer leadership training), design, implementation and evaluation" and the creation of "a system in which service recipients manage the dollars allocated to their care, either on their own or in consultation with a peer specialist trained in shared decision making." Other items on the wish list include creating alternatives to the traditional mental health system; fostering wellness and recovery instead of illness and maintenance; and promoting community integration and the expansion of workforce development.

12.15 Conclusion

The efforts of all the TACs have been critical in helping the consumer/survivor movement develop and have an impact in the mental health arena. "Sometimes it's hard to see systemic changes when you're doing it day to day," said Dianne Shenton, formerly of NCSTAC. "But, looking back, the progress that the consumer movement has made in the past few years is just amazing. It's always great to be a part of that."

However, there is a lot more to be done. "I think we've been pretty successful in helping consumer/survivors develop a voice – a voice for transformation – but there remain elements in the system that are resisting change and transformation," Fisher said. "In some ways, our successes lead to new challenges."

---

[7] Ibid., For example, the evaluation found that 1,113 individuals contacted the TACs in one month and made 1,586 requests for technical assistance. TAC users made 1,964 topical requests of which 54.5% were about clinical issues. Of the 329 organizations that requested technical assistance, 29% were consumer-run organizations or groups; 17% were NAMI or Mental Health America (MHA) affiliates; 12.8% were state, county or local mental health authorities; 11.6% were provider organizations; and 11.2% were academic institutions.

Table 12.1 Consumer and consumer supporter technical assistance center wish list

---

Category:
- Wish list item.

Promote self-determination:
- Achieve a paradigm shift to a system of care that puts treatment planning squarely in the hands of service recipients, and that includes their meaningful involvement in mental health services policy, planning, training (including peer leadership training), design, implementation and evaluation.
- Affirm the promise of the President's New Freedom Commission on Mental Health of a consumer-driven systems transformation by guaranteeing the significant participation of consumers on the policy-making advisory boards of all the major government agencies involved in community integration, such as the Social Security Administration, the Centers for Medicare & Medicaid Services, the Substance Abuse and Mental Health Services Administration, the National Institute on Disability and Rehabilitation Research, the Department of Housing and Urban Development, and the National Institute of Mental Health. Also, guarantee the fulfillment of the Commission's mission and goal by publishing the subcommittee reports on Consumer Issues and on Rights and Engagement.
- Create a system in which service recipients manage the dollars allocated to their care, either on their own or in consultation with a peer specialist trained in shared decision making.
- Reform entitlement programs to allow more choice.

Create alternatives to the traditional mental health system:
- Develop a comprehensive array of voluntary, effective and attractive alternatives, such as peer-run respite services and other peer-delivered services and supports. These alternatives to hospitalization and other traditional treatment models would allow the opportunity for positive disengagement from the formal treatment system.
- Fund a comprehensive, comparative economic analysis of the current mental health system that can be used by policy-makers to justify implementing peer-support services and programs that promote self-determination, and to ensure that such effective models are accepted as evidence-based practices.
- Fund consumer-run statewide organizations in every state and territory and six consumer-run regional technical assistance centers.

Foster wellness and recovery instead of illness and maintenance:
- Create a holistic and well-funded approach to health and mental health care that encourages personal responsibility and self-determination and that does not tell service recipients that they are damaged and incapable but instead builds on their strengths and wellness.
- Fund efforts to provide interested individuals with opportunities to more intensively experience recovery, healing, integration and wellness practices, such as occur at conferences and similar venues.
- Develop a national engagement campaign for peer recovery leaders to interact with leaders in such domains as medicine, social work, psychology and nursing in order to transform the medical/illness model into the recovery/wellness model.

Promote community integration:
- Fund and develop peer leadership activities in underserved communities that resonate with various cultural/ethnic/community beliefs and values, and which may or may not use mental health/illness language.
- Involve individuals who "don't use mental health services" in activities that promote wellness/health/resilience in their communities, such as faith communities, social networks, peer communities, and others.

Promote the expansion of workforce development:
- Identify and develop more employment opportunities for service recipients, both inside and outside of the mental health arena.
- Create a mandate for states to address the gaps in certifying peer specialists as a workforce investment priority.

References

Andre, L. (2009). *Doctors of deception: What they don't want you to know about shock treatment.* Piscataway, NJ: Rutgers University Press, 2009, pp. 236–240.

Campbell, J. (2005). *Emerging research base of peer-run support programs.* Retrieved from http://www.power2u.org/emerging_research_base.html

Chamberlin, J. (1978). *On our own: Patient-controlled alternatives to the mental health system.* New York: Hawthorn Books.

Goode, E. (1999, Oct. 6). Federal report praising electroshock stirs uproar. *The New York Times,* Page A18.

Kaplan, K., Kottsieper, K., Scott, J., Salzer, M., & Solomon, P. (2009). AFSA state statutes regarding parents with mental illnesses: A review and targeted intervention. *Psychiatric Rehabilitation Journal, 33*(2), 91–94.

Kentucky Center for Mental Health Studies and The Evaluation Center at HSRI. (2006). *Assessing the dream: The third annual evaluation of the consumer and consumer supporter national technical assistance centers.* Georgetown, KY: Kentucky Center for Mental Health Studies.

Missouri Institute of Mental Health. (2002). *Trauma among people with mental illness and/or substance use disorders.* Retrieved from http://mimh200.mimh.edu/mimhweb/pie/reports/MIMH%20Fact%20Sheet%20Nov%202002.pdf

National Consumer Supporter Technical Assistance Center (n.d.). *How to establish a 501c3.* Retrieved from http://www.ncstac.org/content/materials/501c3.pdf

National Summit of Mental Health Consumers and Survivors. (1999). *Plank reports – Executive summary.* Retrieved from http://www.mhselfhelp.org/pubs/view.php?publication_id=119

President's New Freedom Commission on Mental Health (2003). Achieving the promise: Transforming mental health care in America. Rockville, MD: Substance Abuse and Mental Health Services Administration. Retrieved from www.mentalhealthcommission.gov

PRNewswire (2005, Sept. 19). *MHA of SE/PA goes to Texas to support Katrina evacuees.* Retrieved from http://www.redorbit.com/news/health/244233/mha_of_sepa_goes_to_texas_to_support_katrina_evacuees/index.html

Rogers, S. (1992). SHARE wins prestigious NIMH grant to fund national information center. *Lines of Communication,* Spring-Summer 1992, Page 1.

Sabin, J. E. & Daniels, N. (2002). Strengthening the consumer voice in managed care: IV. The leadership academy program, *Psychiatric Services, 53,* 405–406, 411.

Salzer, M. (2003). *Disaster community support network of Philadelphia.* Retrieved from http://www.mhselfhelp.org/resources/view.php?resource_id=130

Substance Abuse and Mental Health Services Administration. (n.d.). *Consumer and consumer supporter technical assistance centers (TACs) program historical background.* Retrieved from http://mentalhealth.samhsa.gov/cmhs/CommunitySupport/consumers/background.asp

Whitaker, R. (2002). *Mad in America: Bad science, bad medicine, and the enduring mistreatment of the mentally ill.* Cambridge, MA: Perseus Publishing.

Chapter 13
A Statewide Collaboration to Build the Leadership and Organizational Capacity of Consumer-Run Organizations (CROs)

Oliwier Dziadkowiec, Crystal Reinhart, Chi Connie Vu, Todd Shagott, Ashlee Keele-Lien, Adrienne Banta, Scott Wituk, and Greg Meissen

Abstract Mental health consumer-run organizations (CROs) are a heterogeneous group of recovery-oriented settings founded on peer support and mutual aid. This chapter focuses on consumer-run organizations in Kansas. The discussion begins with the history of the consumer movement on a national level, followed by the history of CROs in Kansas. The next section consists of an in-depth commentary about the collaborative relationship between the Center for Community Support and Research (CCSR) and Kansas CROs and is followed by a brief overview of research studies conducted by CCSR to assess impact and capacity needs of CROs. The chapter concludes with a focus on the future of CROs and the future of the consumer movement in Kansas.

The President's New Freedom Commission on Mental Health report, *Achieving the Promise: Transforming Mental Health Care in America* (2003) recognized consumer-run organizations as an "emerging best practice," in mental health care. While not yet considered an evidence-based practice due to the absence of rigorous evaluation research regarding their direct benefits, consumer-run organizations are gaining a momentum in the mental health field with high levels of member satisfaction and low-cost operations.

The Center for Community Support and Research (CCSR, formerly known as the Self-Help Network) at Wichita State University has provided evaluation as well as organizational and leadership development assistance to Kansas CROs for the last 10 years. This strong and mutually beneficial relationship between Kansas CROs and CCSR has resulted in a substantial growth in the number and membership size of CROs as well as expanded the knowledge base about their benefits through a number of reports and peer-reviewed publications.

The purpose of this chapter is to examine the history and function of CROs in Kansas, as well as their partnership with CCSR. We first set the stage with a discussion of the consumer movement and then explain how CROs fit in the consumer

O. Dziadkowiec (✉)
Center for Community Support and Research, Wichita State University, Wichita, KS, USA
e-mail: oliwier.dziadkowiec@wichita.edu

movement. This is followed by an in-depth discussion of the collaborative relationship between the CCSR and Kansas CROs as well as an overview of research studies conducted by CCSR to assess the impact and capacity needs of CROs. The last section is dedicated to the future of CROs and the consumer movement in Kansas with emphasis on leadership development as a vehicle for promoting sustainability and further growth of CROs and the consumers who attend them.

13.1 What Are CROs and What Do They Do?

Initially developed in the late 1960s as an alternative to traditional mental health services, consumer-run organizations (CROs) have been an integral part of the consumer empowerment movement on the local as well as the national level (Zinman, Harp, Budd, 1987). Grounded in peer support, CROs (also referred to as consumer-operated services) demonstrate the possibilities of mutual support by moving beyond the "drop-in center" paradigm, and working in the capacity of nonprofit organizations that are staffed and governed by mental health consumers (Brown, Shepherd, Merkle, Wituk, & Meissen, 2008; Brown, Shepherd, Wituk & Meissen, 2007).

An important aspect of CROs is their ability to complement services provided by the current mental health system (Brown et al., 2008, 2007). Some CROs, such as the Michigan-based drop-in centers, choose to partner more closely with local community mental health centers (Mowbray & Tan, 1993) while others such as the CROs in Kansas (Brown et al., 2007) or Ontario, Canada (Nelson et al., 2006a, 2006b) work more independently. CROs provide a variety of common services and activities including increasing awareness about mental illness, advocacy, outreach, social support, and opportunities for leadership within the CRO (Brown et al., 2007; Mowbray & Moxley, 1997; Silverman, Blank, & Taylor, 1997). Research by Trainor, Shepherd, Boydell, Leff, and Crawford (1997) found that members, who used a wide range of services, considered their CRO the single most helpful component of the mental health system. Outcomes associated with CROs include a decrease in the use of crisis services, along with a decrease in institutionalization, substance abuse, and the use of community mental health center services (Young & Williams, 1987; Mowbray & Tan, 1993).

13.2 History and Background of CROs in Kansas

Caring Place, the first CRO in Kansas, was founded in 1971 in Newton. Project Acceptance in Lawrence and Living, Inc. (LINC) in Shawnee followed soon after in 1975 and 1978, respectively. CCSR began as a self-help group clearinghouse in 1984. The center advocated and publicized CROs by listing them in a statewide database that provided referrals and resources regarding self-help groups. In 1990, the Substance Abuse and Mental Health Services Administration (SAMHSA) awarded a federal grant to the Kansas Department of Social and Rehabilitation Services (SRS) to strengthen and establish a statewide consumer organization, the Kansas Mental Illness Awareness Council, Inc. (KMAIC). CCSR became involved as the evaluators for this initiative.

Even though new CROs had been established and funded by SRS by the late 1990s, many struggled as their budgets were small and they had little local community support and it was difficult for SRS as a state bureaucracy to provide assistance to these small grassroots, self-help organizations. Therefore, the SRS Office of Mental Health and Substance Abuse, the CROs, and CCSR began a collaboration to provide organizational and leadership development to both established and new CROs. The CCSR began providing workshops regarding the operation of these self-help organizations as nonprofits, which included strategic planning, board development, and grant writing. While the workshops were well received, the impact was limited because the CROs faced several organizational challenges including being new, under-funded, and having relatively inexperienced staff and boards.

The KMAIC disbanded in 1998, and during the effort to restart a statewide consumer organization, local CROs stated their dissatisfaction regarding the technical assistance KMAIC provided to CROs and instead asked for a partnership with SRS and CCSR to build the capacity of existing CROs and to develop new CROs in parts of the state with high need. It was agreed by CRO members and SRS that the CROs were under-funded and under-supported. In 1999, additional financial and organizational support became available for CROs and CCSR was asked to provide more in-depth organizational and leadership development assistance to the seven existing CROs. This transition marked a pivotal point in time for Kansas CROs, beginning a 10-year period of substantial growth and positive organizational capacity development of Kansas CROs (Fig.13.1).

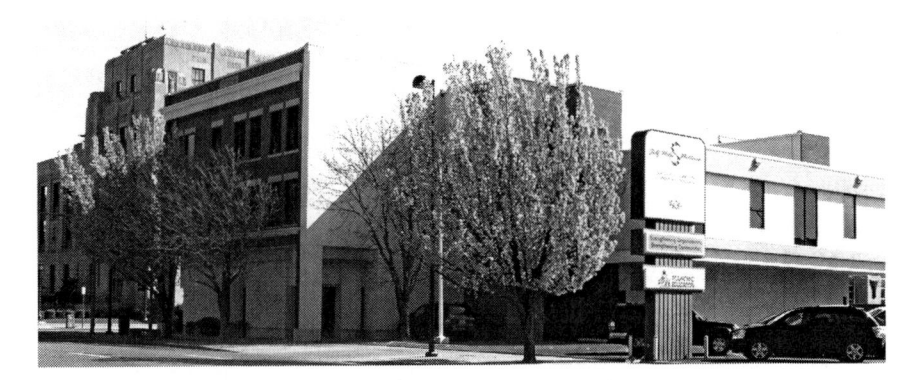

Fig. 13.1 Center for community support and research

13.3 The Center for Community Support and Research: Program Description

Currently CCSR, CROs, and SRS collaborate to provide organizational and leadership development support to the 22 consumer-run organizations in Kansas. The CCSR staff involved in the work on this initiative includes both consumer and non-consumer employees from different backgrounds and disciplines, including community psychology, social work, education, and business, as well as graduate and undergraduate students at Wichita State University. Additionally, the "Consumer to Consumer" initiative connects experienced members and staff from one CRO to another CRO which would benefit from their technical and experiential expertise. Much like other nonprofits, CROs face a variety of management and organizational challenges. Having such close ties with CROs across Kansas and with expertise in nonprofit capacity building, CCSR is able to assist CROs in various areas of organizational development. CCSR's support in this area includes helping CROs obtain their nonprofit 501c (3) status, grant writing, board development, as well as business and financial management.

The CCSR develops Memorandums of Understanding (MOU) with each CRO on an annual basis, which outlines the specific support and services to be offered during the year. This MOU development is based on data from quarterly reports to SRS, grants and organizational goals, organizational assessments, and through use of a checklist for capacity development.

The CCSR also conducts research with CROs through a joint grant from the National Institute of Mental Health (NIMH) and the Substance Abuse and Mental Health Services Administration (SAMHSA). This research is intended to help develop best practices for CROs and help move these emerging best practices to evidence-based practice. CCSR's research activities are centered on finding the benefits of attending CROs for individual members as well as determining the organizational capacity needs of CROs.

13.4 The Growth of CROs in the Kansas Mental Health System

In Kansas, CCSR has tracked the progress and success of CROs from 1999 to the present. In 1999, a total of 11 CROs existed, with an average annual budget of $17,000. Average membership for these CROs was 20. Currently there are 23 CROs operating in Kansas, with an average membership of 60 individuals, with some of the larger CROs having memberships as high as 250 individuals. Operating budgets range from $31,430 to $112,111 annually.

It is important to note that CROs in Kansas are recognized by SRS as a legitimate and integral part of the statewide mental health care system. It is also important to note that CROs in Kansas are not only in the two primary urban centers of the state, Kansas City and Wichita, but are dispersed throughout Kansas. This includes many rural communities where professional services are not readily available, especially during evenings and weekends. With access to services in rural areas being a crucial factor for the mental health delivery system in Kansas, the success of CROs in these areas is especially significant. Evidence of this recognition is the role SRS has asked CROs to play as community transition peer support providers for mental health consumers as they are discharged from inpatient facilities.

13.5 Organizational-Level Changes: CROs Developing Organizational Capacities

Kansas CROs have changed and developed new organizational capacities over the last decade. Examining trends in the services provided to CROs, as well as the satisfaction of CRO leaders and members with their own organization's functioning assist in documenting this increased capacity.

13.5.1 Tracking Organizational Development

Examining the changes in types of service and support that CCSR has provided to CROs over the years offers insight into how CROs in Kansas are developing over time. Through tracking quarterly reports of the existing CROs from 2001 to 2003 (Shepherd, 2003), it was found that CROs were seeking assistance for financial reporting and management at a higher rate than any other form of assistance; 65% more than the two other most requested forms of assistance: grant writing and help with SRS quarterly reports. In a June 2004 report (Shepherd & Brown, 2004a) however, it was noted that there was a drop in the rate that financial reporting and management assistance (from 37% in the 2003 report to 30% in the 2004 report), as well as an increase in the request for grant writing assistance (from 24% in 2003 to 32% in 2004).

One factor that seems to have contributed to this change was the burgeoning practice by many CROs of using external accountants for their financial matters, which is a practice used by many nonprofits to insure greater financial accountability. In addition, CROs became cognizant of their need for improved financial management and took appropriate action, thereby increasing their overall organizational health, as well as allowing for more focus on other organizational capacity issues.

Another shift in support and assistance needs of CROs also indicates an overall improvement in organizational capacity. A study conducted by CCSR (2007) found that while capacity building needs such as grant writing, quarterly reporting, board development, and business management continued to remain the most common requests, there was also a gradual decrease in requests typical of start-up nonprofits, such as increasing membership and achieving nonprofit status. This decrease suggests that "start-up activities" were no longer a focus of most of these CROs, suggesting increased organizational maturity.

13.5.2 Involvement and Satisfaction of CRO Leaders and Members

CRO members regularly attend their CROs, participating several days per week on average and generally participating for more than 3 h per visit. Thus, it appears that CRO participation is a significant part of how members spend their time.

Involvement and satisfaction of CRO leaders and members is also a relevant indication of organizational capacity. During late 2003 and early 2004, the CCSR collected survey information from 250 members, volunteers, and leaders of all Kansas CROs (Shepherd & Brown, 2004b). Results indicated high organizational involvement, with 59% reporting that they had voted in an election for board members, 69% reporting they had taken part in deciding what activities would be held, and 64% reporting that they volunteered on a regular basis. A sense of pride in their organization was also indicated with 78% reporting that they had helped with the daily operation of the CRO, and 71% reporting they had been responsible for preparing meals or bringing refreshments.

The study also indicated that participants' sense of community was high, with a majority of the members responding that they "Agree A Lot" with statements such as "I feel like I belong to the community here" or "The friendships I have with people here mean a lot to me." Besides the high scores on the sense of community scale, the scores on the organizational climate scale were also high, with most members indicating that they either "Strongly Agree" or "Agree" with statements such as "This place promotes learning, striving and growth" and "This place helps people feel valued and respected." (Fig.13.2).

Reinhart, Meissen, Wituk, and Shepherd (2008) examined setting-level characteristics associated with CROs to determine which were related to positive outcomes among 250 participants in 20 CROs. Interviews were conducted with participants to gauge their perception of setting-level characteristics and personal outcomes of

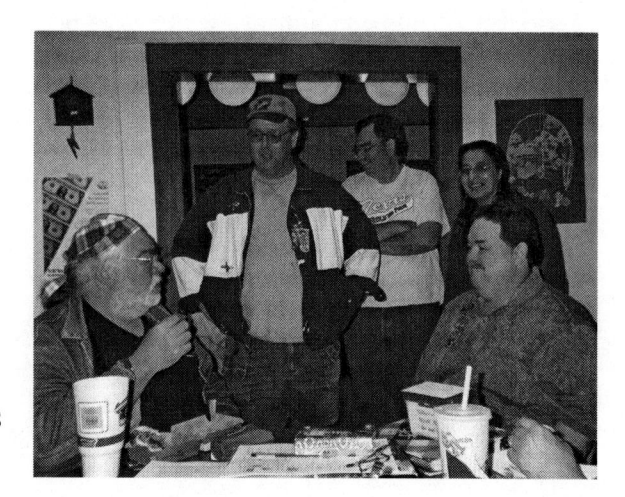

Fig. 13.2 Members of the PS Club CRO enjoying lunch and conversation

services. Similar to the aforementioned study by Shepherd and Brown (2004b), the results from this study indicated that the setting-level characteristics of organizational climate and sense of community were related to a measure of improved outcomes, which included questions about members satisfaction and other outcomes related to attending CROs.

13.6 Individual-Level Changes: Social and Psychological Integration

The final and perhaps most vital aspect of CROs to consider are the individual-level changes that occur for mental health consumers who become involved in CROs. Participation in CROs can help strengthen coping skills, enhance personal empowerment, and increase social support and networking, which are important elements of recovery (Brown et al., 2008). One of the most important needs addressed by CROs is social support, which is a basic need for recovery. The vital role of social support in recovery from mental illness is powerfully articulated by the executive director of Sunshine Connection CRO:

> ...when I finally started getting better I realized that to me folks with mental illness did not have a place to go in Topeka to hang out, to be with other friends, to learn the resources in the community and such...my mom had schizophrenia so I grew up with her and I just really saw people struggle and lose hope and so I wanted to do something to give people hope again...

13.6.1 Impacts of CRO Experiences

The CCSR has conducted a number of studies that examined individuals' experiences and benefits when participating in CROs. In a 2004 study (Shepherd & Brown, 2004b) based on data from 250 CRO members reported that the CRO experience helped them feel better about themselves (81.4% agreed or strongly agreed) and feel more confident (81% agreed or strongly agreed). CRO members also reported improvements in their use of both crisis (54.7% agreed or strongly agreed) and non-crisis mental health services (53% agreed or strongly agreed).

Another study conducted with 100 participants from eight Kansas CROs (Shagott, Vu, Reinhart, Wituk, & Meissen, 2006) found that participating in a CRO contributes to higher levels of psychological well-being and a greater sense of belonging to their community. First-time attendees were compared with established members who had attended their CRO for 18 months or more. Results showed that established members reported socializing and talking more with other members outside of the CRO, borrowing things and exchanging favors with others more often, and also feeling more able to rely on others in an emergency. Established members also reported attending more meetings and engaging in more activities than first-time attendees. What these results show is well captured by a response from the executive director of the CRO SIDE regarding the impact of being a CRO member on her recovery:

> ...being involved in a CRO I had more friends and relationships that I could ever ask for and in a lot of ways, my life is better than before because not only did I learn more about mental health, I learned about having healthy relationships

When examining the social networks of 132 CRO members it was found that other CRO members were the largest single contributor to a participant's social network, making up almost 27% of their social networks, more than mental health professionals and family members (Shagott, Vu, Reinhart, Wituk & Meissen, 2009). Over 85% of participants also reported having at least one other CRO member in their social network in which they felt a close relationship. These findings are supported by other studies that found that consumer-operated settings contribute to development of social networks, which appear to have a positive relationship with recovery (Brown et al., 2008; Mowbray, Robinson, & Holter, 2002; Nelson et al., 2006b; Solomon, 2004).

Knowing that consumers develop broader social networks through CRO involvement, CCSR researchers utilized the qualitative photovoice research method and set out to examine the nature of interactions between people in Kansas CROs. Photovoice, a photography-based research methodology (Wang & Burris, 1997; Wang & Redwood-Jones, 2001), was used to examine the impact of daily activities and peer interactions on psychological and social integration of CRO. Results showed that members engaged in numerous activities offered by their CRO which led to the development of friendships, which enriched their lives (Brown, Collins, Shepherd, Wituk & Meissen, 2004).

CRO participation may also help prevent unneeded mental health service use. A study conducted by Shagott and colleagues (2008) of 132 participants from eight Kansas CROs indicates that for 20% of CRO members, their CRO was the only mental health service utilized within the last 60 days. Nearly 95% of members reported no hospitalization within the last 60 days for psychiatric reasons, and 86% reported not utilizing services from a day program or treatment center in the past 60 days. While these results do not demonstrate a direct causal relationship between CRO participation and a decrease in the use of other mental health services, they do suggest CRO members are generally low in the need for intensive use of mental health services.

Research findings from other states lead to similar conclusions about mental health service use by members of peer-run organizations. In one recent longitudinal study from Canada, Nelson et al. (2007) reported that only 3.6% of active CRO members received psychiatric hospitalization during a 36-month period. According to Trainor et.al. (1997), CRO participants reported that their use of inpatient services decreased by 91% after joining the CRO. Further, Ochocka et al. (2006) found that participation in CROs facilitates community integration, and Corrigan et al. (2005) found participation in CROs was positively related to improvement in the process of recovery both of which are likely to decrease service use.

13.7 Putting CROs in Perspective: Other Consumer Movement-Related Activities in Kansas

The impact of CROs, especially the leadership efforts of CRO directors, reaches far beyond the CROs themselves and their membership. CRO leaders in conjunction with CCSR staff, some of whom are consumer leaders, have been a critical part of two other statewide initiatives driving the consumer movement in Kansas: the Adult Mental Health Consumer Advisory Council (CAC) and the Mental Health Consumer Run Organizations Network of Kansas (MHCRONK).

13.7.1 The Adult Mental Health Consumer Advisory Council

The Adult Mental Health Consumer Advisory Council (CAC) was instituted in 2001 as a statewide advocacy group for consumers of mental health services in Kansas. Its mission includes aiding consumers "through education, advocacy, collaboration, feedback, and equal representation." The Council consists exclusively of mental health consumers from throughout Kansas, and it offers a variety of programs and events for mental health consumers, families, and providers.

One of these programs is the Leadership Academy, which is a leadership capacity building/training program for Kansas consumers, who apply and are selected by the CAC based on their ability to positively impact the mental health consumer movement in Kansas and nationally. The Leadership Academy provides a peer support context that emphasizes shared learning from classmates, Leadership Academy graduates, and established Kansas consumer leaders. The program focuses on grassroots advocacy at the local and state level, awareness of the mental health policy system, individual leadership skill development, and further developing a support structure for consumer leaders. Su Budd, the matriarch of the Kansas consumer movement and a pioneer in the national consumer movement is the primary faculty for the Leadership Academy, which has been one of the major reasons the number of recognized consumer leaders has grown from a handful in the 1990s to dozens across Kansas today.

The CAC is the lead partner with CCSR and SRS in hosting the annual Kansas Recovery Conference, which routinely draws between 750 and 900 participants from across Kansas. While there are plenty of professional providers in attendance, close to 90% of attendees are consumers. Nationally recognized keynote speakers (e.g., Dan Fisher, Shery Mead, and Mark Davis) highlight the conference but the bulk of sessions, workshops, and discussion groups are designed and offered by Kansas consumers on such topics as peer support, spirituality and recovery, taking charge of your treatment, advocating for yourself and others, and numerous other topics related to recovery. The CAC is also involved in facilitating quarterly statewide CRO Network gatherings, and organizing an annual statewide leadership retreat for CRO staff, board members, and CAC members (Fig.13.3).

The Mental Health Consumer Run Organizations Network of Kansas, Inc. The Mental Health Consumer Run Organization Network of Kansas, Inc. (MHCRONK),

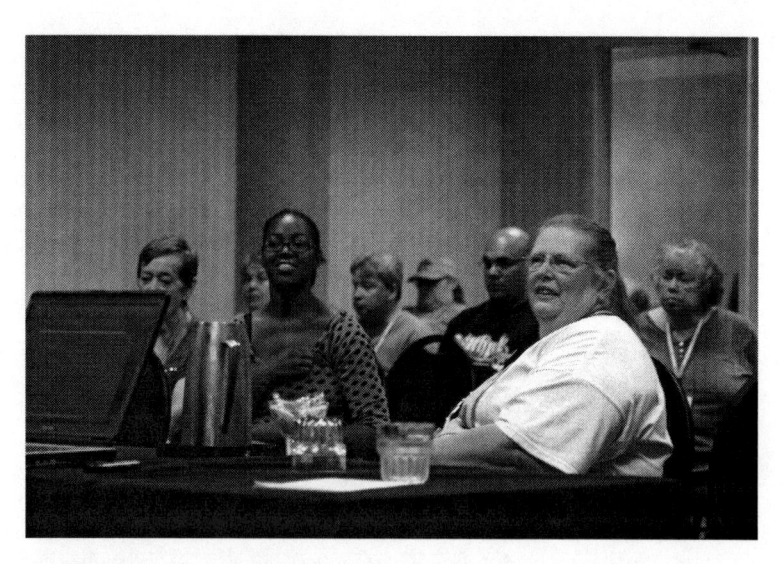

Fig. 13.3 2009 Kansas Recovery Conference

previously known as the CRO Network, is a statewide membership association that was established in 2005 to provide mutual support to consumer-run organizations in Kansas. Its mission states that it will "provide technical assistance, peer support, and advocacy to strengthen, empower, and unify CROs of Kansas." The MHCRONK meets on a quarterly basis and its primary business revolves around assisting member CROs, sharing information regarding legislation and state policy that could impact CROs, and facilitating a unified voice to SRS regarding issues important to member CROs. The CCSR provides technology and support for the MHCRONK Web site (www.kansascro.org) which continues to be expanded as a resource for emerging practice materials, announcements, consumer empowerment training curricula, communication through forums/chat rooms, calendar of events, bulletin board, links, news and information about individual CROs, and the MHCRONK.

The success of the MHCRONK and the CAC are positive indicators of the growth and maturity of the consumer movement in Kansas. These two groups not only provide other resources and outlets for consumers to get involved in Kansas mental health policy and programs, but also provide a collective voice for the thousands of people receiving public mental health services in Kansas. These two organizations are actively involved in advocating for consumers as members on Kansas Governor's Mental Health Services Planning Council, with SRS staff, with the public mental health managed care organization, Kansas Health Solutions, and with other state-level health care administrators and state legislators.

13.8 Discussion: Lessons Learned and Future Directions

The future of the CRO movement in Kansas will continue to rely on the leadership of mental health consumers and the collaborations they have developed in and outside the mental health system. Based on the above experiences and research, several insights emerged that may be useful to consumer advocates, researchers, mental health administrators, policy makers, and others in a position to support consumer-operated services.

13.8.1 Developing the Capacity of Consumer Leadership

The past 10 years in Kansas would have not been possible without consumers who are interested and passionate about providing support to others. Recognizing this interest and passion, the CCSR was able to collaborate with consumers to provide leadership development to assist CROs and the consumer movement across the state. A number of collaborative leadership development opportunities were offered each year, including a 2-day consumer leadership retreat, a consumer leadership academy, and leadership workshops at the Recovery Conference, as well as numerous leadership development opportunities at local CROs. The CCSR was able to provide organizational capacity building support to hundreds of nonprofits in Kansas and, it was found that the types of organizational needs of CROs are not unlike many other nonprofits, especially those similar in size and organizational development. This "normalizing" approach to nonprofit capacity building based on leadership development allowed the focus to be about the organization and not mental illness.

13.8.2 CROs as a Setting to Exercise Leadership

Leadership needs a setting or place in which to be exercised and CROs provide a supportive and safe place for leadership to develop. Expanding the CROs across Kansas provides additional opportunities for consumers to participate in leadership roles, whether as a director, staff, board member, or volunteer. Opportunities for leadership within the mental health system by mental health consumers are relatively few but if such settings exist new leadership opportunities for mental health consumers emerge. The range of inclusiveness and participation in organizational leadership is powerfully captured by the executive director of Bridge to Freedom:

> I would say 95% in the CRO are actively involved in Leadership. One of the things that I think is the most important is the programming and every month, the whole membership sits down and plans out what we want to do and because of that, you know, like maybe this person is really good at art or crafts, maybe this person over here is good at cooking, maybe this person is good at something else, it really focuses on their interests, they can participate, they can help run that particular program.

Additionally, as explained by the executive director of High Plains Independence CRO, the value of inclusive participatory leadership is especially important in difficult situations such as medical emergencies and organizational transitions:

> Most of the tasks that run the center are done by paid staff. But if the paid staff doesn't take care of them then everybody just pitches in and does what needs to be done. I know we have had staff in the hospital at times and they will just have something where they pull a task out of a bowl and just say this is your task for the night.

Another vehicle for developing strong statewide consumer leadership is MHCRONK, which provides assistance to CROs and advocates for consumer-run services to the state legislature. Their efforts have helped Kansas CROs gain recognition for their larger role in outreach for Medicaid and other services. As a result of their contributions, CRO leaders are also being asked to assist in Medicaid-funded program planning and policy development for the improvement of coordination and delivery of medical and mental health services to individuals and families at the state and national level.

13.8.3 Fostering a Mental Health System that Prioritizes Consumer Leadership

Wider recognition and understanding of the importance of leadership in the consumer movement in Kansas has been created by providing opportunities for consumer leaders to connect with each other through the MHCRONK, the Recovery Conference, Adult Mental Health Consumer Advisory Council (CAC), and the Leadership Academy. Rather than operating as isolated nonprofits with issues central to their CRO, CRO leaders and members have the ability to connect with one another, gain advice, insight, and support. With many of the CROs in Kansas being in rural areas, the MHCRONK helps counteract feelings of isolation and creates a collective identity for the CROs. MHCRONK's educational role regarding state legislators and mental health care administrators is also normalizing because it is based not on the experience of mental illness but on the experiences of leading a nonprofit.

13.9 Conclusion

CROs have been central to the consumer movement in Kansas. Although CROs started as small grassroots self-help organizations, through their own growth and development, they have had significant and beneficial impact on the mental health system, as well as the individual members involved. These important changes were possible because of the collaborative work between CROs, CCSR, and SRS. CCSR, an intermediary between SRS and CROs has played an important role in facilitating and maintaining this 10-year partnership, which has helped in creating strong consumer leaders, strong CROs, and a stronger mental health system.

Acknowledgment The authors wish to thank the Kansas Department of Social and Rehabilitation Services (SRS), the National Institute of Mental Health (NIMH), and the Substance Abuse and Mental Health Services Administration (SAMHSA) for their support throughout the years for this work.

References

Brown, L. D., Collins, V., Shepherd, M. D., Wituk, S. A. & Meissen, G. (2004). Photovoice and consumer-run mutual support organizations. *International Journal of Self Help and Self Care,* 2(4), 339–344.

Brown, L. D., Shepherd, M. D., Merkle, E., Wituk, S. A., & Meissen, G. (2008). Understanding how participation in a consumer-run organization relates to recovery. *American Journal of Community Psychology,* 42(1), 167–178.

Brown, L. D., Shepherd, M. D., Wituk, S. A., & Meissen, G. (2007). Goal achievement and the accountability of consumer-run organizations. *The Journal of Behavioral Health Services & Research,* 31(4), 73–82.

Center for Community Support and Research (2007). *2007 Track and trend report.* WSU Center for Community Support and Research, Wichita, KS.

Corrigan, P. W., Slopen, N., Gracia, G., Phelan, S., Keogh, C. B., & Keck, L. (2005). Some recovery processes in mutual-help groups for persons with mental illness; II: Qualitative analysis of participant interviews. *Community Mental Health Journal,* 41(6), 721–735.

Mowbray, C., & Moxley, D. (1997). Future for empowerment of consumer role innovation. In C. Mowbray, D. Moxley, C. Jasper, & L. Howell (Eds.), *Consumers as Providers in Psychiatric Rehabilitation* (pp. 518–525). Columbia, MD: International Association of Psychosocial Rehabilitation Services.

Mowbray, C. T., Robinson, E. A., & Holter, M. C. (2002). Consumer drop-in centers: Operations, services, and consumer involvement. *Health and Social Work,* 27, 248–261.

Mowbray, C. T., & Tan, C. (1993). Consumer-operated drop-in centers: Evaluation of operations and impact. *Journal of Mental Health Administration,* 20(1), 8–19.

Nelson, G., Ochocka, J., Janzen, R., & Trainor, J. (2006a). A longitudinal study of mental health consumer/survivor initiatives: Part I. *Journal of Community Psychology* 34(3), 247–260.

Nelson, G., Ochocka, J., Janzen, R., & Trainor, J. (2006b). A longitudinal study of mental health consumer/survivor initiatives: Part 2 – A quantitative study of impacts of participation on new members. *Journal of Community Psychology,* 34(3), 261–272.

New Freedom Commission on Mental Health (2003). *Achieving the promise: Transforming mental health care in America. Executive summary* (Publication No. SMA-03-3831). Bethesda, MD: U.S. Department of Health and Human Services.

Ochocka, J., Nelson, G., Janzen, R., & Trainor, J. (2006). A longitudinal study of mental health consumer/survivor initiatives: Part 3 – Impacts of participation on new members. *Journal of Community Psychology,* 34(3), 273–283.

Reinhart, C., Meissen, G., Wituk, S., & Shepherd, M. (2008). Setting level characteristics in consumer-run organizations that enhance member outcomes. *International Journal of Self-Help and Self-Care,* 4(1–2), 137–147.

Shagott, T., Vu, C., Reinhart, C., Wituk, S., & Meissen, G. (2009). Member characteristics of consumer run organizations and service utilization patterns. *International Journal of Self-Help and Self-Care,* 4(3), 221–238.

Shagott, T., Vu, C., Reinhart, C., Wituk, S., & Meissen, G. (2006). Evaluating the impact of participation in consumer run organizations. WSU Center forCommunity Support and Research, Wichita, KS.

Shepherd, M. D. & Brown, L. (2004a). Technical assistance provided to consumer run organizations in 2003. WSU Center for Community Support and Research, Wichita, KS.

Shepherd, M. D., & Brown, L. (2004b). The organizational health of consumer run organizations in Kansas. WSU Center for Community Support and Research, Wichita, KS.

Shepherd, M. D. (2003). Assistance provided to consumer run organizations by self help network: Center for Community Support and Research. WSU Center for Community Support and Research, Wichita, KS.

Silverman, S. H., Blank, M. B., & Taylor, L. C. (1997). On our own: Preliminary findings from a consumer-run service model. *Psychiatric Rehabilitation Journal, 21*(2), 151–159.

Solomon, P. (2004) Peer support/ Peer provided services underlying processes, benefits, and critical ingredients. *Psychiatric Rehabilitation Journal. 27*(4), 392–401.

Trainor, J., Shepherd, M., Boydell, K. M., Leff, A., & Crawford, E. (1997). Beyond the service paradigm: the impact and implications of consumer/survivor initiatives. *Psychiatric Rehabilitation Journal*, 21(2), 132–140.

Wang, C. & Burris, M. A. (1997). Photovoice: Concept, methodology, and use for participatory needs assessment. *Health Education and Behavior, 24*(3), 369–387.

Wang, C. & Redwood-Jones, Y. (2001). Photovoice ethics: Perspectives from Flint Photovoice. *Health Education and Behavior, 28*(5), 560–572.

Young, J. & Williams, C. L. (1987). An evaluation of GROW, a mutual-help community mental health organization. *Community Health Studies, 11*(1), 38–42.

Zinman, S. Harp, H. T., & Budd, S. (1987). *Reaching across: Mental health clients helping each other.* California Network of Mental Health Clients, CA.

Part VI
Self-Help/Professional Collaboration

Chapter 14
Helping Mutual Help: Managing the Risks of Professional Partnerships

Deborah A. Salem, Thomas M. Reischl, and Katie W. Randall

Abstract This chapter addresses the recent trend for mutual-help organizations to form collaborative partnerships with professionally run organizations. The focus of the discussion is a multi-method case study of a partnership between Schizophrenics Anonymous (SA) and the Mental Health Association of Michigan (MHAM) over a 14-year period. This study explores how the evolution of a formal partnership between SA and MHAM influenced the organizational expansion and development of SA. The partnership resulted in increased access to SA groups throughout Michigan. It also resulted in changes in how new SA groups were started, with more new groups in traditional mental health service settings and more groups led by professionals. New groups established with professional leaders had significantly lower survival rates than new groups established with consumer leaders. Qualitative analyses of interviews with SA's consumer leaders suggested that, while SA became a more stable organization, there was an accompanying loss of consumer leadership opportunities, ownership, and control over organizational functions. These results are discussed with regard to the lessons learned for managing mutual-help/professional partnerships. We draw on organizational theories and risk management principles to discuss strategies by which mutual-help organizations can benefit from partnerships with other types of organizations, while minimizing unintended changes to their basic beliefs, processes, and structures.

14.1 Helping Mutual Help: Managing the Risks of Professional Partnerships

Mutual-help organizations for persons with serious mental illness, once characterized by their independence from the traditional mental health system, have become increasingly involved with professionals and with professionally run organizations

---

D.A. Salem (✉)
Department of Health Behavior & Health Education, University of Michigan School of Public Health, Ann Arbor, MI, USA
e-mail: debbysalem@gmail.com

(Ben-Ari, 2002; Shepherd, Schoenberg, Slavich, Wituk, Warren, & Meissen, 1999; Nelson, Janzen, Trainor, & Ochocka, 2008). Originally viewed as alternatives to traditional care (Zinman, 1987), mutual-help organizations are increasingly becoming partners and collaborators with more formal mental health services (Davidson, Chinman, Kloos, Weingarten, Stayner, & Tebes, 1999). Goldstrom and colleagues (2006) conclude from their national survey of mutual-help and consumer-run organizations that "mental health self-help has evolved from its de facto status into the mainstream of the mental health delivery system" (p. 100).

The development of collaborations between mutual-help organizations and professional settings can be attributed to the increased demand for mutual-help groups by consumers and to increased knowledge of and comfort with these groups by professionals. As interest in mutual-help groups grow, there is a natural desire on the part of mutual-help organizations and professional organizations to increase the number of groups available to consumers. For mutual-help organizations, which typically start as small, voluntary organizations (Bargal, 1992), increased demand for groups can create expansion pressure or desire that is beyond the organization's administrative capacity and can stress the resources of both the organization and its leaders. Partnering or collaborating with professionally run organizations is often seen as a viable option for mutual-help organizations that want to expand.

Increased interaction with professionals and with traditional service organizations has many potential implications for the mutual-help experience. Some of these are positive for consumers. Increased acceptance by and integration with the mental health system may increase consumers' exposure and access to mutual-help settings. It may also lead to the adoption of some of the empowering and destigmatizing principles of mutual help by more traditional settings (Davidson et al., 1999). The increased presence of consumers as board members, advisors, and peer counselors in mental health settings is evidence of this effect. Unfortunately, the risks of institutionalization and cooptation for mutual-help settings through interaction and partnerships with professionals, is also great (Borkman, 1999; Gidron & Hasenfeld, 1994; Hasenfeld & Gidron, 1993; Traunstein, 1984).

In this chapter, we summarize a multi-method case study of a partnership between a consumer-run, mutual-help organization and a professionally run organization. Based on lessons learned from this study and others, we also discuss the risks of such partnerships for mutual-help organizations and risk management strategies that could minimize or mitigate some of the risks for mutual-help organizations. We acknowledge partnership risks for professionally run organizations (e.g., liability risks), but our focus is on the risks and risk management strategies for mutual-help organizations. We hope that professionals interested in collaborating with mutual-help organizations and researchers will also find our analysis helpful for understanding the risks to mutual-help organizations and for seeking ways to support consumer leaders in mitigating these risks.

To date, most of the published literature on professional/mutual-help interaction has focused on the interactions between individual professionals and mutual-help groups or organizations (e.g., Hasenfeld & Gidron, 1993). Scholars have explored professionals' roles in mutual-help groups (e.g., Kurtz, 1990; Shepherd et al., 1999;

Stewart, Banks, Crossman, & Poel, 1994; Toseland & Hacker, 1982), professionals' views of mutual-help groups (e.g., Kurtz, Mann & Chambon, 1987; Meissen, Mason, & Gleason, 1991; Stewart et al., 1994), mutual-help members' views of professional involvement (e.g., Chinman, Kloos, O'Connell, & Davidson, 2002; Lotery & Jacobs, 1994; Stewart et al., 1994), and mechanisms of successful collaboration with professionals (e.g., Chinman et al., 2002; Gartner, 1997; Olson et al., 2005; Toseland & Hacker, 1982).

The few studies that have explored the effects of professional involvement on mutual-help groups have found clear differences between mutual-help groups that do and do not have professional involvement with regard to group process (Cherniss & Cherniss, 1985; Toro et al., 1988), activities (Shepherd et al., 1999; Yoak & Chessler, 1985), associations with other organizations (Shepherd et al., 1999), and survival (Maton, Leventhal, Madara, & Julien, 1989).

While it is clear that professional involvement may strongly influence the nature of mutual-help groups, past debate on whether professionals should be involved in mutual-help is being replaced by a focus on the nature and effects of professional involvement (Ben-Ari, 2002).

In order to understand the implications of this involvement, we must move beyond our past focus on the interactions between individual professionals and mutual-help groups, to study the more extensive collaborations and partnerships between mutual-help organizations and professionally run organizations (e.g., social service agencies, advocacy organizations, HMOs). These relationships are often more direct and more sustained and have the potential to transform mutual-help settings.

Organizational theories have directed our attention to how the beliefs and demands in the organizational environment can influence the values, structures, practices, and life course of organizations (Gidron & Hasenfeld, 1994). Institutional theorists have long argued that in order to increase their legitimacy and access to resources, organizations within the same organizational sector come to look and behave like other organizations in that sector (DiMaggio & Powell, 1983; Meyer & Rowan, 1977). Drawing from institutional theory, Salem (1996) argued that as mutual-help organizations interact closely with organizations in other sectors (e.g., mental health); they are subject to the same institutional pressures and may experience significant changes in their structures, ideologies, and activities. Simply managing a cooperative relationship with a traditionally structured organization requires a structural predictability and stability that is not typical of mutual-help organizations (Gidron & Hasenfeld, 1994). Bargal (1992) argued that, unlike more formal (professional) organizations, mutual-help organizations often aspire to remain forever at the *collectivity* stage of development, which is characterized by informal communication and structure. This informality is incompatible with the structures required for inter-organizational collaborations. Although the nature of interactions between mutual-help organizations and professionally run organizations is changing, our knowledge of how such collaborations develop or influence the ideology, growth, or structure of mutual-help organizations is limited.

To explore the effects of professional partnerships on mutual-help organizations, we draw on almost two decades of collaboration with Schizophrenics Anonymous (SA), a mutual-help organization for individuals with a schizophrenia-related illness. We had the opportunity to observe and study an evolving partnership between SA and the Mental Health Association in Michigan (MHAM), a not-for-profit, professionally run mental health advocacy organization that supported SA's development. Guided by institutional (Meyer & Rowan, 1977) and resource dependence (Pfeffer & Salanick, 1978) theories, we used a combined qualitative/quantitative methodology to study the intended and unintended consequences of this collaboration. We were interested in understanding the evolution of the partnership and its effects on SA and MHAM (for more details, see Salem, Reischl, & Randall, 2008).

14.2 Case Study: Schizophrenics Anonymous (SA) and the Mental Health Association of Michigan (MHAM)

Our study of a partnership between SA and MHAM was part of a larger evaluation study of the SA organization. It began 12 years after the founding of the first SA group, when MHAM received a grant that allowed them to devote full-time equivalent staffing to assist SA with organizational expansion and new group development and to evaluate that effort. Our initial intention was to study the process and outcome of this 3-year expansion effort. One year into the study, however, we became aware that SA was changing its approach to expansion and new group development as a result of working with MHAM. After discussions with leaders from SA and MHAM, we decided to study the newly funded expansion in the context of SA's history of development and partnership with MHAM. In our qualitative and quantitative case study, we collected retrospective data (through archival records and interviews) on SA's development during its first 11 years and then followed SA's expansion and development prospectively for three additional years (years 12–14). These methods allowed us to study a naturally evolving partnership and to compare SA's organizational growth and development before and after formalizing their partnership with MHAM.

14.2.1 Methods

Data came from four sources: (a) interviews with SA organizational leaders, (b) interviews with MHAM staff, (c) archival data, and (d) attendance at organizational meetings and events.

14.2.1.1 Interviews with SA Organizational Leaders

Based on our previous association with SA, we generated a list of SA members who we had observed to be involved in organizational development (e.g., regularly attended organizational leadership meetings, involved in organizational-level decision-making). The leaders on our list independently identified the same four people as SA's primary leaders, or in their words – "Central SA leaders."[1] The Central SA leaders participated in two telephone interviews, a year apart. A fifth SA leader, who was later hired by MHAM to work on SA expansion, was interviewed once. These semi-structured interviews focused on interviewees' roles as SA leaders and SA's organizational structure, leadership, and expansion efforts. All five also participated in more in-depth interviews regarding their personal experience in SA as part of the larger study. Interviews were audio taped. All of the leaders were middle aged and white. Three were female.

14.2.1.2 Interviews with MHAM Staff

Beginning in year 6, one MHAM staff member took primary responsibility for working with SA on group and organizational development. Over a 3-year period, he participated in 21 interviews regarding these efforts. The executive director of MHAM participated in one interview regarding the history of the development of MHAM's relationship with SA. Both were white men with professional training. Neither was a mental health consumer.

14.2.1.3 Archival Data

We reviewed SA literature (e.g., newsletters, correspondence, brochures, training manuals, grant proposals) in order to better understand expansion and leadership support activities. In addition, all letters written by MHAM in response to inquires for information about SA for years 8 through 13 were coded for *type of request* and *recipient*.

14.2.1.4 Attendance at Organizational Meetings and Events

Over a 3-year period, research team members attended and wrote field notes about organizational meetings and events related to SA's expansion and development. We attended three annual conferences, an organizational planning retreat, 23 of 30 organizational leadership meetings, and SA community and conference presentations.

14.2.1.5 Qualitative Analysis of Interview Data

Interview transcripts were transcribed verbatim, checked for accuracy, and then formatted and imported into NU*DIST, a computer software package for qualitative

---

[1] At this stage of SA's organizational development the term "Central SA" leader was used to refer to a self-identified group of SA leaders who formed the leadership core of SA. This was the group who saw themselves as responsible for SA's programmatic and organizational development. The term "Central SA" took on a different meaning later in SA's development, referring to SA's national leadership group.

research. We used inductive content analysis to identify descriptive codes across participants (Patton, 2002). One research team member, who was very familiar with the interviews, read each document and constructed a preliminary set of content codes. Two other research team members reviewed and helped revise the code categories and the data was recoded. The team then worked together to identify higher order themes. We reviewed the final content themes and example quotes with MHAM staff and SA leaders to ensure the credibility of the analysis (Patton, 2002).

14.2.1.6 Documenting Group Development

To track new SA group development, we studied archival documents that referenced the status of specific SA groups (e.g., all SA newsletters) and interviewed SA organizational and group leaders and MHAM staff. From these sources, we recorded four variables reflecting each group's longevity and geographic location: *start date, closing date, distance in miles from original SA group*, and *county*. We also recorded two variables describing the group's connection to the traditional mental health system: *type of group leader*[2] (mental health service consumer, professional service provider, or co-led by consumer and professional) and *type of group setting* where the group met (community non-service settings, community-based mental health service settings, or institutional settings). Finally, we recorded *leader experience with a "Central SA group."* Central SA group was a term used early in SA's development for groups led by one of SA's self-identified leadership core. The Central SA groups formed the core of the organization. Prior to formal leadership training initiated by MHAM, these groups served as the training ground for new SA leaders.

Using all data sources, we verified that 64 SA groups had operated for some period during SA's first 14 years. Forty-two groups were active during years 12–14 when we conducted the study. Data for these 42 groups was collected from either the group's leader ($n = 34$) or from archival records that were then confirmed by one of SA's organizational leaders ($n = 8$). We collected retrospective data on the 22 groups that closed before our study began. Due to missing data, sample sizes for different study questions varied between 56 and 60 groups.

Our case study focused on four questions: (a) How did the partnership relationship between SA and MHAM develop? (b) How did the partnership affect SA's strategy for group development and SA group survival? (c) How did the partnership affect SA's organizational development? (d) How did the partnership affect MHAM?

---

[2]Professionals were used at times to start groups, with the goal of developing consumer leadership over time. For some this was part of paid employment at their service agency/institution; others volunteered their time. All consumer leaders were volunteers.

14.2.2 The Development of the SA – MHAM Partnership

The seed for a relationship between SA and MHAM was planted a year before the start of SA, when Joanne Verbanic[3] (SA's founder) became a volunteer for MHAM. She explained

> I knew what it was like to be ... so sick and I knew what it was like to be well. I wanted to share that experience .... I had no idea of starting a group. I thought I'd just stuff envelopes. After a few meetings [with the MHAM executive director] ... I was asked to appear on [*The Sally Jesse Raphael Show*] .... I went public to help erase the stigma.

Soon after "going public," Joanne decided to start a self-help group. Using her own money, she advertised in a local newspaper stating that she was starting a self-help group for persons with schizophrenia. Two people responded and the first meetings occurred around tables at a local restaurant and a public park. Even though Joanne had gone public with her illness, the group decided to maintain anonymity in the Alcoholics Anonymous tradition. They named the group Schizophrenics Anonymous. When the colder autumn weather came, the executive director of MHAM suggested that the group meet in the board room of the MHAM building on Sunday afternoons. A member of the first group recalls, "The whole time, he was taking a real risk. He's giving us the keys to the building .... Here we have, you know, 15, 20 people with this illness which has got a bad rep [reputation]."

With the assistance of MHAM, Joanne publicized the group. She recruited an MHAM staff member to help her write a pamphlet and MHAM paid for the printing. Joanne used her own money to mail the pamphlets to all of the psychiatrists in the Detroit telephone book. She continued to speak publicly about schizophrenia and about the new SA group. Attendance at the SA meetings was sporadic during the first year, but after several local TV appearances and newspaper articles featuring Joanne and the SA group, attendance grew and became more stable. This first group remained the only SA group for 2 years. As organizational needs arose, a larger leadership group began to form. Driven by the desire to reach out to more people with schizophrenia, several members of this original group started new groups in nearby communities. During the next 3 years, eight new SA groups were started – six of the new group leaders were members of the first SA group.

During the 5th year, MHAM provided financial support to produce a video about SA. As Joanne described, it was an important event in the development of SA's partnership with MHAM

> I asked [the MHAM executive director] ... I was nervous ... I said, "What would you think if I did a video and it cost $3,000?" I wanted it professionally done ... and he liked the idea .... We had to prove to him that people with schizophrenia could have their own group .... He was society, and most people in society think people with schizophrenia can't do anything. You know, they're vegetables. So he bought into the situation.

---

[3] With her permission, Joanne Verbanic is the only person identified by her real name. All other persons are identified with pseudonyms.

During these early years, SA was in what Quinn and Cameron (1983) identify as the *entrepreneurial* stage of organizational development, characterized by innovation, resource mobilization, lack of planning and coordination, power in the hands of a prime mover, and niche creation. Joanne, the prime mover, coordinated the development of new groups and new member recruitment.

As SA continued to grow and develop, it entered the *collectivity* stage, characterized by informal communication and structure, a sense of collectivity, investment of long hours, commitment, a sense of mission, and continued innovation. Joanne continued to lead the original group and became SA's primary organizational leader. Most of the other group leaders had stayed in regular contact with members of the original group. They held periodic organizational leader meetings to discuss issues related to their SA groups and to write the organization's first publication. They called these gatherings "group consciousness meetings." Some of the participants became SA's organizational leaders. Joanne recalled the development of this leadership group in spiritual terms

> You know how God works? People just come to your life ... I believe in serendipity ... Bill comes to a meeting, he hears about it. And Bill said, "When I came to SA ... I knew this is where I belonged." I had no idea he had talents to write. And then Janine ... said we need to, you know, we just had a mimeograph sheet of paper with the steps [SA's six-step program] on it. We needed to get a booklet or something .... So I suggested to Bill and his eyes lit up .... And so we met for 8 months in group consciousness meetings every 2 weeks, and they weren't just leaders [SA members contributed as well].

Bill described the cooperation among SA members involved in these efforts

> A lot of people were involved. We met every 2 weeks .... I would tape the discussions, take it home, and write drafts and Ted wrote some very important parts ... .And then ... [we] would go back with what we had written. It was kind of a group process ... there were a lot of people involved in the ideas .... There was Missy and Jack and Ned, who isn't around anymore ... about five or six people at [each] meeting.

After finishing the SA booklet in 1988, Bill assumed the responsibility for editing a SA newsletter. Started as a single-issue publication, with the approval of other members, Bill continued to edit and write most of the copy for a newsletter that was published twice a year.

During this period, MHAM had an informal, but supportive relationship with SA. MHAM provided space for group meetings and social events and paid for the production of the SA literature and videos. As the publication projects became more involved, MHAM donated staff time to assist in these productions. Perhaps most importantly for SA's expansion, MHAM provided members with opportunities to speak at public events and to the media.

These opportunities to publicize SA led to a pivotal event. During SA's 5th year, an article on schizophrenia appeared in the popular magazine, *Cosmopolitan*, featuring SA's founder (Joanne) and her recovery story. It included a telephone number and address for contacting SA – the telephone number and address of MHAM. The article elicited a large number of calls and letters requesting information and support for starting SA groups.

Both MHAM and the SA leaders recognized the limits to SA's capacity to respond to this sudden demand for information and assistance. Joanne requested that MHAM staff share the responsibility for supporting the development of new groups with SA. During this time, SA and MHAM leaders made several decisions that shaped the partnership between SA and MHAM. First, SA would retain its independent status; it would not become one of MHAM's programs. Second, SA's founder and SA leaders would continue to make programmatic decisions (e.g., those regarding the structure and content of SA meetings). MHAM staff members, however, began to assist directly in responding to information requests and assisting with the development of new groups and new leaders. While SA maintained its independence with regard to the content of its program, this marked *the beginning of a more formal partnership* between SA and MHAM and a division of responsibilities that would influence the future development of SA.

Over time, MHAM's increased role created pressure to solicit external funding for the staff time, travel, and materials needed to assist SA. This funding (coupled with increased interest in SA from around the State of Michigan) created external pressure on SA and MHAM to focus on expansion. This focus was consistent with SA's mission to reach out to others (Schizophrenics Anonymous, 1992) and SA welcomed MHAM's support securing funds for expansion. SA's leaders decided that they did not have the capacity to become an effective non-profit corporation. They decided to have MHAM become the fiduciary body for SA because MHAM had grant writing ability, accounting, and administrative capacity that SA did not. The collaboration continued to grow after MHAM started to obtain external grants targeted to the expansion of SA groups throughout Michigan in SA's 6th year. These grants allowed MHAM to devote more staff time to assisting SA in responding to requests for information and helping support the development of new SA groups (see Table 14.1).

Starting in SA's 12th year, the Ethel and James Flinn Family Foundation awarded MHAM a 3-year grant of nearly $300,000 for the purpose of developing new SA groups throughout Michigan and building consumer leadership capacity in SA. The large amount of this award allowed MHAM to assign increased professional staff time, as well as part-time clerical support, to the development of SA. In addition to paying for MHAM staff time, MHAM hired SA consumer leaders (through personal contracts) to provide part-time organizational development assistance. Finding SA leaders to serve in this role proved to be challenging, as it was somewhat inconsistent with their previous emphasis on volunteer leadership. Most leaders preferred to maintain their status as volunteers.

14.2.3 Impact of the Partnership on Group Development

The influx of external funding created both the capacity and the demand to start more SA groups, leading to a shift in SA's approach to new group development. Prior to receiving external funding, SA had expanded primarily through a process

Table 14.1 The association between MHAM external funding and involvement with SA and the development of SA groups in Michigan

Year	Total grant amounts	Changes in MHAM's involvement with SA	New groups	Closed groups	Ongoing groups[a]
1		First SA group starts meeting at MHAM office	1		1
2					1
3		Publishes SA pamphlet	2		3
4		Publishes SA booklet	4		7
5		Produces SA video presentation Fields *Cosmopolitan* article inquiries	2		9
6[b]	$7,000	**Formal collaboration begins** Part-time MHAM staff assigned to SA	5		14
7	$7,000		3	3	14
8	$21,500		4	3	15
9	$39,866	MHAM staff time increased Convenes group consciousness meetings	9	2	22
10	$41,624	MHAM staff time increased to .50 FTE	4	3	23
11	$18,400		9	5[c]	27
12	$97,605	MHAM staff time increased to 1.00 FTE[d] Hires SA member part-time Starts hosting annual leadership conference	7	3	33
13	$99,169	Begins exploring national expansion strategies	7	6	32
14	$98,592		3	10	25[e]
		Totals	60	35	

[a] A group was counted as ongoing if it met at any time during the year
[b] Bold denotes start of more formal partnership
[c] One of the groups included in this total closed in either year 10 or year 11
[d] At this time MHAM staff starts to focus on leadership support and development as well as expansion
[e] Four of these groups closed at some point during this year

of internal leadership development. As existing SA members developed leadership skills, a desire to test their wings, and a desire to reach out to others with schizophrenia, they started their own SA groups. As described by one leader

> I went to [the first SA group] for 2 years and by that time I decided that I was ready to start my own group, after being in a group for 2 years and listening to Joanne lead. I was [in school] at the time ... and I said, you know, it'd be really good practice for me to lead a group.

With the increased involvement of MHAM, SA's expansion strategy became both more targeted and more reactive. Potential locations for new SA groups were identified either through the expression of outside interest or MHAM's targeting of geographic locations without an SA group. New leaders came primarily from outside of SA – consumers or professionals who had not attended SA groups before. MHAM supplied new leaders with guidelines and training materials in order to start groups.

In partnership with MHAM, SA began a new period of rapid organizational expansion. Table 14.1 summarizes the number of new groups established in Michigan during each year, the number of groups that were closed during each year (a group was considered closed if it had no meetings during the entire year), and the number of ongoing or continuing SA groups.[4] It is clear from the tabulation of new groups in Table 14.1 that increases in external funding and in the level of MHAM's involvement were associated with larger numbers of new SA groups established in Michigan. Following the start of the formal collaboration (year 6), 51 new SA groups (with known start dates) were established. While the number of group closings also increased over the years, the number of ongoing groups more than tripled during this period.

To understand the effect of the formal collaboration with MHAM on SA's expansion, we conducted cross-tabulations comparing SA groups that were established before and after the collaboration began (year 6) on geographic expansion (distance in miles from original SA group and county), type of group setting, and type of group leader. Year 6 marked the start of the formal partnership between SA and MHAM, when MHAM designated a portion of a staff member's time to work with SA and received external grant funding to support this work. As seen in Table 14.2, SA and MHAM were successful in increasing the availability of SA groups throughout Michigan. Before year 6, all but one of the new groups established were in close proximity (within 25 miles) of the first SA group. After year 6, there was a statistically significant difference in the percentage of SA groups established more than 25 miles away from SA's first group (the MHAM office). Before year 6, SA groups met in only four counties. After year 6, SA groups met in 25 Michigan counties.

While SA and MHAM were successful in spreading SA over a much broader geographic area, there were accompanying changes in the nature of the groups. There was a statistically significant difference in the type of settings where groups were established. Before year 6, 44% of the group meetings met in community (non-service) settings (e.g., community building, church). After year 6, the percent of groups meeting in community (non-service) settings dropped to 12%. The percent of groups meeting in community-based, mental health service settings (e.g., community mental health center, drop-in center) increased slightly and the percent

---

[4]While the primary focus of SA's expansion was in Michigan, between years 6 and 14, SA and MHAM also responded to requests from outside Michigan. In the latter years of this study, an increasing amount of MHAM staff time was devoted to group development outside of Michigan.

Table 14.2 Comparison of SA groups started before and after formal collaboration

| | SA groups started | | |
Group variable	Before collaboration	After collaboration	χ^2 Test (df)
Proximity to first SA group/MHAM office[a]			
Less than 25 miles	6 (75%)	15 (29%)	6.27* (df = 1)
More than 25 miles	2 (25%)	36 (71%)	
Type of group setting			
Community (non-service)	4 (44%)	6 (12%)	6.08* (df = 2)
Community-based mental health service	4 (44%)	28 (56%)	
Institutional	1 (11%)	16 (32%)	
Type of group leader			
Consumer leader	7 (88%)	29 (60%)	2.19 (df = 1)
Professional leader or co-leader	1 (12%)	19 (40%)	
Group leader's association with Central SA groups			
Former leader or member of a Central SA group	7 (78%)	14 (28%)	8.24** (df = 1)
Never member Central SA group	2 (12%)	36 (72%)	

[a]The first SA group met at the MHAM office and was excluded from this analysis
*$p < 0.05$, **$p < 0.01$

of groups meeting in institutional settings (hospitals, correctional facilities) almost tripled.

Although the increase of new SA groups in mental health treatment settings provided access for more persons with schizophrenia, it resulted in an increased involvement with mental health professionals. The number of groups that had a professional leader or co-leader went from 12 to 40%. The chi-square test for this difference, however, was not statistically significant. The expansion into new geographic regions was also associated with starting more groups with leaders who had never attended a Central SA group. This was the primary leadership training ground prior to year 6, when seven of the nine groups (78%) had leaders who had attended or led one of the Central SA groups. After year 6, significantly fewer (28%) of the new groups had a leader with any experience with one of the Central SA groups.

14.2.4 SA Group Survival Analysis

Because over half of the Michigan SA groups eventually closed and because all of the closings occurred after year 6, we conducted survival analyses to explore whether the partnership with MHAM and the increased use of professional leaders and professional service settings affected how long groups survived. Survival analysis can model the timing of a discrete change. It can be used for predicting change events (i.e., group closing) even if the event has not yet occurred for a substantial number of groups (see Luke, 1993). The dependent measure in the survival analysis was the amount of time between the start date and the closing date scaled in months[5]. The predictor variables for these analyses included: *whether the group start date was before or after MHAM increased its involvement in year 6, type of group setting*, and *type of group leader*. Group comparisons in survival were estimated using the Kaplan-Meier method and the log-rank test of group differences (Kaplan & Meier, 1958; Mantel, 1966).

The range of survival times for the sample of 59 SA groups included in these analyses was 2–160 months. The median survival time was 34 months (95% CI: 28.0–40.0). The survival function and hazard function curves revealed (a) a high rate of group closings during their first 3 years and (b) groups lasting more than 3 years had a much slower rate of closings.

The comparative survival analyses revealed a wide variability of the estimated median survival times (see Table 14.3). Groups that started before year 6 had a longer median survival period than groups started after year 6, but the confidence intervals were overlapping and the difference was not statistically significant. Likewise, the median survival period for SA groups started in the community (non-service) settings was shorter than SA groups started in community-based, mental health service settings or in institutional settings, but the differences were not significant. Only the comparison of SA groups led by consumers vs. groups with professional leadership revealed a statistically significant difference: groups led

Table 14.3 Comparisons of Survival Time of SA Groups

Group variable	Median survival time (in months)	95% CI	Log-rank test
Group start date			
Before collaboration ($n = 8$)	48	27.7–68.3	$\chi^2 = 1.97$
After collaboration ($n = 51$)	31	20.0–42.1	
Type of group setting			
Community (non-service) ($n = 10$)	24	17.9–30.1	$\chi^2 = .52$
Community-based mental health service ($n = 32$)	36	28.6–43.4	
Institutional ($n = 17$)	34	18.4–49.7	
Type of Group Leader			
Consumer leader ($n = 36$)	36	21.6–50.5	$\chi^2 = 4.21^*$
Professional leader or co-leader (20)	26	8.5–43.4	

*$p < .05$

---

[5] For the groups that had not closed by the end of year 14, the group survival time was the amount of time between the start date and the end of year 14.

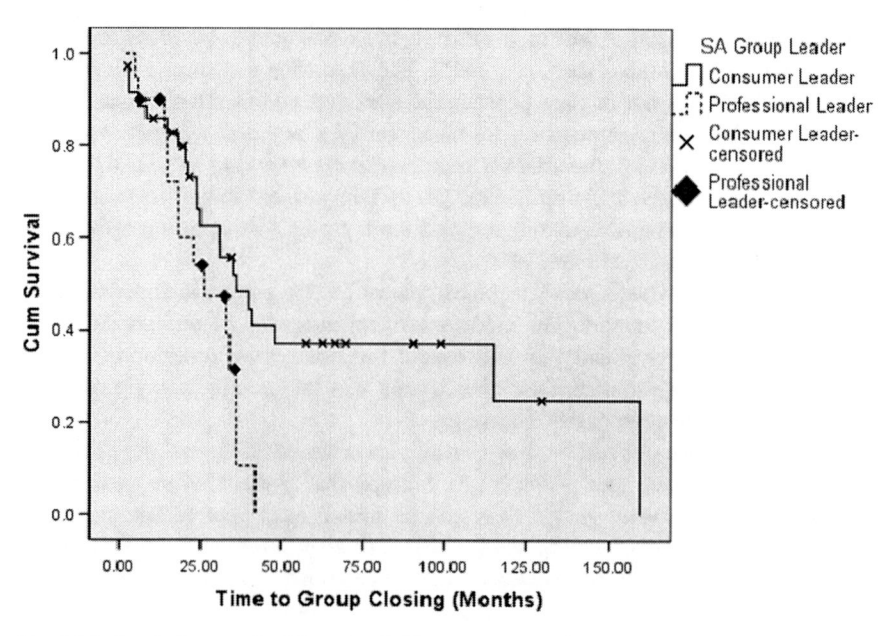

Fig. 14.1 Survival curves for SA groups led by consumers or by professionals

by a consumer were more likely to survive longer than groups led or co-led by professionals.

The survival curves for the SA groups led by consumers and by professional leaders are illustrated in Fig. 14.1. The curves suggest that the group survival probabilities are similar for the first 3 years, but that consumer-led SA groups have a greater probability of surviving beyond 3 years.

14.2.5 Impact of the Partnership on Organizational Development

We studied the influence of the partnership on organizational development using qualitative methods. By year 12, the organizational structure of SA had changed substantially. Joanne Verbanic was still leading SA's first group and continued to be the most influential consumer leader in SA. A professional MHAM staff member was working full-time on SA's development, however, and had taken over much of the leadership responsibility for SA's organizational functions. The MHAM office received and responded to all inquiries about starting SA groups. MHAM now initiated efforts to generate funding, start new groups, and support existing leaders. In essence, while the SA members continued to control the SA program (e.g., the structure and content of the meetings), MHAM was now responsible for the administration of SA's organizational development.

While SA members and leaders still had an important voice in the organization, the nature of their contribution began to change. The monthly group consciousness meetings continued to be the setting for SA leaders to provide input and to volunteer for organizational tasks, but the meetings were now facilitated by the MHAM staff member. In addition, MHAM hired a few SA leaders to assist the MHAM staff with organizational development. At this point SA could be described as moving into the life-cycle stage of *formalization and control* (Quinn & Cameron, 1983). During this stage, there is the development of a stable structure and the formalization and institutionalization of rules and procedures.

In our qualitative analysis, a grounded theory approach (Corbin & Strauss, 2008) was used to identify changes experienced by SA's organizational leaders. Themes emerged regarding, both (a) observed changes to SA's structure and (b) leaders' concerns about these changes. Leaders described five key changes to the structure of SA, all of which were consistent with movement to the stage of formalization and control: (a) *increased control in the hands of one individual*, (b) *a more bureaucratic structure*, (c) *greater consistency*, (d) *greater administrative capacity*, and (e) *greater response capacity*.

All of the SA leaders noted that there was *increased control in the hands of one individual*, the MHAM staff member. One described him as "the most influential person ... the hub of SA ... the leader, who works with Joanne and Bill." Another said, "He is our unity and strength. He keeps it together ... He keeps it all organized."

SA also developed a *more bureaucratic structure*, compared by one leader to a business

[The MHAM staff member] would be the chief administrative officer, Joanne would be the chief executive officer and primary decision maker, Wendy would be like the executive assistant or the chairman of the board of directors – whoever it is who does the administrative work and would answer to [MHAM staff member]. The Group Consciousness Meeting would be like the board of directors.

This new structure had a variety of influences on the SA organization, which SA leaders viewed positively. The partnership provided SA with *greater consistency*, helping leaders to overcome feelings of discouragement and burnout. As one leader described the MHAM staff member, "He is our guiding light. We rely on him for organizing actual stuff. [I am] glad he is there to help keep it going." Another described her sense of relief in having someone to count on

There are 2.5 million people [in the U.S.] with schizophrenia and there are so many people out there that need help.... And so Bill and I starting thinking...how are we going to distribute? It was just Bill and I mostly...and then Bill got tired. You know, it seemed like it was Bill and I all the time that had all the responsibility. And Ted too...you get burned out. You can't do everything...We gotta have people to take over.

The increased involvement of the MHAM staff member also helped SA to develop a *greater administrative capacity*. One member explained

It was good for the administration of the program because [the MHAM staff member] had administrative skills that I never wanted to have.... And it became more of a polished organization because really, we used to laugh...that the organizational file system of SA existed within Joanne's purse.... She had, you know, a bunch of stuff in a big purse.... [The MHAM staff member's] contribution pretty early was to develop administrative capacity for SA.

Finally, the involvement of MHAM gave SA *greater response capacity*. It enabled SA to respond to the high level of interest and requests for information. During years 8–13[6] MHAM staff provided written responses and/or literature to 752 individuals and organizations in Michigan, the rest of the United States, and around the world. In addition, they answered an untold number of phone inquiries. SA could never have responded to this level of interest on their own. As one leader said, this would have been particularly true outside of Michigan

> One of [the MHAM staff member's] real accomplishments has been to coordinate the development of the out-of-state groups and include their leaders in a sort of cadre of SA leadership. It's not just a Detroit area thing anymore.

Unfortunately, this administrative relief and enhanced capacity to respond to inquiries had associated costs. SA's organizational leaders expressed mixed feelings about MHAM's increasing responsibility for managing SA's development. They expressed concerns about: (a) *the more formal, hierarchical structure of SA*; (b) *increased professional involvement*; (c) *decreased consumer control*; and (d) *too much focus on group development and not enough on supporting existing groups*. One leader described the changes in idealism he experienced as SA *developed a more formalized, hierarchical structure*

> I was worried it was getting too big time ... I was concerned, there was kind of a group [who] were kind of pining for the early days, I guess. Kind of, there was less, maybe it was less polished, still more of that old idealism.

Another leader noted his relief after giving up a paid position working for MHAM to support SA and returning to a volunteer role, "I feel a lot better, more like the old idealism, now that I'm not getting a paycheck."

Leaders expressed dissatisfaction with their experience of *increased professional involvement* in SA. This included the growing power of the MHAM staff member

> The group consciousness meeting was nothing but [the MHAM staff member] reporting to the rest of us what he's doing and what he's going to do. There's no real involvement .... I wonder why I go sometimes. Sometimes I'm angry when I leave the meetings .... I try to go because I want to be involved and I'm interested. But then when I leave, I think what did I come here for?

They were also concerned about the increased presence of professionals as SA group leaders

> [The MHAM staff member] likes to deal with professionals. And this is supposed to be a self-help, support group and professionals have never had the illness and the grass roots, the consumers are the ones that should be starting groups and leading them.

As illustrated in the quote above, SA leaders linked increased professional involvement to *decreased consumer control*. They noted the lack of consumer involvement in central SA leadership.

---

[6]In year 8, MHAM started to keep copies of all correspondence they sent out concerning SA.

> When we got together and wrote that blue book and nobody from MHAM helped us with that, except for funding. You know, and there was a big group of people working on it. I mean, right now there's very few people [involved].

One raised the question: "After 11 years, Joanne should have an entourage of recovered schizophrenics willing to help and do what, like Sara is. Why after 11 years isn't there more Saras willing to help? I don't understand."

A decreased role for consumer leaders was echoed in the MHAM staff member's description of the "SA leadership core"

> It's never been defined. And it's kind of loose, but it's referring to the people that have input or offer input into decisions affecting the program whether it be developing guidelines, you know the group consciousness meeting, and that's probably the closest thing to that leadership core right now. I'd say anybody who has come to a group consciousness meeting is part of that leadership core.

This loose description contrasts sharply with the SA leader's ability to clearly identify their "Central SA" leadership core in the early years of SA.

Finally, leaders expressed their concern about *focusing too much on group development and not enough on supporting existing groups*

> In a relatively short period of time, we doubled the number of groups in Michigan .... I had a feeling ... you should really be focusing on, really beefing up, the groups that already exist and as these groups would begin to flourish ... then the word would get around and groups would just be all over the place .... I was really interested in what's happening to the people who are in the groups right now.

While leaders focused on different aspects of the changes in SA, all recognized a less collective, consumer-controlled organization. Most saw both costs and benefits to the partnership.

14.2.6 Reciprocal Influences on MHAM

The influence of organizational partnership was not one-sided. The evolving relationship also shaped MHAM in some unanticipated ways. Based on interviews with the executive director and staff member at MHAM, we identified key ways that the partnership influenced both the internal functioning and external perception of MHAM. Internally, the partnership assisted MHAM in working towards its' own mission of wellness promotion for persons with mental illness by increasing consumer access to SA. MHAM began to *view consumers as resources* for promoting MHAM's mission. It became *more attuned to consumer issues and needs* and developed *increased roles for consumers* within MHAM (e.g., serving on the board of directors, public speaking, involvement in legislative activities). In addition, the grant funding generated by the partnership helped to *support the internal operations* of MHAM.

The partnership also influenced MHAM's relationship with external organizations, increasing MHAM's external *visibility, credibility,* and *access to resources.* The partnership increased MHAM's visibility in Michigan and with the National

Mental Health Association. It improved their relationship with other consumer-run organizations and with all levels of the mental health system in Michigan. MHAM's access to external funding also increased because their role supporting SA made them eligible for service delivery funds.

14.3 Changes in SA

While the partnership accomplished much of what SA had hoped for, it was not without costs to SA's independence from the mental health system or its ability to maintain and develop consumer leadership and control. Consistent with SA's goals, the rate of growth of SA groups increased rapidly and the accessibility of SA to persons in Michigan increased dramatically. In order to accomplish this, however, the new SA groups were more likely to be started in traditional mental health settings and to have professional leaders. Similar changes were evident at the organizational level. SA moved rapidly from the *collectivity* stage of development that characterized its early years, to the *formalization and control* stage (Quinn & Cameron, 1983). This allowed SA to expand and to respond to outside interest in forming groups without overwhelming the consumer leadership. Unfortunately, these changes were accompanied by increased professional control and disenfranchisement of consumer leaders.

The ability of consumer-run organizations, like SA, to create the empowering conditions that facilitate leadership development among consumers is based on their alternative organizational values and structures. Two of the key characteristics of mutual-help organizations that make this possible are (a) an opportunity role structure that is egalitarian, provides permeable and flexible access to valued roles and activities, and provides opportunities to be involved in organizational decision-making (Maton & Salem, 1995; Weaver-Randall & Salem, 2004) and (b) a group-based belief system that is strengths based, recovery inspiring (Maton & Salem, 1995), and values experiential knowledge (i.e., knowledge based on lived experience, Borkman, 1976). The development of a more formal partnership with MHAM appears to have significantly altered these key characteristics of mutual help in SA.

At the group level, the presence of professionals in leadership roles has been found to change the dynamics of mutual-help groups. In a study comparing consumer led GROW groups with groups that were being led by professionals (with the intention of transitioning to consumer leadership), Toro et al. (1988) found significant differences in the social climate of the groups. In our own study of SA's efforts to start groups in forensic settings where a staff "facilitator" was present at all meetings, we found that although staff did not identify themselves as the group leaders, they described themselves as performing most of the leadership functions of the group (Salem & Hughes, 2003). The presence of professional leaders changes the egalitarian and permeable nature of group leadership and introduces a different knowledge base (i.e., professional expertise) to the group (Powell, 1990). The experiential knowledge of members, which is valued in mutual-help groups

(Borkman, 1976; Salem, Reischl, Gallacher, & Randall, 2000), is not possessed by or as highly valued by professionals. Key characteristics that facilitate consumer empowerment are lacking in this context, making the development of consumer leadership extremely difficult. Given staff mobility and limited organizational resources, it is not surprising that SA groups were more likely to close if consumer leadership failed to materialize. This is consistent with Maton et al.'s (1989) findings that, for affiliated mutual-help groups, professional involvement was related to higher closure rates.

At the organizational level, the presence of a professional director and the development of paid consumer jobs also changed the opportunity role structure of the setting – decreasing the egalitarian access to valued roles and responsibilities and diminishing consumer leadership, ownership, and control (Chamberlin, 1990; Zinman, 1987). The permeability of SA's leadership was diminished as the organization's capacity to separate leadership responsibilities from defined leadership roles declined. Access to empowering leadership processes is fundamental to members' experience of mutual-help (Brown, Shepherd, Merkle, Wituk, & Meissen, 2008).

At both the group and the organizational level, the presence of professional leaders, staff, and resources, and the accompanying stability and capacity building, may in and of itself decrease the motivational press for involvement that occurs in under-populated settings (Barker, 1968). The lack of sufficient people to do the needed work can act as a mechanism of empowerment in mutual-help organizations, motivating members to take on new roles and develop new skills (Rappaport, Reischl, & Zimmerman, 1992). While professional leadership and assistance may relieve stress and prevent burnout, it may also decrease the press for this type of leadership engagement among consumers.

While the changes we observed can be attributed, to some extent, to the presence of individual professionals in the groups and organization, organizational theorists argue that settings are also influenced by the resource dependencies (Pfeffer & Salanick, 1978) and beliefs (Meyer & Rowan, 1977; Scott, 1995) in their environments. Both of these appear to be true for SA's partnership with MHAM. Some of the changes SA experienced may have been caused by the complex effects of resource dependencies. For example, when it was decided that MHAM should play a larger role in assisting SA, there was a need to secure external resources to support that effort. As it is easier to obtain external grant money for the development of new initiatives, than for the support of existing programs, the grants SA received funded new group development and the geographical expansion of SA. The internal leadership development process that SA had depended on up until that time was not fast enough, nor geographically diverse enough, to meet this expectation. In response, SA and MHAM developed an expansion strategy that drew on the professional leadership resources available in traditional mental health settings to start new groups throughout the state. This decision changed the nature of SA's relationship to the traditional mental health system from one of being an alternative setting (Cherniss & Deegan, 2000), which viewed itself as an adjunct to traditional care, to a more direct and sustained interaction.

Not all of the changes that occurred in SA were caused by resource dependencies, however. For example, there was no direct expectation from its funders that SA itself become more bureaucratic or that the organizational role of consumer leaders be diminished. In fact, the opposite was true; the foundation that provided most of SA's funding valued the consumer-run nature of SA. These changes were more likely due to the influences of unspoken environmental beliefs and norms that surround the MHAM and the more traditional mental health settings with which SA was now closely aligned. Institutional theorists argue that the values, structures, practices, and life course of organizations are strongly affected by the belief systems in their external environments. These environmental beliefs constitute the shared social reality of an institutional sector (in this case mental health) and are taken for granted by the organizations in that sector (Oliver, 1991). According to institutional theory, organizations come to look like the other organizations that they associate with, because they are rewarded for conforming to unspoken environmental norms with increased resources, legitimacy, and viability (Meyer & Rowan, 1977; Scott, 1995). Although not a service provider, MHAM functioned within the mental health sector. When SA became a partner with MHAM it became subject to pressure to conform to the beliefs, values, and norms of its new environment, the mental health sector. DiMaggio & Powell (1983) suggest that several characteristics of SA's context – high dependence on another organization, limited organizational models, and high levels of professionalism in the organizational environment – increase the likelihood of isomorphism (i.e., becoming more like the other organizations in the organizational environment).

It is difficult to isolate the impact of the partnership on these changes from other organizational decisions and changes. SA had already started the process of expanding before the increased involvement of MHAM, as evidenced by the increased effort to develop new groups, leadership structures, and organizational literature. Growth and changes in SA's organizational structure and processes likely would have occurred even if MHAM had not become more involved. However, because MHAM had a more bureaucratic structure, a history of connection with the traditional mental health system, and was positioned to solicit grant funding, it is likely that the types of changes we observed in SA were influenced by its partnership with MHAM. The views of the SA leadership further corroborated this perspective, increasing our confidence that the differences in structure, organizational sector, and perspective of these two organizations were influential in just how SA expanded and developed following the formalized partnership. While we must be careful in overgeneralizing from SA's experience, we believe that it provides some important lessons that can inform future collaborations.

14.4 Lessons Learned

In seeking to understand what we learned from SA's experience, it is important to note that this partnership was an example of a well-intentioned, careful collaboration, intended to support SA's development while maintaining its independence and integrity. Unlike many traditional mental health service organizations (Anthony, 2000; Deegan, 1988; Nelson et al., 2008), MHAM's internal belief system was not incompatible with that of SA. MHAM describes itself as a "voluntary membership citizens' organization representing a broad base of people working together as an advocate for the mentally ill" (Mental Health Association in Michigan, 2009). Its director and staff respected the capabilities and the experiential knowledge that mental health consumers brought to the organization. From the start, both organizations were conscious of the potential for SA to lose its independence, as evidenced in their decisions that SA would not become a program of MHAM and that SA would maintain full programmatic control. The collaboration was based on mutual trust and respect between SA's founder and the MHAM director. MHAM staff members involved understood the nature of mutual help and were open to evaluation and feedback about the effects of the collaboration. In spite of this, the partnership appears to have changed SA in significant ways.

It is important for mutual-help organization leaders to recognize that, even in the most favorable circumstances, close collaboration with professional organizations is likely to lead to change in the unique structures and processes of mutual-help groups. The more extensive the collaboration and more divergent the organizations, the greater the potential change. For mutual-help organizations, risk and opportunity go hand in hand when collaborating with professional organizations. Indeed, risk may be essential to certain types of progress. The goal for partnerships between mutual-help organizations and professional organizations is not necessarily to avoid all of the risks associated with opportunities, but to learn to anticipate risks, determine which risks are worth taking, and develop strategies for dealing with those risks.

The practice of risk management has long been the domain of for-profit industries, especially the insurance industry (Couchman & Fulop, 2002; Crouhy, Galai, & Mark, 2006). The general principles of risk management, however, are applicable to non-profit organizations (Herman, Head, Jackson, & Fogarty, 2004; Jackson, 2006) and, we argue, to mutual-help organizations as well. Below, we integrate principles of institutional theory with some of the basic principles of risk management and describe how they may apply to managing successful partnerships between mutual-help and professional organizations. In order to protect themselves from unanticipated changes mutual-help organizations should (a) expect change, (b) actively engage in self and environmental assessment, (c) prioritize risk, (d) act to minimize and mitigate risk, and (e) engage in ongoing risk assessment and management (see Table 14.4)

14.4.1 Expect Change

Perhaps the most important lesson to be drawn from SA's experience is that although many of the changes SA underwent were unintended, they were not unpredictable. Organizational theories and past experiences with the institutionalization of alternative settings (e.g., Traunstein, 1984) have taught us that exposure

Table 14.4 Summary of lessons learned about managing partnership risks

Lessons Learned
1. Expect change
2. Actively engage in self-assessment and environmental assessment
3. Prioritize risk
4. Act to minimize and mitigate risk
a. Engage in *compromise* (i.e., bargaining)
b. Engage in *avoidance* (i.e., buffering or escape)
c. Build/strengthen value compatible external environment
d. Build internal capacity
5. Engage in ongoing risk assessment and management

to new environmental beliefs and resource dependencies change organizations. This is particularly true when, like many mutual-help organizations, an organization is lacking in formal structures and strategies for managing institutional influences (Oliver, 1991) and when an organization is highly dependent on another organization for resources or legitimacy (DiMaggio & Powell, 1983). We should assume that mutual-help organizations will be influenced by close and extended interactions with professional organizations.

It is also clear that good intentions alone do not mitigate the powerful forces of institutional beliefs, resource dependencies, and professional training. Given the taken-for-granted nature of many institutional beliefs, individuals and organizations are often not aware of the institutional processes they follow (Oliver. 1991). Mutual awareness that an organization might be changed by a new partnership and a general commitment to try to be sensitive to this, is likely not enough to mitigate it. A more active process of self and environmental assessment and risk management is required to help mutual-help organizations manage these relationships.

14.4.2 Actively Engage in Self-Assessment and Environmental Assessment

Oliver (1991) points out that an organization's ability to exercise strategic choices in the face of institutional pressure can be preempted when the organization is blind to the organizational processes to which it adheres. In order to evaluate the threats that partnerships which alter environmental pressures may hold, mutual-help organizations must first have a clear vision of their own internal belief systems, as well as the structures and processes that support them. As institutional theorists point out, these beliefs and structures can be taken for granted and those involved in the organization can be unaware of them. In order to protect key characteristics, such as consumer leadership or respect for the lived experience of consumers (i.e., experiential knowledge), organizations must be able to articulate their importance. Mutual-help organizations with well-developed mission statements, literatures, program guides, and training materials are more likely to be aware of these organizational characteristics. Those that have not engaged in the process of articulating their mission, processes, and structures should think seriously about engaging in these self-definition activities prior to partnering with other organizations.

In addition to self-assessment, organizations should actively assess the beliefs and structures of both the partnering organization and of the sector it is associated with. Identification of the incompatibilities with partnering organizations and their organizational environments can alert mutual-help organizations to the challenges they face. This can be achieved by exploring the mission statements, literature, and annual reports of the organizations, as well as by observing organizational activities. One of the most important organizational activities to assess is the process by which the partnership itself is developed or negotiated. For example, as part of SA's initial partnership negotiations with MHAM, MHAM developed a set of job descriptions that outlined the roles of MHAM staff and paid SA leaders. SA was concerned that the primary SA leadership job was titled as a "liaison." They expressed this concern to MHAM, suggesting that if the goal of the partnership was to support SA, that the MHAM staff member might more appropriately be considered the liaison. This concern led to a reconsideration of job titles, although in the end, neither the SA leader nor MHAM staff member role was labeled as a liaison.

Nelson et al. (2008) suggest that consumer-run organizations should engage in values clarification and renewal activities, asking themselves: "Who are we and what do we stand for? ... and How are we different from mainstream ... organizations?" (p. 196). After engaging in this assessment process, mutual-help organizations will be better positioned to decide whether or not to proceed with the partnership arrangement. If they proceed, they should be more effective in assessing and managing the associated risks.

14.4.3 Prioritize Risk

Managing risk requires consideration of the severity of risks and the evaluation of their importance. Some risks will have severe consequences, other risks will not. The consumers and professionals responsible for managing the partnership should make these judgments. From our case study, we might conclude that prior to the partnership the risks of losing control over organizational and group development was deemed less severe than other partnership risks (such as losing control of the SA program content) and other risks to SA (such as being overwhelmed by consumer interest in SA groups).

When some of the costs of giving up control over SA's organizational and group development became clear over time, SA and MHAM were again faced with evaluating the importance of these costs and determining a new course of action. SA leaders' feelings of powerlessness over new group development was outweighed, for some leaders, by the relief of increased organizational capacity and decreased stress in their own lives. While efforts to support leadership development were continued and increased (e.g., annual leadership conferences, increased support to group leaders), no significant changes to SA's structure or decision-making processes were made to address SA leaders' sense of disenfranchisement. The survival of new groups, however, was a high priority for everyone involved. When it became clear that new groups were closing more rapidly, decisions were made to change the expansion strategy and minimize the role of professional leaders.

14.4.4 Act to Minimize and Mitigate Risk

While we should anticipate that mutual-help organizations will be influenced by increased interaction with the professional service sector, in some cases changes can be minimized by conscious efforts to manage them. Oliver (1991) describes a variety of strategic responses that organizations employ in response to institutional pressures that are inconsistent with their internal values or functioning. Two of these responses are particularly applicable to mutual-help settings that choose to interact with more professional settings. The first is *compromise*, in particular, *bargaining*. If the organization is aware of the potential changes it will be facing or recognizes unanticipated changes as they occur, it can negotiate to minimize unwanted change. The second approach is *avoidance* (i.e., attempts to preclude conformity). Both *buffering* and *escape* from institutional pressures are avoidance strategies that are potentially applicable to mutual-help/professional partnerships. Buffering refers to the decoupling (i.e., separating) of internal activities from formal structures so they are less available to external influence. Escape refers to an organization exiting the interaction altogether.

Organizations can also mitigate some of the influence of external pressures that are inconsistent with their internal values by strengthening external ties that support their values. Strong links to settings that support a mutual-help organization's mission, such as other consumer-run organizations and self-help networks, can counterbalance incompatible pressures. In a study of how collective advocacy organizations maintained their innovative character, Salem, Foster-Fishman, & Goodkind (2002) found that these organizations worked proactively to create supportive external environments by seeking out individuals, settings, and organizations that supported their mission and philosophy. They did not limit themselves to their local context, going beyond the geographical boundaries of their local communities to create networks that included like-minded individuals, settings, and organizations.

Finally, mutual-help settings can work to build internal capacity with regard to identified risks. Capacity building refers to activities that improve an organization's ability to achieve its goals (De Vita & Fleming, 2001). These can be directed towards improving the skills of individuals and towards strengthening the processes and resources of organizations.

Effective risk management requires planning for prioritized risks. Some risks are unavoidable and their effects should be mitigated. Mutual-help leaders and professionals should develop a set of strategies for preventing or minimizing risks that they believe will have the most severe negative consequences. SA and MHAM made a sincere effort to do this. They recognized that SA's capacity to help its members lay in its consumer-based and controlled program. They understood the risks that SA faced if consumers did not retain control of that program or if their experiential knowledge ceased to guide its development.

SA and MHAM sought to address the risks through bargaining (i.e., negotiation), separating control of the SA program from control of SA's organizational growth and development. The partnership was defined by this separation of responsibilities and everyone seemed to understand that SA leaders, who had been empowered to develop and support new groups, would need to let MHAM staff take over this responsibility. In maintaining control over SA's program, both SA and MHAM believed that the heart of SA was being left in the hands of consumers and the logistics were being turned over to MHAM. The interdependency between organizational program and development and the extensive changes to the structure of SA were not anticipated however.

Given the depth of this partnership, negotiation was not enough. Efforts to buffer SA from the pressures of partnership with MHAM would likely have been more successful. While we believe that, given the goals of the SA–MHAM partnership, to some extent SA's leaders feelings of powerlessness over organizational operations was an unavoidable cost, more careful risk management might have helped to mitigate the extent of disenfranchisement. For example, efforts to maintain consumers' sense of control within SA might have been more successful if clear organizational structures had been attached to the decision for SA leaders to maintain programmatic control and if these structures were clearly separated from the structures that supported organizational expansion. As an example, if the group consciousness meetings had remained a setting where only SA leaders met to make program decisions, they might have remained a setting that functioned based on the values, processes, and structures of the collectivity stage of organizational development. While the set of responsibilities that SA leaders addressed at these meetings may have changed, their sense of power and responsibility might have remained more intact. It is likely that leaders still would have experienced some level of dissatisfaction with the changed emphasis on and approach to expansion, but the overall feelings of disenfranchisement they experienced might have been somewhat mitigated.

We should not underestimate the resources required for anticipating and preventing risks and for addressing costs when they arise. For example, MHAM and SA were aware of the need to support existing SA groups. They hosted conferences for SA group leaders and members and hired experienced leaders to provide support to other SA group leaders. The resources required to quickly establish new SA groups in geographic regions beyond SA's first groups in southeast Michigan may have left too little, however, to more effectively monitor and support new groups.

14.4.5 Engage in Ongoing Risk Assessment and Management

Managing risk requires both a commitment to identifying potential risks prior to the development of the partnership and to the ongoing assessment of risk as the partnership progresses. In the case of the SA–MHAM partnership, those involved were aware of potential risks, such as the SA leaders and group members losing control of the SA program. They developed what they believed was an adequate plan to protect both the integrity of the SA program and the leadership role of SA members, while relieving them of what was starting to feel like an overwhelming burden. The SA leaders who had been responsible for developing new groups (before the separation of responsibilities) and the MHAM staff did not, however, anticipate the negative consequences of SA leaders giving up these responsibilities. The decision to develop new groups in formal mental health service settings and to involve professional leaders influenced both the nature of the groups and their survival. Several of the SA leaders reported feeling powerless and discouraged by these developments, feeling that too much organizational attention was directed to growth and not enough to supporting existing groups. Unfortunately, the influence of these changes on group survival and on consumer leadership was not carefully assessed by those managing this partnership. Only though our case study methods, and the resources of the evaluation study, were we able to identify these consequences. These risks could have been monitored on a more consistent basis and identified earlier. For example, when in a similar situation, GROW also utilized professionals to start groups. They set a 6-month limit on professional leadership, however, and assigned consumer fieldworkers to monitor the process and work with groups that failed to meet the deadline (Zimmerman, Reischl, Seidman, Rappaport, Toro, & Salem, 1991).

14.4.6 Partnership Risks and Risk Management

In Table 14.5 we describe a range of typical ways that mutual-help and professional organizations may partner with each other, some examples of the potential risks that should be assessed, and possible strategies for minimizing/mitigating those risks. While all partnerships are unique, this provides a starting point for thinking about managing collaborative relationships. In the first type of partnership, a professional organization provides operational support for the mutual-help organization (e.g., resources, services). This might take the form of financial support, meeting space, paying for materials, publicizing or making referrals to groups, or providing financial (e.g., bookkeeping or grant writing expertise) or other technical services. This may be the most common type of partnership and may have the fewest risks to mutual-help organizations. Risks will typically result from the imposition of overt policies or practices that are incompatible with a mutual-help philosophy. For example, the professional organization may have concerns about legal liability or the capabilities of consumer leaders that would lead them to require the

Table 14.5 Risks and management of different types of partnerships

Type of partnership	Examples of potential risks	Minimizing/mitigating strategies
Professional organization provides operational support (meeting space, referrals, technical assistance, fiduciary services, funding) for the mutual-help organization	Legal liability (P[a]) Loss of control over who can attend or lead meetings (MH[b]) Loss of organizational capacity (MH)	Bargaining Liability waivers Cooperative agreements Escape
Professional organization becomes the fiduciary for the mutual-help organization	Accountability (P, MH) Excessive or inconsistent reporting requirements (MH) Loss of control over who can attend or lead meetings (MH) Change in organizational operations and norms (MH)	Bargaining Cooperative agreements Buffering Continuous risk management Escape
Professional and mutual-help organizations collaborative program	Loss of control over program content and operations (P, MH) Loss of control over program management (P, MH) Change in organizational operations and norms (MH)	Bargaining Cooperative agreements Buffering Building/strengthening value compatible external environment Capacity development Continuous risk management

[a]P denotes professional organization; [b]MH denotes mutual-help organization

presence of a staff member in the group. They might have concerns about fair access or accountability that would lead them to influence or track who attends group meetings. These risks can likely be minimized through bargaining (Oliver, 1991) and the negotiation of agreed upon procedures and legal documents (e.g., waivers, agreements). For example, when GROW, a mutual-help organization for persons living with serious mental illness, was offered state funding, it came with the requirement that the leaders count how many service hours they "provided" to "chronically mental ill" individuals. GROW felt that this method did not reflect the type of support they provided and that the label was incompatible with their group philosophy. They negotiated an alternative accountability system that focused on time members spent at GROW meetings and used the label "recovering GROWer" instead of chronically mentally ill (Zimmerman et al., 1991). GROW's power to effectively negotiate this change lay in their willingness to turn down the funding if an alternative reporting mechanism could not be agreed upon. While this may sound like semantics, we should not underestimate the consequences for a mutual-help organization of engaging in even small behaviors that are in conflict with their internal beliefs. If these types of issues cannot be resolved, the mutual-help organization can opt at this point to avoid these influences by seeking support or partnership from a more compatible source.

When a professional organization takes on the role of serving as the fiduciary (i.e., having legal authority to hold assets and make decisions regarding financial matters) for a mutual-help organization, the level of partnership risk increases considerably. There is great power, whether desired or not, in controlling the financial resources of an organization. At a minimum, the mutual-help organization will feel pressure to follow financial protocols established by the professional organization, including: financial reporting, limits on spending, accountability procedures, etc. Although the partnership itself may not involve other organizational responsibilities, financial dependency on the professional organization will make the mutual-help organization highly susceptible to the pressures of resource dependencies. This type of partnership will likely have more risks and will require more conscientious identification, continuous assessment, and prioritization of risk along with risk minimization and mitigation. Efforts to negotiate minimally invasive procedures for managing financial manners and to buffer the organization by decoupling organizational structures involved in financial management tasks from other aspects of the organization's internal functioning may be useful risk management tools. For example, decisions regarding program content need not be made at the same organizational meetings or by the same organizational players as those regarding financial issues.

The final type of partnership is one where, like in the case of SA, the two organizations share the responsibility for the operations of the mutual-help organization. In these instances, changes to the processes and structures that epitomize mutual help are a very real risk, with potentially severe consequences. If mutual-help organizations decide to undertake this form of partnership, it will require significant attention and resources devoted to risk management principles. While negotiation can certainly help, structural solutions that buffer valued internal characteristics of mutual help from external pressures (e.g., protect experiential knowledge by limiting professional access to consumer-run aspects of the setting), build internal capacity (e.g., develop internal capacity to manage funds, write grants, or actively engaging in financial decision-making) and strengthen compatible external connections are more likely called for. Continuous monitoring is also needed to avoid the creation of dependencies and loss of organizational capacity that will make it difficult for the mutual-help organization to disengage from the partnership if the costs become too great.

14.5 Conclusions

While mutual-help organizations are likely to value their independence, professional involvement and collaboration with formal service delivery systems have become a reality for many. It is important to recognize that, even in the most favorable circumstances, close collaboration is likely to lead to change in the unique structures and processes of mutual-help organizations. Awareness that such changes are to be expected is the first step to avoiding or mitigating them. Through an active process of self and environmental assessment and risk management the changes mutual-help organizations face may be minimized. These efforts go beyond simple awareness, to process, structural and network changes that buffer and strengthen key characteristics of mutual help, such as consumer leadership and control.

The risks of extensive partnerships, such as the one between SA and MHAM, appear to be great and potentially severe. Mutual-help organizations might choose to minimize their engagement in collaborations that integrate them into the service sectors to which they played an alternative or adjunct role, diminish their independence, or turn over significant leadership responsibilities to non-consumers, if there are alternative ways to achieve their desired goals. Future research aimed at studying the process and outcomes of naturally evolving partnerships will help us to better understand the types of partnerships in which mutual-help organizations are engaging, the types of risks and benefits that are associated with these partnerships, and the efficacy of the strategies that organizations use to mitigate the risks.

14.6 Epilogue

After our study was completed, SA's partnership with MHAM continued to grow in terms of cooperation and involvement. In order to more effectively respond to the increasing demands for assistance with SA groups, MHAM and the staff member who had supported SA during the time of our study established a new non-profit organization, the National Schizophrenia Foundation (NSF), to assume the MHAM's support functions for SA. NSF grew to employ six professional and consumer staff who administered SA and worked on issues of stigma and public awareness with regard to schizophrenia. In 2007, NSF was dissolved due to fiscal insolvency, leaving SA without the administrative structure that supported their organizational development and leadership support activities.

In 2008, a new organization, Schizophrenia and Related Disorders Alliance of America (SARDDA) was formed. Part of its mission is to provide support to SA and to support persons who live with schizophrenia and related disorders, by "providing materials and information that will assist people in their own personal journey in living with their illness" (SARDAA, 2009). SARDAA is a young organization with no paid staff. It does not have the resources to replace all of the functions provided by MHAM and NSF. The SARDAA board of directors and SA leaders are working together to regroup in order to support current SA groups and to respond to external interest in SA. They face the challenge of rebuilding SA's organizational capacity. The future of SA and nature of this new partnership is an evolving story.

Acknowledgement The authors wish to express our appreciation to Joanne Verbanic, Eric Hufnagel, the Mental Health Association in Michigan, The National Schizophrenia Foundation, and the leaders and members of SA who contributed to this study. We would also like to thank

Fiona Gallacher who assisted in data collection and Doug Luke for assistance with data analysis. This research was supported in part by a grant from the Ethel and James Flinn Family Foundation.

References

Anthony, W. A. (2000). A recovery oriented service system: Settting some system level standards. *Psychiatric Rehabilitation Journal, 24*, 159–168.

Ben-Ari, A. T. (2002). Dimensions and predictions of professional involvement in self-help groups: A view from within. *Health and Social Work, 27*, (2), 95–103.

Barker, R. G. (1968). *Ecological psychology: Concepts and methods for studying the environment of human behavior*. Stanford, CA: Stanford University Press.

Borkman, T. J. (1976). Experiential knowledge: A new concept for the analysis of self-help groups. *Social Science Review, 50*, 445–456.

Borkman, T. J. (1999). *Understanding self-help/mutual aid*. New Brunswick, NJ: Rutgers University Press.

Brown, L. D., Shepherd, M. D., Merkle, E. C., Wituk, S. A., & Meissen, G. (2008). Understanding how participation in a consumer-run organization relates to recovery. *American Journal of Community Psychology, 42*, 167–178.

Chamberlin, J. (1990). The ex-patients' movement: Where we've been and where we are going. *Journal of Mind and Behavior, 11*, 323–336.

Cherniss, C., & Cherniss, D. S. (1987). Professional involvement in self-help groups for parents of high-risk newborns. *American Journal of Community Psychology, 15*, 435–444.

Cherniss, C., & Deegan, G. (2000). The creation of alternative settings. In J. Rappaport & E. Seidman (Eds.), *Handbook of Community Psychology* (pp.359–378), New York: Plenum.

Chinman, M., Kloos, B., O'Connell, M., & Davidson, L. (2002). Service provider's views of psychiatric mutual support groups. *Journal of Community Psychology, 30*, 349–366.

Corbin, J., & Strauss, A. (2008). *Basics of qualitative research: Techniques and procedures for developing grounded theory* (3rd ed.). Los Angeles, CA: Sage.

Couchman, P. K., & Fulop, L. (2002). The meanings of risk and interorganizational collaboration. In Clegg, S. R. (Ed.), *Management and Organization Paradoxes* (pp. 41–65). Amsterdam: John Benjamins Publishing.

Crouhy, M., Galai, D., & Mark, R. (2006). *The essentials of risk management*. New York: McGraw-Hill.

Davidson, L., Chinman, M., Kloos, B., Weingarten, R., Stayner, D., & Tebes, J. K. (1999). Peer support among individuals with severe mental illness: A review of evidence. *Clinical psychology: Science and practice, 6*, 165—187.

Deegan, P. E. (1988). Recovery: The lived experience of rehabilitation. *Psychosocial Rehabilitation Journal, 11*, 11–19.

De Vita, C. J., & Fleming, C. (Eds.) (2001). *Building capacity in nonprofit organizations*. Washington, DC: The Urban Institute.

DiMaggio, P. J., & Powell, W. W. (1983). The iron cage revisited: Institutional isomorphism and collective rationality in organizational fields. *American Sociology Review, 48*, 147–160.

Gartner, A. (1997). Professionals and self-help: The uses of creative tension. *Social Policy, 27*(3), 47–52.

Gidron, B., & Hasenfeld, Y. (1994). Human service organizations and self-help groups: Can they collaborate? *Nonprofit Management and Leadership, 5*, 159–172.

Hasenfeld, Y., & Gidron, B. (1993). Self-help groups and human service organizations: An interorganizational perspective. *Social Service Review, 67*, 217–235.

Herman, M. L., Head, G. L., Jackson, P. M., & Fogarty, T. E. (2004). *Managing risk in nonprofit organizations: A comprehensive guide*. Hoboken, NJ: Wiley.

Kaplan, E. L., & Meier, P. (1958). Nonparametric estimation from incomplete observations. *Journal of the American Statistical Association, 53*, 457–481.

Kurtz, L. (1990). The self-help movement: Review of the past decade of research. *Social Work with Groups, 13*, 101–115.

Kurtz, L. F., Mann, K. B., & Chambon, A. (1987). Linking between social workers and mental health mutual-aid groups. *Social Work in Heath Care, 13*, 69–78.

Luke, D. A. (1993). Charting the process of change: A primer on survival analysis. *American Journal of Community Psychology, 21*, 203–246.

Mantel, N. (1966). Evaluation of survival data and two new rank order statistics arising in its consideration. *Cancer Chemotherapy Reports, 50*, 163–170.

Maton, K. I., Leventhal, G. S., Madara, E. J., & Julien, M. (1989). Factors affecting the birth and death of mutual-help groups: The role of national affiliation, professional involvement, and member focal problem. *American Journal of Community Psychology, 17*, 643–671.

Maton, K. I., & Salem, D. A. (1995). Organizational characteristics of empowering community settings: A multiple case study approach. *American Journal of Community Psychology, 23*, 631–656.

Meissen, G. J., Mason, W. C., & Gleason, D. F. (1991). Understanding the attitudes and intentions of future professionals toward self-help. *American Journal of Community Psychology, 19*, 699–714.

Meyer, J. W., & Rowan, B. (1977). Institutional organizations: Formal structure of myth and ceremony. *American Journal of Sociology, 83*, 340–363.

Nelson, G., Janzen, R., Trainor, J., & Ochocka, O. (2008) Putting values into practice: Public policy and the future of mental health consumer-run organizations. *American Journal of Community Psychology, 32*, 192–201.

Oliver, C. (1991). Strategic response to institutional processes. *Academy of Management Review, 16*, 145–179.

Olson, B. D., Jason, L. A., Ferrari, J. R. & Hutcheson, T. D. (2005). Bridging professional and mutual-help: An application of the transtheoretical model to the mutual-help organization. *Applied and Preventive Psychology, 11*, 167–178.

Patton, M. Q. (2002). *Qualitative research and evaluation methods*. (3rd ed.). Thousand Oaks, CA: Sage.

Pfeffer, J., & Salanick, G. R. (1978). *The external control of organizations*. New York: Harper Collins.

Powell, T. J. (1990). Self-help, professional help, and informal help: Competing or complementary systems? In T. J. Powell (Ed.), *Working with self-help*. Silver Spring, MD: NASW Press.

Powell, T. J., & Cameron, M. J. (1991). Self-help research and the public mental health system. *American Journal of Community Psychology, 19*, 797–805.

Quinn, R. E., & Cameron, K. (1983). Organizational life cycles and shifting criteria of effectiveness: Some preliminary evidence. *Management Science, 29*, 33–51.

Rappaport, J., Reischl, T. M., & Zimmerman, M. A. (1992). Empowerment mechanisms in the empowerment of former mental patients. In D. Saleebey (Ed.), The strengths perspective in social work practice (pp. 84–97). New York: Longman.

Rappaport, J., Seidman, E., Toro, P.A., McFadden, L.S., Reischl, T.M., Roberts, L.J., Salem, D.A., Stein, C.H., & Zimmerman, M.A. (1985). Collaborative research with a mutual help organization. *Social Policy, 15*, 12–25.

Salem, D. A., Foster-Fishman, P. G., & Goodkind, J. R. (2002). Adoption of innovation in collective advocacy organizations. *American Journal of Community Psychology, 30*, 681–710.

Salem, D. A., Gant, L., & Campbell, R. (1998). The introduction of mutual-help groups in group homes for the mentally ill: Barriers to participation. *Community Mental Health Journal, 34*, 419–429.

Salem, D., & Hughes, B. (2003, June). *The development of SA groups in forensic settings*. Paper presented at the ninth biennial conference on Community Research and Action, Las Vegas, New Mexico.

Salem, D. A., Reischl, T. M., Gallacher, F., & Randall, K. W. (2000). The role of referent and expert power in mutual help. *American Journal of Community Psychology, 28*, 303–324.

Salem, D. A., Reischl, T. M. & Randall, K. W. (2008) The effect of professional partnership on the development of a mutual-help organization. *American Journal of Community Psychology, 42*, 179–191.

Schizophrenics Anonymous (1992). *Schizophrenics Anonymous: A self-help support group.* Southfield, MI: Mental Health Association in Michigan.

SARDAA. (n.d.) *SARDAA: About us.* Retrieved March 14, 2009 from http://www.sardaa.org.

Schubert, M. A., & Borkman, T. J. (1991). An organizational typology for self-help groups. *American Journal of Community Psychology, 19*, 769–788.

Scott, W. R. (1995). *Institutions and organizations.* Thousand Oaks, CA: Sage.

Stewart, M. (1990). Professional interface with self-help mutual aid groups. *Social Science and Medicine, 31*, 1143–1158.

Stewart, M., Banks, S., Crossman, D., & Poel, D. (1994). Partnerships between health professionals and self-help groups: Meanings and mechanisms. In F. Lavoie, T. Borkman, & B. Gidron (Eds.), *Self-help and mutual aid groups: International and multicultural perspectives* (pp. 199-240). New York: The Hawthorne Press.

Toro, P. A., Reischl, T. M., Zimmerman, M. A., Rappaport, J., Seidman, E., Luke, D. A., et al. (1988). Professionals in mutual help groups: Impact on social climate and members' behavior. *Journal of Consulting and Clinical Psychology, 56*, 631–632.

Traunstein, D. M. (1984). From mutual-aid self-help to professional service. *Social Casework: The Journal of Contemporary Social Work, Dec.*, 622–627.

Scott, W. R. (1995). *Institutions and organizations.* Thousand Oaks, CA: Sage.

Shepherd, M. D., Schoenberg, M., Slavich, S., Wituk, S., Warren, M., & Meissen, G. (1999). Continuum of professional involvement in self-help groups. *Journal of Community Psychology, 27*, 39–53.

Weaver-Randall, K., & Salem, D. A. (2004). Mutual-help groups and recovery: How settings influence participants' experience of recovery. In P. W. Corrigan & R. O. Ralph (Eds.), *Recovery and mental illness: consumer visions and research paradigms.* Washington, DC: American Psychological Association Press.

Yoak, M., & Chessler, M. (1984). Alternative professional roles in health care delivery: Leadership patterns in self-help groups. *Journal of Applied Behavioral Science, 21*, 427–444.

Zimmerman, M. A., Reischl, T. M., Seidman, E., Rappaport, J., Toro, P. A. & Salem, D. A. (1991). Expansion strategies of a mutual help organization. *American Journal of Community Psychology, 19*, 251–278.

Zinman, S. (1987). Is the "partnership model" self help? In S. Budd, H. T. Harp, & S. Zinman (Eds.), *Reaching across: Mental health clients helping each other* (pp. 16–18). Riverside, CA: California Network of Mental Health Clients.

Chapter 15
The Contribution of Self-Help Groups to the Mental Health/Substance Use Services System

Thomas J. Powell and Brian E. Perron

Abstract Self-help groups provide an immense amount of service, which mental health professionals do not adequately understand or coordinate with their services. Epidemiological surveys have documented the profiles of self-help users, the amount of self-help use, and the association between self-help use and professional services. The large majority of self-help users use professional services sometimes as a gateway into professional services, other times concurrently with professional service or as aftercare following a course of professional services. The hallmark features of self-help groups: their use of the experiential perspective, referent power, and reciprocal helping relationships are contrasted with professional mental health services. The essential elements of effective referrals to self-help groups are discussed. At another level, the chapter also discusses the organizational supports necessary for effective collaboration between self-help groups and professional services. While the boundaries between mental health services and self-help groups must be respected, both parties have much to gain by entering into more extensive community partnerships.

Self-help groups are responsible for an immense amount of service to the larger M/SU[1] system. Nonetheless, this contribution tends to be underestimated and its experiential nature poorly understood. Self-help services are complementary to professional services, and yet professionals often do not coordinate with them. Moreover, the reluctance of professionals to support self-help groups in the community is part of the reason the contribution of self-help groups is not fully realized (Salzer, Rappaport, & Segre, 1999). To help address these problems, this chapter (1) Documents the volume and demographics of self-help utilization including the racial/ethnic characteristics of the participants using epidemiologic

---

T.J. Powell (✉)
School of Social Work, University of Michigan, Ann Arbor, MI, USA
e-mail: tpowell@umich.edu

[1]M/SU refers to "mental and/or substance use" following the practice of the: Committee on Crossing the Quality Chasm: Adaptation to Mental Health and Addictive Disorders (2006). *Improving the quality of health care for mental and substance-use conditions: Quality chasm series.* Washington, D.C.: Institute of Medicine, National Academies Press.

data; (2) Describes the nature of self-help in terms of its experiential perspective, distinctive base of power, and the reciprocal nature of its helping relationships; (3) Highlights challenges associated with and provide recommendations for coordinating self-help and professional services; (4) Addresses the potential of the M/SU services system to enhance the acceptance and growth of the self-help sector by engaging self-help groups in organizational exchanges and in collaborative community projects.

15.1 Service Utilization

15.1.1 Volume

In comparison with the mental health/addictive specialty sector of the M/SU system, self-help groups provide services to fewer people. Of the 13% using outpatient services in a 12-month period, 5.8% accessed the mental/addictive sector while 3.2% accessed unspecified groups in the self-help sector (Kessler et al., 1999). Although the proportion served by the self-help sector is large by any measure, the professional mental health/addictive specialty sector serves more people than the self-help sector. However, if the measure is visits and not people, the ranks are reversed. Forty percent of all outpatient visits for psychiatric problems are to self-help groups according to the National Comorbidity Survey (NCS) (Kessler et al., 1999). The 40% to self-help compares to 35% to the mental health/addictive specialty sector, 16% to the human services sector, and 8% to the general medical sector (Kessler, Mickelson, & Zhao, 1997).

Additional details are available from a later national survey. The Midlife Development in the United States (MIDUS) survey is based on interviews conducted in 1995–1996 following the 1990–1992 NCS interviews. More than one-third of the MIDUS self-help attendees were in groups for substance use problems, accounting for nearly 70% of the self-help visits. People with substance use problems are more likely to go to self-help groups, attend more frequently, and attend for longer periods than those with other mental health problems. Participants in substance use self-help groups average 76 visits a year while those in other self-help groups such as NAMI, Recovery, Inc. and DBSA (Depression and Bipolar Support Alliance) average 24 visits. Fifty percent of those attending substance use groups, mostly 12-step groups, also participate in professional treatment services. The proportion using professional services among non-substance use groups is even higher at 75% (Kessler et al., 1997).

15.1.2 Demographics

The MIDUS survey provides information about the age, income, gender, and marital status of self-help participants. Younger people participate more than older people.

However, the participation of all age groups has continued to increase since WWII. Assuming a continuation of the trend, the 1996 figure of 18% of the population using self-help services over the life course has already been eclipsed. Participation also varies by income – it is inversely related to income, especially for those with substance use problems (Kessler et al., 1997).

Women participate in self-help groups more often than men. Even in substance use groups such as AA or NA, which are sometimes thought of as male preserves, women participate more often in proportion to their level of substance use problems. Unmarried adults and those with less supportive networks also participate more often in self-help according to the MIDUS survey.

The MIDUS survey is the source of some finely nuanced findings about race: "Blacks are only half as likely as Whites to participate in self-help groups overall, but this difference is largely due to an extremely low rate of participation in groups for people with eating problems. There are no significant race differences in participation in groups for substance use problems or emotional problems" (Kessler et al., 1997, p. 33). This is consistent with a treatment follow-up study by Humphreys and colleagues (1991, 1994). They found that African Americans were at least as likely to attend and benefit from 12-step groups as Whites. These findings, which some might think run counter to conventional wisdom, might be more easily assimilated if it is understood that African Americans have a lower prevalence rate for substance use problems than Whites.

The National Epidemiologic Survey on Alcohol and Related Conditions (NESARC) interviews 2001–2002 is a more recent source of information about Black participation in 12-step groups. Examining those with drug use disorders (DUDs), the findings suggest that African Americans participate in 12-step groups at a higher level than Whites. The participation pattern for Latinos is lower than that for Blacks and similar to that of Whites (Perron, Mowbray, Glass, Delva, Vaughn, & Howard, 2009). However, the use of self-help services should be considered in relation to the total treatment package. For example, the NESARC data suggests that Blacks tend to use private practitioners (physicians, social workers, psychiatrists, and other professionals) less than other racial and ethnic groups, though they are somewhat more frequent users of outpatient and drug rehabilitation services. However, this finding needs to be considered in the context that other studies suggest that 12-step groups may be more effective than professional services (Humphreys & Moos, 2007; Seligman, 1995). Therefore, a preference for 12-step involvement may be wise. But not to be lost sight of, other studies have found that the combination of 12-step participation and professional treatment is best (Fiorentine & Hillhouse, 2000; McLellan, 2008)

Still there is much about these rates that need clarification and it is best to think of these figures as rough estimates. One puzzling piece of information is that the Alcoholics Anonymous Membership Survey (2007) shows much lower rates of Black and Hispanic participation than one would expect from the national surveys. Delving into this issue is beyond this paper but worthy of examination.

Aside from the rates of relative participation, the more significant meta-finding is that both minorities and non-minorities are under-enrolled in self-help groups and under-treated in professional services. Using the MIDUS data set, Wang and colleagues (2000) found under-treatment in that even among persons with severe mental illness, only 25% were receiving guideline-concordant, evidence-based treatment. Using the more recent (2001–2003) National Comorbidity Survey Replication (NCS-R), Wang et al. (2005) found under-enrollment in that the people with substance use and impulse control disorders were least likely to connect with treatment. Based on NESARC data, less than 15% of those with alcohol use disorder receive treatment, whether self-help or professional in nature (Cohen, Feinn, Arias, & Kranzler, 2007). For mental and substance use problems as a whole, only a fraction of those who could presumably benefit from self-help services actually receive them (Kessler et al., 1997). Based on the NCS-R data, the authors conclude, "Unmet need for treatment is greatest in traditionally underserved groups, including elderly persons, racial-ethnic minorities, those with low incomes, those without insurance, and residents of rural areas" (Wang et al., 2005, p. 629). For other serious mental disorders, as well as substance use disorders, concurrent participation in self-help groups and professional treatment can be a way to address this unmet need. Considerable support exists for combining professional treatment and self-help services for serious mental illness as well as substance use (Davidson et al., 1999; Freimuth, 2000; Humphreys et al., 2004; Magura, 2007; Magura, Laudet, Mahmood, Rosenblum, & Knight, 2002; McLellan, 2008; Moos & Timko, 2008; Pistrang, Barker, & Humphreys, 2008; Powell, 1990; Powell, Yeaton, Hill, & Silk, 2001).

15.1.3 Financial Implications

The question of whether self-help services can offset costly professional services is probably premature given the prevailing under-treatment of severe mental illness. Since people with mental illness struggle with too widely spaced and time-pressured medication reviews, scarce supportive housing, work, and education services, and limited access to wraparound services such as ACT, it is hardly surprising that self-help groups seek more of these services for their members (Wang et al., 2005). As long as professional services are weak and lack appropriate intensity, initiatives to substitute self-help services for professional services should be considered potentially counterproductive. Yet, it should be acknowledged that there are already areas where substitution is less concerning. In the area of substance use disorders, Humphreys & Moos (2007) found that participation in 12-step groups improved post-treatment outcomes while it also reduced the cost of continuing professional care.

But narrow cost-effectiveness considerations shouldn't be the only concern. Cost-benefit analyses are needed to estimate the costs of lost workforce productivity and losses of disability-adjusted life years (DALYS) associated with M/SU disorders. M/SU disorders are high on the list of all diseases and injuries contributing to DALYS (USPHS, 2000; WHO, 2001). The huge costs of DALYS compared to the minimal costs of self-help services suggest a very favorable cost-benefit ratio – assuming of course some level of self-help effectiveness. With regard to cost, it should also be considered that self-help use produces more self-help resources. More use generates more pairs of givers and receivers, more personal models, more recovery stories, and more resource networks. To raise awareness of this multiplier effect, Riessman (1995) referred to prosumers rather than consumers of self-help services.

15.1.4 The Timing of Self-Help and Professional Services

Concurrent participation in self-help and professional treatment is only one of several ways self-help and professional services relate to one another (Meissen, Wituk, Warren & Shepherd 2000). Self-help participation may take place before, during, and after professional treatment. And of course it can take place independent of any connection to professional treatment. When it comes before professional treatment it can serve as a mechanism that informs, motivates, reduces barriers, and provides encouragement to engage professional services. Self-help participation may also reconnect participants who earlier were dissatisfied with professional services, or for a variety of reasons experienced a disruption in treatment. Self-help groups also facilitate access to professional services since they tend to be a source of reliable information about who the best providers are and how to access them (Warner et al., 1994). Informal conversations about the benefits of professional treatment tend to enhance motivation. Barriers may be reduced as self-help peers locate possible sources of funding for professional services and assist with everyday problems related to transportation and child care. Considering the prominence of professional services on the agenda of self-help groups and the frequency with which it is a topic of side conversations, it would seem likely that self-help participation encourages participation in professional treatment (Aron, Honberg & Duckworth et al. 2009). But of course it could have the opposite effect. Stories about self-help members who discourage the use of professional services are ubiquitous (Chesler, 1990). No doubt discouragement takes place but it needs to be considered against the backdrop that many more self-helpers participate in professional services than the reverse (Kessler et al., 1997). A more specific allegation is that self-help groups discourage taking prescribed medications. No doubt this occurs in contravention to AA policy. However, the extent to which this occurs may be more limited than supposed. A study based on interviews with AA contact persons suggests that they were open to members taking prescribed psychiatric medications (Meissen, Powell, Wituk, Girrens, & Arteaga, 1999). Yet a single study is not enough and the ongoing debates suggest that it should be a priority area for study. Meanwhile, there are variant 12-step groups, including Dual Recovery Anonymous, that should be considered for persons with co-occurring disorders (Ries, Galanter, & Tonigan, 2008).

Whether self-help is included in aftercare plans largely depends on professional views about the efficacy of self-help (Salzer, Rappaport, & Segre, 2001). When the views are strongly positive, self-help may be seen as the main engine of recovery (Moos, 2007). Professionals subscribing to this view seek to prepare clients and patients for full and productive participation in the recovering community which might be thought of as loosely made up of the members and friends of 12-step groups (Project MATCH Research Group et al., 1998). However, many professionals see self-help as a second best resource, to be accessed only when professional treatment is not an option (Salzer, Rappaport, & Segre, 1999). In the worst case scenario, some professionals seem to make so called referrals to self-help groups to detach themselves from unwanted clients (Powell & Perron, 2010).

A contrasting and appropriate use of self-help is to maintain or amplify the gains of professional treatment and to sustain them over time. This approach would be consistent with an understanding that the nature of the task changes as individuals move from acute to continuing care status or from treatment to rehabilitation services. Simultaneously, they may be moving from a practicing to a recovering person, and from victim to survivor. As individuals move along these continua the balance shifts toward increasing self-help participation as professional care decreases or is stepped down.

Unfortunately, few data are available to document the relative frequency of these patterns. That which is available suggests that participants in self-help are likely to also participate in professional services. This is less true of participants in professional services, as suggested by NCS data: "63% of those in self-help were also in some other sector, compared with 42–50% of those in other sectors" (Kessler et al., 1999, p. 121). It seems that self-help users are more aware of the added value of professional services than those using professional services are aware of the potential additive value of self-help services.

15.2 Nature of Self-Help

Self-help is enormously diverse. Some part of this diversity is reflected in their different names: mutual help groups, mutual aid groups, support groups, 12-step groups, and fellowships. But even this list omits the increasingly important online groups (Murray, Burns, See-Tai, Lai, & Nazareth, 2005) whose special features are discussed in more detail in Chapter 5 of this book. Differences in names, however, do not reference some of the fundamental differences among self-help groups. One example is how they view the origin of the problem. Some assume the problem resides in the individual, e.g., 12-step groups. Other groups assume the problem resides in society's lack of acceptance, e.g., LGBTQ groups. Still others assume that the problem is located in both the individual and society, e.g., NAMI (Sagarin, 1969). The perceived locus of the problem is in turn related to the different positions groups take on advocacy.

Self-help groups also vary on a variety of organizational dimensions. Some self-help groups have national and local affiliate structures, e.g., DBSA, Recovery Inc. whereas others operate as unaffiliated local groups. Some have well-defined formats, e.g., 12-step and GROW groups, while others use less structured formats, e.g., NAMI and DBSA (Schubert & Borkman, 1991).

And then there are the uses of "self-help" that are different from its use here. Self-help, as used here, is not seeking guidance and inspiration in "self-help" books, which are often written by professionals (Norcross, 2006). Self-help is not the use of self-administered therapies often derived from professional therapies (Watkins & Clum, 2008). Agencies employing consumers to provide services are not self-help groups as they are understood here (see comments below about reciprocal helping roles) (Hardiman & Segal, 2003). Nor are cooperative residences that are built on self-help ideas such as the 12 steps (Majer et al., 2008). Most decidedly, self-help is not be confused with pulling oneself up by one's bootstraps. Self-help isn't done alone; it is done in groups and involves mutual help.

Despite the diversity, self-help groups share a basic appeal. People, anxious or in difficulty, share a universal desire to associate with others in similar situation (Schacter, 1959). These associations lead to comparisons and self-appraisals (Brown, 2009; Davison, Pennebaker, & Dickerson, 2000; Festinger, 1954). These in turn can result in a number of supportive conclusions such as, "I'm not alone; I'm liked in this community of respectable people. In some ways, I'm doing comparatively well and can help others do better. In other respects, I could do better and I can learn from people who will work with me." This is the group context in which mutual aid is exchanged. This mutuality is less typical of professionally facilitated or led support groups (Salem, Reischl & Randall, 2008; Toro et al., 1988) though professionals often play helpful secondary roles in self-help groups (Gitterman & Shulman, 2005; Shepherd et al., 1999; Wituk, Shepherd, Slavich, Warren, & Meissen, 2000). Moreover, this doesn't include the important role professionals play in the formation of self-help groups (Borman, 1979). However, excluding professionally led support groups is consistent with the practice of national epidemiological surveys (R. Kessler et al., 1997) and consistent with a potentially insightful understanding of the "self" in self-help groups. The term self refers to a group of *ourselves* who share common experiences, challenges, and identities.

Identifying with these shared attributes is the basis of group cohesion and the mutual exchange of help (Mowrer, 1984). Thus a more accurate, though more cumbersome, name might be self-help/mutual help groups. Shedding the cumbersome, self-help groups share three fundamental properties: (a) the experiential perspective, (b) a distinctive form of social power, and (c) a behavioral pattern of giving and receiving help. The experiential perspective highlights the nature of sharing in the self-help group. The basis of power speaks to who is an authority in self-help groups. And giving as well as receiving help refers to a behavioral pattern linked to positive outcomes.

15.2.1 Experiential Perspective

Experience is the currency of the realm or the thing that is exchanged in self-help groups. Sharing goes something like: My experience is . . . . What is your experience? What has worked for you? What has worked for me is . . . . The process of contending with the condition or situation is the basis of the experiential perspective. It differs from the perspective of the professional that is rooted in scholarly, scientific study (Borkman, 1990; Mowrer, 1984).

15.2.2 Referent Power

What moves people to action? To whom do we grant the power to move us? Action might be taken because we're rewarded, forced, or persuaded by the logic of the proposed action (French & Raven, 1959; Raven, Schwarzwald, & Koslowsky, 1998). We might also be moved by expert power because of the formal educational credentials of the person making the recommendation (Raven, 1988). This is the predominant form of power in professional mental health services. In self-help groups, referent power is the prevailing form of social power (Powell, Hill, Warner, Yeaton, & Silk, 2000; Salem, Reischl, Gallacher, & Randall, 2000). Referent power is visible in its effects. By definition, referent power is evident when the focal individual is under the influence of those he or she admires and wants to be like. The individual is moved to change because of his or her desire to be liked and approved by the referent individual or group.

15.2.3 Reciprocal Giving and Receiving Roles

In self-help groups, participants help others as well as themselves. In so doing the helper benefits as Riessman (1995, 1965) laid out in the helper-therapy principle. It's a case of, for example, the tutor benefiting as much or more than the tutee. Other studies of the principle have shown surprising benefits, e.g., increased longevity (Brown, Nesse, Vinokur, & Smith, 2003). Obviously, the client of a professional provider should not endeavor to help the provider. Yet help giving as well as help receiving occurs in self-help groups. And research in these groups suggests there are benefits to giving as well as receiving help (Maton, 1988; Roberts et al., 1999). The self-help participant who gives help may begin to see him- or herself as increasingly competent and powerful instead of deficient and helpless. The giver, then, seems to be rewarded with increased self-efficacy.

The foregoing analysis is intended to enable M/SU professionals to recognize authentic self-help and to more effectively relate to its healing properties. In the period leading up to the landmark Surgeon General's Workshop on Self-Help and Public Health (1988) anything labeled self-help was swept up in an attractive social movement. But the period was also marked by the overly inclusive and indiscriminate use of the term self-help. The counter move was to ridicule the self-help movement for harboring trivial groups such as Messies Anonymous. Nonetheless the purifying criticisms combined with the popularity of self-help set the stage for including questions about self-help services in important national epidemiological surveys in the 1990s, the Epidemiological Catchment Area Survey (ECA) (Narrow,

Regier, Rae, Manderscheid, & Locke, 1993) and the NCS (Kessler et al., 1999). This inclusion marked self-help's entry into the legitimate mainstream of mental health services. These surveys also revealed self-help groups to be a significant source of help for the U.S. population. Yet much remains to be done to integrate self-help services into the larger M/SU services system while preserving and enhancing their essential autonomy. Progress along these lines will depend on a better understanding of how the properties of self-help differ from those of professional services. It will also depend on developing enlightened professionals who appreciate that self-help is neither a mere adjunct to professional service nor something that is interchangeable with it (White, 1998).

15.3 Coordinating Professional Services with Self-Help

The fundamental reason to coordinate professional services with self-help services is to create a service system that takes advantage of the complementary strengths of each approach. Each compensates for elements that are in short supply in the other. The scholarly/scientific perspective of the professional, while long on expert wisdom is relatively short on experiential wisdom. Self-help members, and this means seasoned and successful ones, have potentially a great deal to offer about how to negotiate the practical, everyday issues stirred up by the troubling condition or situation. Examples of these practical concerns can be seen in the following questions: How do you remember to take your medication? What do you do when you don't want to take them? How do you deal with the side effects? How do you explain the gaps in your work history to potential employers? How do you resist the temptations of alcohol or drugs? How do you say no to old buddies? How do you quiet the troubling voices, and control the suspicions that rise and recede in your thoughts? These "how" questions imply a type of anxiety that is especially responsive to the care of those who have been there. And on a different heading, there are questions like the following: What did you have to do to get SSDI (Social Security Disability Insurance) benefits? These questions address completing practical tasks without which there can be little quality in one's life.

Taken together these questions connect with issues that both the self-help and professional sector deal with. The essential idea is that conversations in both sectors about these issues can enrich both modalities. The professional can enrich therapy by asking about prevailing ideas, suggestions, or sources of practical assistance in the self-help group. Proceeding in the reverse direction, the professional can ask the client to solicit the opinions of self-help members on some topic of interest to therapy.

15.3.1 Referral-Competent Counselors

Successful referral requires knowledgeable, self-help competent professionals. This competence is not a common outcome of basic education in any of the M/SU professions (Kurtz, 1997). Indeed, given the epidemiologically documented importance of self-help groups it is disconcerting that graduates of these professional programs are not better prepared to work with self-help groups (Meissen, Mason, & Gleason, 1991; White & Kurtz, 2005). Currently, professionals seeking to acquire self-help competence must do so on a continuing education, self-initiated basis after obtaining their professional degree. To elicit interest in acquiring this competence they might be asked to consider some imaginary or real personal problem. Then they could be asked how they might benefit from both persons who shared their experience and from professional helpers, in other words from those working from an experiential perspective and from those with a scholarly scientific perspective. Professionals might also be asked to reflect on the importance of admired referent individuals in their own lives to appreciate how this power might play out within self-help groups. Finally professionals could be encouraged to contemplate how the dependency associated with client/patient status can be demoralizing. Then they might be asked to consider how transforming oneself from a receiver of help to a giver of help can constitute a self-efficacy preventive intervention against the frequent undermining of confidence associated with extended client status.

15.3.1.1 Personal Knowledge of Self-Help

Successful referral requires first-hand knowledge of self-help groups (Kurtz, 1985). Research shows that personal experience with self-help groups is associated with more effective referral practices (Chinman, Kloos, Maria O'Connell, & Davidson, 2002; Humphreys, 1999). Thus, questions about personal self-help experience may be useful in applications to health and human service professional education programs, just as there are often questions about personal counseling. The idea, of course, is not simply to know whether applicants have had this experience but rather to encourage reflection about how these experiences might inform their professional work. Just as classroom work without a substantive practicum is not enough to learn how to provide professional services, so too book knowledge without hands-on experience is not enough to learn how to work with the self-help sector. Easy ways to begin acquiring this experience is to invite self-help leaders to agencies, visit self-help groups, and develop relationships. All this must be done with respect for group norms, e.g., closed meetings, and in a way that makes one's purpose transparent (Wilson, 1995a).

The term referral is problematic because of its professional connotations. It implies the professional is selective about which clients are referred to self-help groups. Self-help leaders are concerned that professionals should not control entry. Referral, they say, should be universal rather than selective. Every person with an alcohol problem should be encouraged to consider AA; every person with a connection to mental illness should be encouraged to consider NAMI. The professional should not screen out certain individuals but rather let the self-help group and the individual decide about suitability (Wilson, 1995b). Professionals should also be aware that an introduction to a self-help group could be more complicated than many professional referrals. It can be seen as going out of the system to a lesser-known entity. In any event, the encouragement needs to be highly individualized.

Some clients respond best to a low-key discussion of the self-help group; others will need more intensive encouragement. Encouraging participation or putting people in touch with self-help groups suggests a process that should be considered more complicated and requiring more individualization than a routine professional referral.

Only persons knowledgeable about the target self-help program and acquainted with its leaders are in a position to be truly encouraging. Only they have the knowledge-based confidence to discuss the client's fearful, skeptical, hesitant inclinations. This confidence also enables them to engage the client in a detailed conversation about the client's first experiences with the self-help group. The conversation might begin with the question: What was the meeting like? Were there any turn-offs? e.g., people who appeared too sick (or too well) to be in the group; people from a different socioeconomic group who might be difficult to relate to; people who seemed intent on subverting the program; people who appear to be possible predators, etc.? Yes – every intervention has risks, and they must be managed wisely. Still other questions might orient clients to various aspects of the group: Are there options to be selective with respect to the activities? With respect to how you relate to the other participants? Who are the helpful people? Have you thought about who might be helpful to you? What did you learn? Were you a part of any positive conversations?

These conversations may touch on many of the topics included in the Twelve Step Facilitation, a program to encourage active involvement in 12-step groups (Humphreys, 1997; Nowinski & Baker, 1992; Ries, Galanter, & Tonigan, 2008). These and other suggested protocols emphasize the use of available tools: readings, service work, sponsors, and the like (Chappel & DuPont, 1999). Clearly, discussion of their effective use requires a good deal of specific knowledge on the part of the professional counselor (Ries, Galanter, & Tonigan, 2008).

15.3.1.2 Effective Encouragement Strategies

The research on referrals (read encouragement) is unambiguous. The strongest and most effective referrals connect the self-help prospect with seasoned, welcoming self-help members. This connection to an experienced trained greeter is best if it occurs before the prospect's first meeting. The connection may be by phone, or in person, and preferably include an offer to accompany the newcomer to his or her first meeting. This approach has been successful with 12-step groups and with mental health groups such as the Depression and Bipolar Support Alliance and 12-step groups (Powell et al., 2000; Timko, Debenedetti, & Billow, 2006; Timko & Debenedetti, 2007). The various components of these interventions offer the prospect a personalized, anxiety reducing introduction to the self-help group with the opportunity to debrief after the meeting.

An effective encouragement strategy should also include the option of a companion to accompany the newcomer to meetings at least until he or she feels some degree of comfort. The spirit of this recommendation is captured in the saying that sometimes people need more than a travel agent, a travel companion. AA provides this kind of companionship but across self-help groups as a whole, too little of it is available. One possible answer to this need resides in the development of peer specialists in M/SU agencies, training for which is provided by the Depression and Bipolar Support Alliance (2009). They also ask potential trainees about their support group leadership experience. Likewise, participation in self-help groups might logically be included among the potential qualifications for peer specialists. Peer specialist job descriptions could then establish the importance of accompanying consumers in a companionable manner to self-help group meetings.

Efforts to encourage participation should recognize that people in certain categories might find it especially beneficial to participate in a self-help group. The MIDUS survey offers clues to these potential beneficiaries with its finding that the not married and those with lower social support from family participated at higher rates in self-help groups (Kessler et al., 1997). Others may also need special attention. Men are generally reticent about asking for help whether it be medical, counseling, or self-help group assistance (Addis & Mahalik, 2003). They may require individualized strategies to normalize their help seeking, perhaps citing the opportunity it would provide to help others whether family or self-help members.

15.3.2 Respecting Boundaries

While much has been made of the need for closer relations between M/SU professionals and self-help groups, it should be understood that differences and distance must be maintained as well. To make the most of the complementarity between self-help and professional services, the integrity and autonomy of both professional and self-help modalities must be maintained. Boundaries must be respected to avoid debasing the distinctive help available from each of the modalities. Often this is framed in threats to the autonomy of self-help groups, but it also applies to the integrity of professional programs. In his insightful and influential work, White (1998) cautions against the tendency to cede professional responsibility to 12-step groups. Professionals must retain responsibility for the treatment component of their own programs. The Minnesota model which encourages 12-step involvement is a good idea but when 12-step group activity substitutes for professional treatment activities, it is a good idea taken too far (Miller, 1994). If fruitful conversations are to take place across helping modality boundaries, they will need to be supported by organizational exchanges between self-help groups and M/SU agencies.

15.4 Organizational and Community Requisites

Service providers are not independent actors. They are firmly attached to their organizational and community environments (Hatch & Cunliffe, 2006; Scott, 2005). If self-help facilitation is to become policy, that is become standard practice or the usual course of action within the professional M/SU service system, the organizational environment must support it. To provide this organizational support, the professional M/SU service system must extend its boundaries to engage in a variety of exchanges with self-help groups (Heracleous, 2004; Schmid, 2004). The M/SU agency must transition from thinking of itself as a self-contained and self-sufficient entity to thinking of itself as an open-system organization in constant exchange with its environment (Scott, 2003). It must engage in adaptive exchanges with self-help groups at all levels of the organization (Donaldson, 2001; Powell & Perron, 2010). Starting with the highest level, self-help leaders need to be represented on the agency's board of directors. This would be a good place to discuss the mutual obligations of self-help leaders and mental health professionals. Self-help leaders also need to be involved in staff development and in-service training. Staff must be given the time and training necessary to visit self-help groups and develop relationships with their leaders (Wituk, Tiemeyer, Commer, Warren, & Meissen, 2003). And here a word needs to be said about going beyond 12-step groups. Because of their numbers, and the extensive literature they have generated, 12-step groups sometimes disproportionately dominate the discussion of self-help. Indeed, it is a limitation not entirely escaped in this chapter. However, there is no scarcity of other highly relevant groups and M/SU agencies should be encouraged to engage them. A recent national survey found that self-help groups and related organizations actually outnumber professional mental health organizations (Goldstrom et al., 2006). Groups affiliated with organizations such as NAMI, the Depression and Bipolar Support Alliance, GROW, and Recovery, Inc. are too little attended to by M/SU agencies.

But it is not enough to engage in adaptive exchanges with self-help groups. M/SU agencies must also partner with self-help groups to enhance their institutional status in the community (Scott, 2001; Wituk, Ealey, Brown, Shepherd, & Meissen, 2005). Self-help groups can become even more significant resources for M/SU agencies as their institutional standing, i.e., as their level of acceptance and approval increases in the community (Baum, 1996; Meyer & Rowan, 1977; Meyer, 1986). M/SU agencies can be a part of bringing this about by including self-help groups in various community events such as media interviews, panel discussions, poster displays, video productions, etc. (Wang et al., 2000). To the extent they do so, M/SU agencies are likely to experience an increase in their own institutional standing owing to the public endorsements and positive references they receive from a stronger network of self-help groups.

15.5 Conclusions

Self-help groups make an immense though somewhat one-sided contribution to the M/SU professional services system. While 12-step groups make an indispensable contribution, a vast range of non-12-step groups remain underutilized to the detriment of the M/SU services system. A great many local NAMIs, DBSAs, and unaffiliated self-help groups receive too little attention from the professional side of the system.

To address underutilization, M/SU professionals need to understand the distinctive complementary properties of self-help groups. They need to understand the experiential nature of self-help, the referent power underlying the helpful influence of self-help leaders, and the unusual opportunity self-help participation offers to experience the benefits of giving help as well as receiving it. M/SU professionals also need to understand the importance of developing relationships with self-help group leaders. These relationships can be built upon to facilitate clients becoming connected to welcoming self-help leaders. With respect to the counseling enterprise, M/SU professionals must learn to create opportunities for synergistic dialogues across professional and self-help boundaries.

To sustain these initiatives, organizational support must be in place. Accordingly, M/SU agencies must enter into organizational exchanges with self-help groups, all the while being careful to maintain and enhance their integrity and autonomy. Simultaneously, M/SU agencies must partner with self-help groups to enhance their institutional standing and acceptance in the community. In undertaking these actions, M/SU agencies can ensure that more people will participate in self-help groups and that they will be able to choose from a wider range of 12-step and non-12-step groups.

References

Addis, M. E., & Mahalik, J. R. (2003). Men, masculinity, and the contexts of help seeking. *American Psychologist, 58*, 5–14.

Alcoholics Anonymous. *Alcoholics Anonymous membership survey 2007*. Retrieved February 7, 2009 http://www.aa.org/pdf/products/p-48_07survey.pdf

Aron, L., Honberg, R., & Duckworth, K. et al. (2009). *Grading the States 2009: A report on America's health care system for adults with serious mental illness*. Arlington, VA: National Alliance on Mental Illness.

Baum, J. A. C. (1996). Organizational ecology. In S. P. Clegg, C. Hardy & W. Nord (Eds.), *Handbook of organization studies* (pp. 77–114). London/Thousand Oaks, CA: Sage.

Borkman, T. J. (1990). Experiential, professional, and lay frames of reference. In T. J. Powell (Ed.), *Working with self-help* (pp. 3–30). Silver Spring, MD: National Association of Social Workers.

Borman, L. D. (1979). Characteristics of development and growth. In M. A. Lieberman, & L. D. Borman (Eds.), *Self-help groups for coping with crisis* (pp. 13–42). San Francisco: Jossey Bass.

Brown, L. D. (2009). Making it sane: Using narrative to explore theory in a mental health consumer-run organization. *Qualitative Health Research, 19*(2), 243–257.

Brown, S. L., Nesse, R. M., Vinokur, A. D., & Smith, D. M. (2003). Providing social support may be more beneficial than receiving it: Results from a prospective study of mortality. *Psychological Science, 14*(3), 320–328.

Chappel, J. N., & DuPont, R. L. (1999). Twelve-step and mutual-help programs for addictive disorders. *The Psychiatric Clinics of North America, 22*(2), 425–446.

Chesler, M. A. (1990). The "dangers" of self-help groups. In T. J. Powell (Ed.), *Working with self-help* (pp. 301–324). Silver Spring, MD: National Association of Social Workers.

Chinman, M. J., Kloos, B. O., Maria O'Connell, M., & Davidson, L. (2002). Service providers views of psychiatric mutual support groups. *Journal of Community Psychology, 30*, 349–366.

Cohen, E., Feinn, R., Arias, A., & Kranzler, H. R. (2007). Alcohol treatment utilization: Findings from the national epidemiologic survey on alcohol and related conditions. *Drug & Alcohol Dependence, 86*(2–3), 214–221.

Committee on Crossing the Quality Chasm: Adaptation to Mental Health and Addictive Disorders. (2006). *Improving the quality of health care for mental and substance-use conditions: Quality chasm series*. Washington, D.C.: Institute of Medicine, National Academies.

Davidson, L., Chinman, M., Kloos, B., Weingarten, R., Stayner, D., & Tebes, J. K. (1999). Peer support among individuals with severe mental illness: A review of the evidence. *Clinical Psychology-Science & Practice, 6*(2), 165–187.

Davison, K. P., Pennebaker, J. W., & Dickerson, S. S. (2000). Who talks? the social psychology of illness support groups: The human asset. *American Psychologist, 55*(2), 205–217.

Department of Health and Human Services Public Health Service. (1988). *Surgeon general's workshop on self-help and public health*. Health resources and services administration, Bureau of maternal and child health and resource development, Publication no. *224–250*. Washington DC.: U. S. Government Printing Office.

Depression and Bipolar Support Alliance (DBSA). *Peer specialist training*. Retrieved 2/13/2009 http://www.dbsalliance.org/site/PageServer?pagename=training_certified_peer_specialist

Donaldson, L. (2001). *The contingency theory of organizations*. Thousand Oaks, CA: Sage.

Festinger, L. (1954). A theory of social comparison processes. *Human Relations, 7*, 117–140.

Fiorentine, R., & Hillhouse, M. P. (2000). Drug treatment and 12-step program participation: The additive effects of integrated recovery activities. *Journal of Substance Abuse Treatment, 18*(1), 65–74.

Freimuth, M. (2000). Integrating group psychotherapy and 12-step work: A collaborative approach. *International Journal of Group Psychotherapy, 50*(3), 297.

French, J. R. P., & Raven, B. (1959). The bases of social power. In D. Cartwright (Ed.), *Studies in social power* (pp. 150–167). Ann Arbor, MI: Institute for Social Research, University of Michigan.

Gitterman, A., & Shulman, L. (2005). *Mutual aid groups, vulnerable and resilient populations, and the life cycle*. New York: Columbia University Press.

Goldstrom, I. D., Campbell, J., Rogers, J. A., Lambert, D. B., Blacklow, B., Henderson, M. J., et al. (2006). National estimates for mental health mutual support groups, self-help organizations, and consumer-operated services. *Administration and Policy in Mental Health, 33*(1), 92–103.

Hardiman, E. R., & Segal, S. P. (2003). Community membership and social networks in mental health self-help agencies. *Psychiatric Rehabilitation Journal, 27*(1), 25–33.

Hatch, M. J., & Cunliffe, A. L. (2006). *Organization theory: Modern, symbolic, and postmodern perspectives*. Oxford: Oxford University Press.

Heracleous, L. (2004). Boundaries in the study of organization. *Human Relations, 57*(1), 95–103.

Humphreys, K., & Moos, R. H. (2007). Encouraging posttreatment self-help group involvement to reduce demand for continuing care services: Two-year clinical and utilization outcomes. *Alcoholism: Clinical and Experimental Research, 31*(1), 64–68.

Humphreys, K., Mavis, B., & Stofflemayr, B. (1991). Factors predicting attendance at self-help groups after substance abuse treatment: Preliminary findings. *Journal of Consulting and Clinical Psychology, 59*(4), 591–593.

Humphreys, K. (1997). Clinicians' referral and matching of substance abuse patients to self-help groups after treatment. *Psychiatric Services, 48*(11), 1445–1449.

Humphreys, K. (1999). Professional interventions that facilitate 12-step self-help group involvement. *Alcohol Research and Health, 23*(2), 93–98.

Humphreys, K., Mavis, B. E., & Stoffelmayr, B. E. (1994). Are twelve step programs appropriate for disenfranchised groups? Evidence from a study of posttreatment mutual help involvement. *Prevention in Human Services, 11*(1), 165–179.

Humphreys, K., Wing, S., McCarty, D., Chappel, J., Gallant, L., Haberle, B., et al. (2004). Self-help organizations for alcohol and drug problems: Toward evidence-based practice and policy. *Journal of Substance Abuse Treatment, 26*(3), 151–158.

Kessler, R. C., Zhao, S., Katz, S. J., Kouzis, A. C., Frank, R. G., Edlund, M., et al. (1999). Past-year use of outpatient services for psychiatric problems in the national comorbidity survey. *American Journal of Psychiatry, 156*(1), 115–123.

Kessler, R., Mickelson, K. D., & Zhao, S. (1997). Patterns and correlates of self-help group membership in the United States. *Social Policy, 27*(3), 27–46.

Kurtz, L. F. (1985). Cooperation and rivalry between helping professionals and members of AA. *Health & Social Work, 10*(2), 104–112.

Kurtz, L. F. (1997). *Self-help and support groups: A handbook for practitioners.* Thousand Oaks, CA: Sage.

Magura, S. (2007). The relationship between substance user treatment and 12-step fellowships: Current knowledge and research questions. *Substance Use & Misuse, 42*(2–3), 343–360.

Magura, S., Laudet, A. B., Mahmood, D., Rosenblum, A., & Knight, E. (2002). Adherence to medication regimens and participation in dual-focus self-help groups. *Psychiatric Services, 53*(3), 310–316.

Majer, J., Jason, L., North, C., Ferrari, J., Porter, N., Olson, B., et al. (2008). A longitudinal analysis of psychiatric severity upon outcomes among substance abusers residing in self-help settings. *American Journal of Community Psychology, 42*(1–2), 145–153.

Maton, K. I. (1988). Social support, organizational characteristics, psychological well-being, and group appraisal in three self-help group populations. *American Journal of Community Psychology, 16*(1), 53–77.

McLellan, A. T. (2008). Evolution in addiction treatment concepts and methods. In M. Galanter, H. D. Kleber, M. Galanter & H. D. Kleber (Eds.), *The American psychiatric publishing textbook of substance abuse treatment* (4th ed., pp. 93–108). Arlington, VA: American Psychiatric Publishing, Inc.

Meissen, G. J., Mason, W. C., & Gleason, D. F. (1991). Understanding the attitudes and intentions of future professionals towards self-help. *American Journal of Community Psychology, 19*(5), 699–714.

Meissen, G., Powell, T. J., Wituk, S. A., Girrens, K., & Arteaga, S. (1999). Attitudes of AA contact persons toward group participation by persons with a mental illness. *Psychiatric Services, 50*(8), 1079–1081.

Meissen, G., Wituk, S., Warren, M., & Shepherd, M. (2000). Self-help groups and managed health care: Obstacles and opportunities. *International Journal of Self-Help and Self-Care, 1 (2)*, 201–210.

Meyer, J. W., & Rowan, B. (1977). Institutionalized organizations: Formal structure as myth and ceremony. *The American Journal of Sociology, 83*(2), 340–363.

Meyer, J. W. (1986). Institutional and organizational rationalization in the mental health system. In W. R. Scott, & B. L. Black (Eds.), *The organization of mental health services.* Beverly Hills, CA: Sage Publications.

Miller, N. S. (1994). *Treating coexisiting psychiatric and addictive disorders: A practical guide.* Center City, MN: Hazelden Educational Materials.

Moos, R. H. (2007). Theory-based processes that promote the remission of substance use disorders. *Clinical Psychology Review, 27*(5), 537.

Moos, R. H., & Timko, C. (2008). Outcome research on 12-step and other self-help programs. In M. Galanter, H. D. Kleber, M. Galanter & H. D. Kleber (Eds.), *The American Psychiatric Publishing Textbook of Substance Abuse Treatment* (4th ed., pp. 511–521). Arlington, VA: American Psychiatric Publishing, Inc.

Mowrer, O. H. (1984). The mental health professions and mutual-help program: Co-optation or collaboration. In A. Gartner, & F. Riessman (Eds.), *Self-help revolution* (pp. 139–154). New York: Human Sciences Press Inc.

Murray, E., Burns, J., See-Tai, S., Lai, R., & Nazareth, I. (2005). Interactive health communication applications for people with chronic disease. *Cochrane Database of Systematic Reviews, 4*, 1–70.

Narrow, W. E., Regier, D. A., Rae, D. S., Manderscheid, R. W., & Locke, B. Z. (1993). Use of services by persons with mental and addictive disorders: Findings from the national institute of mental health epidemiologic catchment area program. *Archives of General Psychiatry, 50*(2), 95–107.

Norcross, J. C. (2006). Integrating self-help into psychotherapy: 16 practical suggestions. *Professional Psychology-Research and Practice, 37*(6), 683–693.

Nowinski, J., & Baker, S. (1992). *The twelve-step facilitation handbook: A systematic approach to early recovery from alcoholism and addiction*. New York: Lexington Books.

Perron, B. E., Mowbray, O. P., Glass, J. E., Delva, J., Vaughn, M. G., & Howard, M. O. (2009). Differences in service utilization and barriers among African Americans, Hispanics, and Caucasians with drug use disorders. *Substance Abuse Treatment, Prevention, and Policy, 4*, 1–10 (electronic).

Pistrang, N., Barker, C., & Humphreys, K. (2008). Mutual help groups for mental health problems: A review of effectiveness studies. *American Journal of Community Psychology, 42*(1), 110–121.

Powell, T., & Perron, B. E. (2010). Self-help groups and mental Health/Substance use agencies: The benefits of organizational exchange. *Substance Use & Misuse, 45*

Powell, T. J. (1990). Self-help, professional help, and informal help: Competing or complementary systems? In T. J. Powell (Ed.), *Working with self-help* (pp. 31–49). Silver Spring, MD: National Association of Social Workers.

Powell, T. J., Hill, E. M., Warner, L., Yeaton, W., & Silk, K. R. (2000). Encouraging people with mood disorders to attend a self-help group. *Journal of Applied Social Psychology, 30*(11), 2270–2288.

Powell, T. J., Yeaton, W., Hill, E. M., & Silk, K. R. (2001). Predictors of psychosocial outcomes for patients with mood disorders: The effects of self-help group participation. *Psychiatric Rehabilitation Journal, 25*(1), 3–11.

Project MATCH Research Group: Allen, J., Anton, R. F., Babor, T. F., Carbonari, J., Carroll, K. M., Connors, G. J., et al. (1998). Matching alcoholism treatments to client heterogeneity: Project Match three-year drinking outcomes. *Alcoholism-Clinical and Experimental Research, 22*(6), 1300–1311.

Raven, B. H. (1988). Social power and compliance in health care. In S. Maes, C. D. Spielberger, P. B. Defares & I. G. Sarason (Eds.), *Topics in health psychology* (pp. 229–244). New York: Wiley.

Raven, B., Schwarzwald, J., & Koslowsky, M. (1998). Conceptualizing and measuring a Power/Interaction model of interpersonal influence. *Journal of Applied Social Psychology, 28*(4), 307–332.

Ries, R. K., Galanter, M., & Tonigan, J. S. (2008). Twelve-step facilitation. In M. Galanter, H. D. Kleber, M. Galanter & H. D. Kleber (Eds.), *The American psychiatric publishing textbook of substance abuse treatment* (4th ed., pp. 373–386). Arlington, VA US: American Psychiatric Publishing, Inc.

Riessman, F. (1965). The helper-therapy principle. *Social Work, 10*(2), 27–32.

Riessman, F., David. (1995). *Redefining self-help*. San Francisco: Jossey Bass.

Roberts, L. J., Salem, D., Rappaport, J., Toro, P. A., Luke, D. A., & Seidman, E. (1999). Giving and receiving help: Interpersonal transactions in mutual-help meetings and psychosocial adjustment of members. *American Journal of Community Psychology, 27*(6), 841–868.

Sagarin, E. (1969). *Odd man in: Societies of deviants in America*. New York: Quadrangle.

Salem, D. A., Reischl, T. M., Gallacher, F., & Randall, K. W. (2000). The role of referent and expert power in mutual help. *American Journal of Community Psychology, 28*(3), 303–324.

Salem, D., Reischl, T., & Randall, K. (2008). The effect of professional partnership on the development of a mutual-help organization. *American Journal of Community Psychology, 42*(1–2), 179–191.

Salzer, M. S., Rappaport, J., & Segre, L. (2001). Mental health professionals' support of self-help groups. *Journal of Community & Applied Social Psychology, 11*(1), 1–10.

Salzer, M. S., Rappaport, J., & Segre, L. (1999). Professional appraisal of professionally led and self-help groups. *American Journal of Orthopsychiatry, 69*(4), 536–540.

Schacter, S. (1959). *The psychology of affiliation*. Stanford, CA: Stanford University Press.

Schmid, H. (2004). Organization-environment relationships: Theory for management practice in human service organizations. *Administration-in-Social-Work, 28*(1), 97–113.

Schubert, M. A., & Borkman, T. J. (1991). An organizational typology for self-help groups. *American Journal of Community Psychology, 19*(5), 769–787.

Scott, W. R. (2005). Institutional theory: Contributing to a theoretical research program. In K. G. Smith, & M. A. Hitt (Eds.), *Great minds of management: The process of theory development* (2nd ed., pp. 460–484). New York: Oxford University Press.

Scott, W. R. (2003). *Organizations: Rational, natural, and open systems*. Upper Saddle River, NJ: Prentice Hall.

Scott, W. R. (2001). *Institutions and organizations* (2nd ed.). Thousand Oaks, CA: Sage.

Seligman, M. (1995). The effectiveness of psychotherapy: The Consumer Reports study. *American Psychologist, 50*(12), 965–974.

Shepherd, M. D., Schoenberg, M., Slavich, S., Wituk, S., Warren, M., & Meissen, G. (1999). Continuum of professional involvement in self-help groups. *Journal of Community Psychology, 27*(1), 39–53.

Timko, C., & Debenedetti, A. (2007). A randomized controlled trial of intensive referral to 12-step self-help groups: One-year outcomes. *Drug & Alcohol Dependence, 90*(2–3), 270–279.

Timko, C., Debenedetti, A., & Billow, R. (2006). Intensive referral to 12-step self-help groups and 6-month substance use disorder outcomes. *Addiction, 101*(5), 678–688.

Toro, P., Zimmerman, M., Seidman, E., Reischl, T., Rappaport, J., Luke, D., et al. (1988). Professionals in mutual help groups: Impact on social climate and members' behaviour. *Journal of Consulting and Clinical Psychology, 56*(4), 631–632.

United States Public Health Service (USPHS), Office of the Surgeon General (OSG), Center for Mental Health Services (CMHS), & National Institute of Mental Health (NIMH.). (2000). *Mental health A Report of the Surgeon General*. Washington, DC: Department of Health and Human Services.

Wang P. S., Lane, M., Olfson, M., Pincus H., A., Wells K., B., & Kessler R., C. (2005). Twelve-month use of mental health services in the United States: Results from the National Comorbidity Survey Replication. *Archives of General Psychiatry, 62*(6), 629–640.

Wang, P. S., Berglund, P., Olfson, M., Pincus, H. A., Wells, K. B., & Kessler, R. C. (2005). Failure and delay in initial treatment contact after first onset of mental disorders in the national comorbidity survey replication. *Archives of General Psychiatry, 62*(6), 603–613.

Wang, P. S., Berglund, P., & Kessler, R. C. (2000). Recent care of common mental disorders in the United States: Prevalence and conformance with evidence-based recommendations. *Journal of General Internal Medicine, 15*(5), 284–292.

Warner, L., Silk, K., Yeaton, W. H., Bargal, D., Janssen, J., & Hill, E. M. (1994). Psychiatrists' and patients' views on drug information and medication compliance. *Hospital and Community Psychiatry, 45*(12), 1235–1237.

Watkins, P. L., & Clum, G. A. (2008). *Handbook of self-help therapies*. New York: Routledge.

White, W., & Kurtz, E. (2005). The varieties of recovery experience: A primer for addiction treatment professionals and recovery advocates. *International Journal of Self Help and Self Care, 3*(1), 21–61.

White, W. L. (1998). *Slaying the dragon: The history of addiction treatment and recovery in America*. Bloomington, IL: Chestnut Health Systems/Lighthouse Institute.

World Health Organization (WHO), (2001). *The world health report 2001 – mental health: New understanding, new hope*. Retrieved online January 23, 2009 from http://www.who.int/whr/2001/en/.

Wilson, J. (1995a). *How to work with self-help groups: Guidelines for professionals*. Hants: Arena/Ashgate Publishing.

Wilson, J. (1995b). *Two worlds: Self-help groups and professionals*. London: Venture Press.

Wituk, S., Ealey, S., Brown, L., Shepherd, M., & Meissen, G. (2005). Assessing the needs and strengths of self-help groups: Opportunities to meet health care needs. *International Journal of Self Help & Self Care, 3*(1–2), 103–116.

Wituk, S., Shepherd, M. D., Slavich, S., Warren, M. L., & Meissen, G. (2000). A topography of self-help groups: An empirical analysis. *Social Work, 45*(2), 157–165.

Wituk, S. A., Tiemeyer, S., Commer, A., Warren, M., & Meissen, G. (2003). Starting self-help groups: Empowering roles for social workers. *Social Work with Groups, 26*(1), 83–92.

Index

A

Accountability, 160, 163–165, 243, 291, 329–330
Addiction (to groups), 64, 68, 88–89
Advantages (of online groups), 91–94
Advocacy, 2, 6–7, 10, 26, 42, 45–46, 48, 50, 62–63, 120, 164, 178–182, 184, 213–233, 237, 244, 247–249, 266, 268–269, 271–273, 276–278, 280–283, 288, 295–296, 305–306, 326, 340
Anonymity, 91–92, 309
Anxiety, 8, 66–68, 70, 73, 76–78, 80, 82, 89, 92, 94, 100, 110, 113, 128, 140, 142, 177, 343, 345

B

Behavior setting theory, 7, 23–26, 30, 32, 34
Bereavement, 8, 68, 70, 74–76, 78–80, 82, 131

C

Center for Mental Health Services (CMHS), 158, 173–174, 231, 236–253, 256–258, 269–270, 272, 274, 277, 284
Certified peer specialist/peer specialist/CPS
  barriers to employment of, 177, 182–183, 185
  employment, 173, 176–177
  job titles, 177–182
  medicaid reimbursement of, 172
  training, 3, 6, 172–176, 186, 196–197, 199–200
  work activities, 9, 177–182, 178–182
Choice and self-determination, 227
Chronic mental illness, 8, 68, 70–77, 80, 82, 134
Code of conduct, 162, 165
Collaboration
  with the professional mental health system, 2, 11

Collaboration, 2, 5, 7–8, 11–12, 40–41, 43–44, 47, 50, 101, 129, 146, 160, 163–165, 221, 229, 231, 238, 241, 250–251, 255, 269, 278, 282–283, 287–298, 303–348
Community
  integration, 4–5, 7, 10, 20–22, 175, 184, 188, 283–285, 294
  physical integration, 22
  psychological integration, 23, 293–294
  relations, 9, 156, 164
  social integration, 22, 294
Community Support Program, 11, 235, 237, 259, 269
Conflict resolution, 156–157, 162
Consumer
  advocacy initiatives, 7
  -delivered services, 2, 6–7, 9–10, 155–165, 169–188, 193–207
  -driven care, 256
  -/family-driven system of care, 268
  involvement, 54, 237–238, 239–241, 243–244, 246–247, 258, 283, 318
  leadership, 238, 244–245, 251, 278, 297–298, 311, 320–321, 324, 328, 331
  movement, 6, 11, 194, 265–285, 295–298
  -operated services, 3, 158, 239–241, 246–248, 253, 257–258, 276, 288
  as providers, 13, 67, 176
  rights, 6, 244
  -run drop-in centers, 2–4, 7, 9, 32, 48, 155–165, 244
  -run services, 2, 67, 245–246, 249, 281, 298
  /survivor initiatives, 2, 44, 158
  /survivor movement, 10, 214–215, 222, 227–229, 232–233, 269–270, 275, 282, 284

Consumer and consumer-supporter national technical assistance centers (TACs), 11, 265–285
Consumer-run organizations (CROs), 2, 5, 7, 11, 228–229, 246, 249, 257, 258, 274–275, 284, 287–298, 304, 320, 325–326
Contracts, 146, 163, 222, 238, 242–243, 251–253, 311
Cooptation, 3, 163–164, 304
Coping, 2, 9, 20–22, 27–29, 32, 34, 65, 74, 79, 107, 109, 113, 120–122, 127–130, 133, 136, 139–140, 146, 148, 158, 163, 182, 184, 194, 236, 293
CPS History, 194, 205
Critical review, process evaluation, 112
Cross-disability, 223, 233
Cyber-harassment, 94

D
Depression, 5, 8, 68–70, 73–74, 76–80, 82, 88, 94–95, 100, 120, 122, 129, 172, 175, 217, 270, 282, 336, 345–347
Disability, 10, 21, 91, 186, 219, 223, 230–233, 249–250, 254–255, 270, 283, 285, 338, 343
Disadvantages/Harm (in online groups), 87, 94–95
Discrimination and stigma, 266
Dissemination, 50–52, 54, 111, 165
Drop-in centers, 2–4, 6–7, 9, 32, 48, 155–165, 178–179, 181, 244, 246, 288, 313

E
Effectiveness, 3, 8–9, 12–13, 35, 49, 65–68, 77–80, 82–83, 94, 111, 124, 131–132, 147, 158–159, 165, 183, 185, 187–188, 225, 231, 239, 256–258, 283–284, 338–339
Empirical support, 35
Employment, 9, 40, 42, 45–46, 63, 77, 158, 173, 176–177, 179–180, 186, 188, 202, 205, 237, 241–242, 249–250, 254–257, 285, 308
Empowerment, 4–7, 9, 23, 25–26, 30, 34, 36, 40–41, 44–46, 48–49, 65, 80, 82, 89, 101, 109, 125–126, 131–133, 155, 159, 163–164, 175, 187, 194–195, 197, 199, 214, 217–221, 248–249, 258, 269, 271–272, 275–277, 279, 281–283, 288, 293, 296, 321
  theory, 7, 23, 25–26, 30, 34, 159
Engagement, 12, 99, 132–133, 136–137, 165, 184, 285, 321, 331

Evaluation, 8–9, 12–13, 39–54, 80, 99, 101, 108, 112, 132–135, 138–140, 146–149, 158, 173, 175, 231, 235, 237–243, 252, 256–259, 271, 275, 283–285, 306, 323, 325, 328
  capacity, 44, 54
Evaluator roles, 52
Evidence-base, 51, 80, 165, 247–248, 251, 253, 285, 290
Experiential knowledge, 8, 21–23, 26–28, 30, 34, 44, 47, 54, 65, 159, 161, 165, 188, 194, 239, 320, 323–324, 327, 330
Extreme communities/sites, 96–97, 99

F
Family caregivers, 9, 107–149
Federal, 6, 10–11, 214, 219, 227, 235–241, 245–247, 252, 254–255, 258–259, 269–270, 276–278, 284, 289
Flame, 94
Friends of, 89, 123, 340
Funding, 3, 6–7, 9–10, 35, 44, 50, 64, 156–158, 163–165, 171–172, 200, 229, 231–232, 235–259, 269, 271, 274, 277–279, 311–313, 316, 319–320, 322, 329, 339
  agencies, 3, 163–165
  support, 9, 156, 163, 165, 240, 252

G
Goal
  achievement, 133, 158, 164
  tracking, 164–165
Government, 10–11, 62, 178, 235–259, 269, 275, 277, 280, 285
Grant(s), 238–247, 250–255, 273, 277, 280, 290, 311, 321, 330
  requirements, 163–164, 276
  writing, 156–157, 161, 165, 281, 289, 290–291, 311, 328
Grassroots associations, 157
Group survival, 308, 314–316, 328

H
Helper-therapy principle, 8, 25–27, 30, 34, 342
Help
  provider, 22, 24, 30, 32–33
  seeker, 22, 24, 30, 32–33
History, 4–6, 11, 40, 43, 47, 51, 135, 193–194, 196–197, 205–206, 222, 229, 240, 246, 248, 269–270, 271, 288–289, 306–307, 322, 343
Hospitalization, 4, 27, 69, 109, 158, 219, 231, 285, 294
Hyperpersonal communication, 90, 92

Index

I
Identity transformation, 31, 33–34
Implementation, 9, 13, 45–49, 53–54, 147, 165, 182–185, 186, 188, 193–208, 238–239, 247, 253, 256, 284–285
Interagency collaboration, 250
Inter-organizational collaboration, 164
Interpersonal processes, 21, 26–30, 35
Interrelate, 232

J
Job Satisfaction, 10, 177–182, 202, 203, 205, 208

K
Knowledge construction, 8, 47–49, 53–54

L
Leadership, 4, 7, 11, 22, 24–27, 32–34, 89–90, 98, 128, 131, 155–161, 165, 185, 228, 232, 238, 244–246, 251, 272–276, 278, 280–281, 283–285, 287–298, 306–312, 314–316, 318–322, 324–325, 328, 331, 346
Listserv, 88
Lurk/lurking, 53, 90, 93, 99

M
Medical condition, 89, 92
Membership, 23, 63, 66, 68, 75–76, 79, 81, 89–90, 93, 97, 160, 186, 229, 246, 249, 253, 277, 287, 290–291, 295–297, 323, 337
Mental health, 1–13, 19–35, 39–54, 61–83, 87–101, 107–149, 155–156, 158–159, 163–165, 172–174, 177, 182–183, 185, 187–188, 194–207, 213–233, 236–258, 269–270, 272–273, 275–285, 288–291, 293–298, 303–308, 313–315, 320–323, 328, 335–348
Mental health consumer/survivor movement, 228–229
Mental health policy, 4, 6, 10, 19, 170, 266, 295–296
Mental health practitioners, 87, 97–99
Mental illness, 4–10, 21–23, 26–29, 31, 34, 40, 53, 66–77, 80, 82–83, 92, 108–131, 134, 137, 141, 147–148, 156, 159, 161, 163–164, 183, 195–202, 205, 214, 217–218, 223–224, 227–228, 236, 239, 245, 250, 254, 257, 279, 282–283, 288–289, 293, 297–298, 303, 319, 329, 338, 344

MHSH (Mental health self-help)
factors influencing the use of, 6–7
funding organizations, 241–242, 259
history of, 4–6
practice, 13, 35
research, 35
Moderated (group), 88, 90, 97–98
Movement for social justice, 265–266
Multi-user online role-playing, 99
Munchausen by Internet, 95
Mutual aid, 2, 8–9, 13, 51, 65, 67–69, 73, 78, 87–101, 141, 145, 172, 340–341
Mutual-help, 2, 8, 11, 303–306, 320–321, 323–326, 328–331
Mutual help group, 2, 8, 61–83, 304–305, 320–321, 323, 340–341
Mutual-help groups for caregivers, 1, 8, 304–305
Mutual help groups for mental health problems, 8, 61–83
Mutual support, 2–3, 5, 9, 43, 65, 67, 69–70, 73, 91, 96, 101, 107–149, 155–156, 200, 247, 249, 258, 270, 288, 296
Mutual support group, 2, 9, 65, 67, 70, 73, 107–149, 258

N
National coalition, 10, 214, 221, 228, 230–232, 258, 277–278, 282
Netiquette, 91, 97
Nonprofits, 156–157, 163–164, 257, 274, 288–291, 297–298

O
Online self-help, 2, 8, 13, 87–101
Online support group, 66–67, 69, 78, 88, 95–96, 99
Organizational capacity needs, 156–157, 290
Organizational collaboration, 164, 305
Organizational decision-making, 159–160, 320
Organizational development of self-help, 235, 244, 248
Organizational exchanges with self-help, 347–348
Organizational focus, 2–4, 164
Organizational goals, 158, 164–165, 290
Organizational networks, 164–165
Organizational structure, 2–3, 9, 100, 156–157, 307, 316, 322, 327, 330
Outcome evaluation, 12, 49
Outcome measures, 35, 68–70, 72, 80, 82, 128, 148, 280

Outcomes, 3, 7–9, 12, 20–23, 25–26, 30, 35, 41–42, 44–50, 53–54, 65–66, 68–83, 93–94, 99–100, 107–149, 158, 171, 173, 175–176, 184, 187–188, 195, 207, 217, 238–240, 244, 256, 258, 280, 288, 292–293, 306, 331, 338, 341, 343
Overpopulation, 23, 34

P

Paradigm, 4–5, 47–49, 53–54, 214, 217–218, 285, 288
Participation, 6–9, 12–13, 20–23, 25–26, 29–32, 40–44, 46–49, 51, 54, 76–78, 80–82, 90–91, 93–94, 96, 99–100, 108, 112, 119–120, 123–125, 128–135, 143–146, 148, 158–159, 161–162, 164–165, 175, 218, 220, 240–242, 244, 246, 275, 281, 285, 292–294, 297, 337–340, 345–346, 348
Participatory action research, 7–8, 39–54
Partnership, 7, 11–12, 40–41, 52, 54, 98, 231, 241, 254, 279, 283, 289, 298, 303–331
Passion, 157, 216, 220–223, 226–228, 231–232, 270, 280, 297
Peer counselors, 162–163, 193, 240, 245, 304
Peer-run services, 280
Peer support, 2, 6, 9, 13, 46, 48–49, 64–65, 67, 69, 109, 112, 116, 119, 129, 170–175, 177–181, 186–188, 194–196, 207, 220, 222, 224, 230, 232, 236–237, 239, 246, 248–251, 256, 258, 278–279, 284–285, 288, 291, 295–296
Peer support specialists, 6, 9, 177, 194, 256, 279
People with mental health problems, 7–9, 40, 47, 64–66, 107–149, 158
Personal change, 49, 54, 89, 125, 164
Personal knowledge of self-help, 344–345
Person-environment interaction, 31, 34, 159
Policy, 4, 6–7, 10–11, 26, 43, 45–46, 48, 50–51, 53, 63, 67, 82, 157, 164, 185, 213–233, 235–259, 269, 271, 273, 277–278, 284–285, 295–298, 339, 346
Power, 3, 6, 8, 35, 40–45, 47–54, 63, 127, 135, 137, 147, 174, 198, 215, 224–226, 228–229, 310, 318, 327, 329–330, 336, 341–342, 344, 348
  -sharing, 40–41, 43–45, 49–51, 54
Practice, 7–8, 10, 12–13, 19–35, 39–54, 87–101, 127–128, 139, 147, 156, 165, 186–187, 195, 207, 221, 247–248, 251, 290–291, 296, 312, 323, 341, 346
Priorities, 160, 221, 229, 231, 238–240, 251–253, 255–258

Professional involvement, 305, 318, 321, 330
Program
  development, 35, 196
  evaluation, 40, 46, 252
  logic model, 45–46, 54
  theory, 45, 53
Psychiatric disabilities, 158, 231, 241, 254–255, 276, 279, 283
Public mental health system, 6, 9, 231, 239

R

Randomized controlled trial (RCT), 12, 65, 69, 71, 79–80, 112, 116–118, 147, 246, 253
Recovery, 2, 4–11, 21, 23, 25, 48–49, 51, 63, 72, 79, 88, 92, 95, 97, 130, 134, 159, 161, 163–165, 172, 174–175, 177, 179–188, 194–199, 204, 208, 214–222, 225, 228–232, 238–241, 248–251, 257–259, 271–272, 273, 275–276, 278–279, 281–285, 293–298, 310, 320, 336, 339–340, 347
Research, 7–13, 19–35, 39–54, 64, 66, 68–69, 80–83, 88, 92–96, 98–101, 111–112, 114, 127–129, 131–132, 134, 136–137, 140–141, 144–145, 147–149, 156–159, 164–165, 183, 185, 187–188, 195–196, 200–201, 205–208, 214, 225, 235–259, 271–272, 277, 281, 283, 285, 288–290, 294, 297, 304, 307–308, 331, 340, 342, 344–345
Resource exchange, 30–34, 269
Roles, 3, 5–8, 10, 22–28, 40–41, 43, 47, 51–52, 54, 76, 91, 100, 109–110, 116, 125–126, 132–148, 159–161, 165, 173–174, 178, 182–185, 188, 194–195, 199–200, 206–208, 215–220, 236, 238, 240, 242–243, 245, 249–250, 256, 270, 272, 279–280, 282–283, 291, 293, 297–298, 304, 307, 311, 318–322, 325–326, 328, 330–331, 341–342
  framework, 8, 30–35, 159

S

Self-appraisal, 30–35, 341
Self-determination, 25, 135, 141–142, 179–180, 194, 227–228, 237, 239, 241, 256, 274, 281, 284–285
Self-help, 1–13, 19–35, 39–54, 62–70, 72, 74–76, 78–79, 81–82, 87–89, 91, 93, 95, 97, 99, 111–112, 130, 148, 155–159, 162, 165, 172, 194, 205, 214, 220, 228, 235–259, 269–272, 282, 288–289, 298, 303–331, 335–348
Self-help and advocacy groups, 266

Self-help as an institution, 347–348
Self-help demographics, 336–338
Self-help and the experiential perspective, 341–342, 344
Self-help groups and professional services, 12
Self-help referrals, 7, 115, 121, 288, 328–329, 340, 344–345
Sense of community, 7, 23, 26, 30–31, 34, 270, 292–293
Service system, 9, 46, 164, 194, 237, 239, 241, 245–246, 248, 269, 343, 346–347
Social comparison theory, 8, 26, 28–29, 34, 109
Social interaction, 22, 29, 162
Social isolation, 109, 155, 157
Social networking, 8, 22, 29, 35, 91, 96–97, 99, 109, 159, 285, 294
Social programming, 8, 45–47, 53–54
Social support (and socially supportive), 5, 8–9, 20–21, 26, 29–30, 34, 42, 45–46, 49, 65–67, 69, 73, 78, 89, 91, 94, 98–99, 109, 118, 127–129, 131–133, 139, 145, 147–148, 155, 158–159, 161–163, 165, 187, 288, 293, 346
12-step group, 63, 72, 77, 336–340, 345–348
Stigma, 4–7, 27, 47, 53, 109, 138, 142, 155, 179–180, 197, 224, 246, 266, 279–280, 309, 331
Stigmatized identity, 89
Strategic planning, 156–157, 273, 289
Substance Abuse and Mental Health Services Administration (SAMHSA), 158, 173–174, 228, 236–237, 242, 246, 250, 252, 254, 269, 285, 288, 290

Substance use, 12, 68, 71–72, 77, 178, 256, 335–348
Support group, 9, 32, 68–69, 73, 78, 81, 88, 91, 96, 99, 108–110, 112, 114, 116–118, 120–121, 123–125, 128–137, 140–148, 222, 318, 346
Sustainability, 10, 12, 229, 238, 279, 281, 288
System transformation, 188, 271

T

Technical assistance, 2, 6–7, 11, 159, 164, 196, 228–229, 241–244, 247–248, 250, 252–253, 258, 265–285, 287–298, 329
Technical assistance organizations, 2
Theoretical frameworks, 8, 35, 39–54
Therapy group, 5, 91
Transformation, 4, 31, 33–34, 48, 188, 220, 227, 239, 242–243, 245, 251, 271, 281, 284–285
Treatment-evaluation perspective, 66

U

Under-population, 23–24, 34
U.S. Department of Health and Human Services, 236, 249
Utilization, 8, 49–51, 54, 113, 127–128, 140, 147, 194, 336–340

V

Values, 8, 21, 25, 40–42, 45, 53–54, 89, 109, 174, 180, 195, 198, 204, 214, 216, 231, 276, 285, 305, 320, 322, 325–327

W

Workplace Integration, 10, 201–202, 205–206